A Special Issue of
Neuropsychological Re...

The assessment and rehabilitation of vegetative and minimally conscious patients

Guest Editor

Martin R. Coleman
*Cambridge University, Cambridge Coma
Study Group, Addenbrookes Hospital, UK*

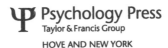

Ψ Psychology Press
Taylor & Francis Group
HOVE AND NEW YORK

Published in 2005 by Psychology Press Ltd
27 Church Road, Hove, East Sussex BN3 2FA

Simultaneously published in the USA and Canada
by Psychology Press
711 Third Avenue, New York, NY 10017

First issued in paperback 2015

*Psychology Press is an imprint of the Taylor and Francis Group,
an informa business*

British Library Cataloguing in Publication Data
A catalogue record for this book is available from the British Library

ISBN 13: 978-1-138-87326-1 (pbk)
ISBN 13: 978-1-8416-9992-9 (hbk)

ISSN 0960-2011

Cover design by Kate Hybert
Typeset in the UK by Techset, Salisbury

Contents*

---

* This book is also a special issue of the journal *Neuropsychological Rehabilitation* and forms Issues 3/4
of Volume 15 (2005). The page numbers used here are taken from the journal and so begin on p. 161.

NEUROPSYCHOLOGICAL REHABILITATION
2005, 15 (3/4), 161–162

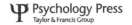

Preface

The assessment and rehabilitation of vegetative and minimally conscious patients

Martin R. Coleman

Cambridge Coma Study Group, Addenbrooke's Hospital, Cambridge, UK

This special edition of *Neuropsychological Rehabilitation*, entitled 'The assessment and rehabilitation of vegetative and minimally conscious patients', consists of 35 invited papers from many experts in this field. These articles cover the definitions and diagnostic criteria relating to the vegetative and minimally conscious states; they describe behavioural assessment techniques and discuss the significant insights functional imaging and electrophysiology are making to both our knowledge of these patients and the physiological basis of human consciousness; they describe the prevalence and life expectancy of patients, and discuss the issue of misdiagnosis as well as the law relating to withdrawal of tube feeding and the many relevant ethical considerations; finally, many articles describe the rehabilitation of these patients, including neurosurgical, pharmacological, mechanical and sensory interventions as well as the use of assistive technology. They highlight the diverse and multidisciplinary background of those treating and investigating these emotive and challenging conditions. I hope the contents of this special edition will pique the interest of health care professionals and scientists alike and encourage further multidisciplinary collaboration.

This special edition grew out of a symposium held at the International Neuropsychological Society Conference in Berlin 2003, which was organised by Professor Agnes Shiel. At the request of *Neuropsychological Rehabilitation*'s editor-in-chief, Barbara Wilson, I was asked as one of the speakers at the symposium to organise a special edition, which would build upon the large interest shown by delegates into the vegetative and minimally conscious states. It was with great pleasure therefore that I was able to invite many of the world's experts to contribute manuscripts reviewing and highlighting the many advances that have been achieved since the term vegetative state was

http://www.tandf.co.uk/journals/pp/09602011.html   DOI:10.1080/09602010443000669

coined in 1972 by Jennett and Plum. To ensure the highest standard, all contributions have been peer-reviewed by at least one of the other contributors and one external reviewer.

I am very grateful to all the contributors for submitting many fascinating papers and to all the reviewers for their timely and detailed reviews. Finally, I would like to express my gratitude to Barbara Wilson who initiated this special edition.

ORGANIZATION OF PAPERS

Part I: Definitions, diagnosis, prevalence and ethics

1. Definitions and current diagnostic guidelines
Giacino & Kalmar; Bates; Beaumont & Kenealy; Ashwal

2. Neuropathophysiology
Graham et al.

3. Neurological assessment
Barker; Pickard et al.

4. Legal issues
McLean; Zasler

5. Ethical issues
Borthwick; Province

Part II: Functional imaging, electrophysiology and mechanical intervention

1. Functional and structural imaging
Beuthien-Baumann et al.; Boly et al.; Owen et al.; Bekinschtein et al.

2. Electrophysiology
Kobylarz & Schiff; Kotchoubey; Guérit; Fischer & Luauté; Schnakers et al.

3. Mechanical intervention
Cooper et al.; Yamamoto & Katayama

4. Pharmaceutical intervention
Matsuda et al.

Part III: Behavioural assessment and rehabilitation techniques

1. Behavioural assessment tools
F. C. Wilson et al.; Rappaport; Kalmar & Giacino

2. Rehabilitation
Andrews; Reimer & LeNavenec; Elliott & Walker; Shiel & B. A. Wilson; Munday; Naudé & Hughes; Magee; Finch; Crawford & Beaumont

NEUROPSYCHOLOGICAL REHABILITATION
2005, 15 (3/4), 163–165

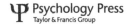

Part I: Definitions, diagnosis, prevalence and ethics

Foreword by Bryan Jennett

The strange and harrowing sight of a person who is awake but unaware, with no evidence of a working mind, provokes intense debate among scientists, health professionals, philosophers, ethicists, and lawyers. The interest provoked by the vegetative state in these professionals and in the general public is out of all proportion to the rarity of the condition. For this is the least common and most extreme form of disability in those who now survive severe brain damage that before modern methods of resuscitation and intensive care would usually have proved fatal. When we first described this state (Jennett & Plum, 1972) we emphasised that persistent did not mean permanent and it is now usual to omit "persistent" and to describe a patient as having been vegetative for a certain time. When there is no recovery after a specified period the state can be declared permanent and only then do the ethical and legal issues around withdrawal of treatment arise.

Because of these issues it is particularly important that there is confidence in the diagnosis. There have been a number of published diagnostic criteria, mostly from the US, but the most recent and authoritative are those from the Royal College of Physicians in 2003 (Bates paper). Moreover the definition of the minimally conscious state in 2002 has made clearer the recognition of awareness in these severely brain damaged patients (Giacino & Kalmar paper). These two contributions should do much to reduce the risk of misdiagnosis. The problem is that the diagnosis depends on expert observation of the patient over a sufficient period of time to discover whether there is any evidence of awareness. This may not always be easy because patients retain a variable range of reflex responses that may mistakenly be interpreted as evidence of awareness, while the limited possible motor responses may impede reactions that might indicate awareness. Misdiagnosis does occur and it is vital that due care is taken to attend to all details when assessing the patient, and that this involves more than one person and discipline (Barker paper in Part I). There is a case for using special assessment scales (Wilson et al., Rappaport, and Kalmar, papers in Part III).

http://www.tandf.co.uk/journals/pp/09602011.html   DOI:10.1080/09602010443000632

Because some of these reflex behaviours seem likely to involve some cortical activity some observers claim that they are incompatible with the vegetative state. However, neuropathological studies reveal that severe cortical damage is less consistent than is damage to subcortical white matter and the thalami (Graham et al. paper). Moreover, recent functional imaging in vegetative patients sometimes shows residual cortical and perhaps cognitive function, sometimes linked to observed isolated fragments of higher level behaviour (papers in Part II). These appear to reflect cortical activity in the primary rather than the associative areas in vegetative patients, while functional responses in minimally conscious patients are different. In vegetative patients there may be survival of islands of cortex no longer part of a sufficient and coherent cortico-thalamo-cortical system to generate awareness. It is therefore no longer valid to require as a diagnostic criterion of the vegetative state that there is no evidence of any cortical activity. Although functional brain imaging is a useful tool in understanding the mechanisms underlying the vegetative state, these investigations are not presently practical as diagnostic aids in the wide range of locations where this diagnosis has to be made. For the moment the diagnosis depends on clinical assessment.

Many patients vegetative a month after an acute insult regain consciousness and some become independent; the probability of recovery depends on the cause of the acute insult and on how long the patient has been vegetative (Ashwal paper). In the UK it is legally accepted that permanence can be declared for non-traumatic cases after 6 months, but not until 1 year after head injury. Almost all alleged later recoveries become only minimally conscious or marginally better than this. Better aids to prognosis may evolve based on results from on-going functional studies (papers in Part II). Once patients have survived the first few months they stabilise and may survive for many years in a vegetative state.

Many studies of how various groups of people regard indefinite survival in the vegetative state indicate that most regard this as worse than death and that they would not want life-sustaining treatment to be continued, including artificial nutrition and hydration (ANH). The opposing vitalist view is against withdrawal of treatment, holding that life of any kind is sacred, regardless of considerations of quality of life or respect for the patient's autonomy. Many secular and theological moral philosophers and institutions have formally rejected this minority view, and the courts in several countries have declared that ANH is medical treatment that may be withdrawn if deemed of no further benefit to the patient. The ethical debate and its legal consequences revolve largely around the decision about whether it is appropriate to withdraw ANH from a permanently vegetative patient. The issues are whether this is consistent with the ethical principles of proportionality in balancing the benefits and burdens of medical intervention, and with respecting the autonomy of the patient. A competent patient has the right to refuse treatment even if this is life-sustaining. The problem is how to discover whether this patient would likely want to refuse continued treatment in a vegetative state. Ideally this would be discovered from a living will or advance directive—but few people have such a document, especially younger patients. In practice it usually depends on the testimony of the family about the known beliefs and values of the patient and on their recalling any verbal statements that the patient might have made about their wishes in the event of vegetative survival. Moralists and lawyers agree that there is no difference between withholding and withdrawing treatment, but that there is a clear distinction between killing and letting die.

There have now been many cases through the courts in the US and the UK and in both countries appeals to the highest courts in the land have confirmed that withdrawal of treatment from a permanently vegetative patients is lawful. The English High Court has also ruled that this does not infringe the recently adopted Human Rights Act. There have been single cases approving withdrawal in Scotland, Ireland, South Africa, New Zealand, Germany and the Netherlands (Jennett, 2002). Only in England, however, is it required to seek court approval before withdrawal of ANH from a vegetative patient, and this is the only condition for which prior court approval is required before withdrawing non-beneficial treatment. There are lawyers in the UK, however, who believe that it is time to review this situation (McLean paper).

REFERENCES

Jennett, B. (2002). *The vegetative state: Medical facts, ethical and legal dilemmas.* Cambridge, UK: Cambridge University Press.

Jennett, B., & Plum, F. (1972). Persistent vegetative state after brain damage: A syndrome in search of a name. *Lancet, 1* (April 1, 7753), 734–737.

PART I: ORGANIZATION OF PAPERS

1. Definitions and current diagnostic guidelines
Giacino & Kalmar; Bates; Beaumont & Kenealy; Ashwal

2. Neuropathophysiology
Graham et al.

3. Neurological assessment
Barker; Pickard et al.

4. Legal issues
McLean; Zasler

5. Ethical issues
Borthwick; Province

NEUROPSYCHOLOGICAL REHABILITATION
2005, 15 (3/4), 166–174

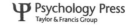

Diagnostic and prognostic guidelines for the vegetative and minimally conscious states

Joseph T. Giacino and Kathleen Kalmar

JFK Medical Center, Edison, NJ, USA

Many individuals who sustain severe brain injury experience prolonged or permanent disorders of consciousness. While these disorders may appear homogeneous, important distinctions exist in prognosis and clinical management. Studies suggest, however, that the incidence of diagnostic inaccuracy is high in both acute care and rehabilitation settings. In this paper, we review consensus-based diagnostic and prognostic criteria for the vegetative and minimally conscious states. We also discuss recent developments and future directions for research in this area.

INTRODUCTION

Diagnostic accuracy and consistency are critical to assuring appropriate clinical management of patients with disorders of consciousness. Important differences exist among specific disorders of consciousness with respect to course of recovery, prognosis, clinical management, and outcome. Diagnostic inaccuracy and non-specificity may lead to an overly pessimistic prognosis, limit accessibility to medical and rehabilitation services and inappropriately influence end-of-life decision-making. For example, an acutely brain-injured patient who retains subtle signs of consciousness but is incorrectly diagnosed with persistent vegetative state (PVS), is less likely to be referred for specialised neurorehabilitative services than if the patient's diagnosis accurately reflected the preserved features of consciousness. In some settings,

Correspondence should be sent to Joseph T. Giacino, Ph.D., New Jersey Neuroscience Institute, 65 James Street, Edison, NJ 08818, USA. Tel: 732-205-1461, Fax: 732-632-1584. Email: jgiacino@solarishs.org

© 2005 Psychology Press Ltd
http://www.tandf.co.uk/journals/pp/09602011.html   DOI:10.1080/09602010443000498

the diagnosis of PVS might also lead to discussion of withdrawal of life-sustaining care which may be premature this early in the course of a patient who retains some degree of self or environmental awareness. Unfortunately, there is published evidence that the incidence of misdiagnosis among individuals with severe disturbances in arousal and behavioural responsiveness is unacceptably high. Estimates of misdiagnosis of the vegetative state (VS) range from 15–45% (Andrews, Murphy, Munday, & Littlewood, 1996; Childs, Mercer, & Childs, 1993; Tresch et al., 1991). Causes of misdiagnosis include poorly specified terminology, lack of familiarity with established diagnostic criteria and use of crude or inappropriate assessment methods. Although there are no empirical studies on diagnostic accuracy concerning patients in the minimally conscious state (MCS), a recent study by Giacino, Kalmar, and Whyte (2004) found that approximately 10% of patients diagnosed with VS according to the Disability Rating Scale (DRS; Rappaport et al., 1982) were actually in MCS. The false negative errors noted in this study were primarily due to the lack of sensitivity of the DRS to specific features of MCS.

This purpose of this paper is to review the clinical features and diagnostic criteria for VS and MCS as defined by the consensus statements of the Multi-Society Task Force on the Persistent Vegetative State (Multi-Society Task Force on PVS, 1994) and the Aspen Neurobehavioral Conference Workgroup (Giacino et al., 2002), respectively. We also discuss the prognostic parameters associated with these two conditions and review the current status of research on patients with disorders of consciousness. For additional discussion concerning diagnostic assessment tests and procedures, the interested reader is referred to the articles by Kalmar and Giacino, Shiel et al., and others in this issue.

CLINICAL FEATURES AND DIAGNOSTIC CRITERIA

Vegetative state

The diagnostic criteria for VS were established by the Multi-Society Task Force (MSTF) of the American Academy of Neurology following a systematic review of the literature from around the world. Although the MSTF's conclusions have been criticised from various perspectives (Childs & Mercer, 1996; Howsepian, 1996), they have been generally well accepted in neurorehabilitation and neurology (AAN, 1995; Giacino et al., 1997).

While there is no "official" definition of VS, this disorder is characterised by the complete absence of behavioural evidence for awareness of self and environment, with preserved capacity for spontaneous or stimulus-induced arousal (Giacino & Kalmar, 1997). According to the MSTF, all of the following criteria must be met to establish the diagnosis of VS:

1. No evidence of awareness of self or environment.

2. No evidence of sustained, reproducible, purposeful, or voluntary behavioural responses to visual, auditory, tactile, or noxious stimuli.

3. No evidence of language comprehension or expression.

4. Intermittent wakefulness manifested by the presence of sleep–wake cycles (i.e., periods of eye-opening).

5. Sufficient preservation of autonomic functions to permit survival with adequate medical care.

6. Bowel and bladder incontinence.

7. Variable preservation of cranial nerve and spinal reflexes.

A reliable diagnosis of VS typically requires serial bedside examination as behavioural responses in patients with disorders of consciousness are usually limited in frequency and complexity and may be difficult to interpret. Neuroimaging and laboratory studies are not sufficient to establish a diagnosis. Roving eye movements may be present in VS and are sometimes misinterpreted as visual pursuit, a behaviour commonly noted in MCS. Generalised physiological responses to pain, such as diaphoresis, abnormal posturing and tachypnoea remain intact in VS but there are no avoidant or localised motor responses. Head and limb movements may be observed but these behaviours are never purposeful. Complex movement patterns (Schiff et al., 2002), vocalisation (Jennett & Plum, 1972) and emotional responses (e.g., crying, smiling) (Jennett & Plum, 1972; Giacino et al., 1997) are sometimes noted in patients who survive longer than three months in VS but these behaviours are not provoked by specific environmental events.

Minimally conscious state

The Aspen Workgroup defined the minimally conscious state as a condition of severely altered consciousness in which minimal but definite behavioural evidence of self or environmental awareness is demonstrated (Giacino et al., 2002). This new diagnostic group was distinguished from patients in VS based on the requirement that there be at least one clear-cut behavioural sign of consciousness, and that the diagnostic term chosen to represent them should emphasise that these patients retain at least some capacity for cognitive processing. The diagnostic criteria for MCS are heavily weighted on intactness of the language and motor systems. Unlike determination of a diagnosis of VS, MCS should be diagnosed when there is clearly discernible evidence of *one or more* of the following behaviours:

1. Simple command-following.

2. Gestural or verbal yes/no responses.

3. Intelligible verbalisation.

4. Movements or affective behaviours that occur in contingent relation to relevant environmental stimuli and are not attributable to reflexive activity. Any of the following examples provide sufficient evidence for contingent behavioural responses:

   • Episodes of crying, smiling, or laughter in response to linguistic or visual content of emotional but not neutral topics or stimuli.

   • Vocalisation or gestures that occur in direct response to the linguistic content of comments or questions.

   • Reaching for objects that demonstrates a clear relationship between object location and direction of reach.

   • Touching or holding objects in a manner that accommodates the size and shape of the object.

   • Pursuit eye movement or sustained fixation that occurs in direct response to moving or salient stimuli.

In view of the absence of a gold standard to "prove" the presence or absence of consciousness, the boundaries that have been established to demarcate VS, MCS and emergence from MCS are necessarily arbitrary. Nevertheless, behaviourally-based operational criteria are required to provide a standard nomenclature for use in routine clinical care and in research. The lower limit of MCS is characterised by patients who demonstrate a single low-complexity behaviour such as pursuit eye movements or localisation following application of noxious stimulation. Emergence from MCS requires reliable and consistent evidence of either functional communication or functional object use. To demonstrate that the patient has regained functional communication, verbal or gestural "yes" and "no" responses must be discernible, accurate and consistent. Functional object use infers that the patient is able to discriminate and demonstrate the use of two or more common objects. Functional communication and object use were selected to mark the boundary between MCS and higher level cognitive functioning as these behaviours are prerequisite for meaningful interpersonal interaction and personal autonomy.

PROGNOSTIC PARAMETERS

Vegetative state

In 1972, Jennett and Plum introduced the term "persistent vegetative state" (PVS) to describe individuals who retained "vegetative" functions and periods of wakefulness after emerging from coma, but exhibited no behavioural evidence of self or environmental awareness. They stressed that the vegetative state should not be considered permanent until reliable prognostic criteria were identified. A little more than a decade later, Plum and Posner (1980) stated that PVS referred to the vegetative state in its permanent form. As a result of the ambiguity surrounding this term, PVS has been interpreted with wide discrepancies among clinicians and medical specialties. The MSTF recommended that PVS be diagnosed one month after brain injury but, in the following year, the American Congress of Rehabilitation Medicine suggested that the diagnosis of VS be deferred until 12 months after the onset of the brain injury (American Congress of Rehabilitation Medicine, 1995). The ensuing controversy between neurology and neurorehabilitation specialists provided the momentum needed to convene the Aspen Neurobehavioral Conference in the mid-1990s. Consisting of delegates from neurology, neurosurgery, neuropsychology, physiatry and bioethics, the charge of the Aspen Workgroup was to develop a consensus statement on the diagnosis and prognosis of VS. Among their recommendations, the workgroup proposed that the term "persistent VS" be abandoned in favour of accompanying the diagnosis with information concerning the cause of injury and length of time post-onset. The rationale supporting this recommendation rests on the premise that both of these variables represent important prognostic indicators that significantly influence outcome. The MSTF calculated average probabilities for recovery of consciousness and degree of functional disability at 12 months post-injury based on type of injury (traumatic vs. non-traumatic) and duration of VS utilising a sample of 434 patients with traumatic brain injury (TBI) and 169 non-TBI patients. The data clearly illustrated that cause of injury is a strong determinant of outcome from VS, with non-TBI patients having a shorter window for recovery and considerably greater severity of disability after one year. In 1995, the American Academy of Neurology (AAN, 1995) published a practice guideline based on the MSTF's recommendations that established parameters for determining when VS should be considered. See Table 1.

It is important to view the temporal cut-offs in Table 1 as probabilities. Recovery of consciousness has been reported after the criteria for "permanence" have been met (Arts et al., 1985; Childs & Mercer, 1996; Haig & Ruess, 1990) although such instances are rare. Of the MSTF's original data pool, only 53 patients were available for follow-up evaluation beyond

TABLE 1
Parameters for determining when VS should be
considered permanent

Cause of injury	Criterion for permanence
Traumatic brain injury	After 12 months
Congenital malformations	After 3–6 months
Non-traumatic brain injury	After 3 months
Metabolic disease	After 1–3 months
Degenerative disease	After 1–3 months
Anencephaly	At birth

12 months post-injury, and long-term outcome data were based on anecdotal reports in 50% of those cases. The generalisability of these parameters is also limited because some of the data were taken from studies completed as long as 20 years ago, at a time when medical care for VS patients was less advanced. The Aspen Workgroup also emphasised that *permanent VS* refers to prognosis and identifies the point after which recovery of consciousness is highly improbable but not impossible.

Minimally conscious state

There are few published studies that directly address prognosis in MCS. There is growing evidence that particular clinical signs may predict outcome following MCS. Several studies have reported that re-emergence of visual pursuit may presage recovery of other signs of consciousness. Giacino and Kalmar (1997) report a significantly higher incidence of visual pursuit among MCS patients admitted for inpatient rehabilitation (MCS = 82%, VS = 20%), independent of time post-injury. Additionally, among the 20% of VS patients who exhibited visual pursuit, 73% went on to recover other clear-cut signs of consciousness by 12 months post-injury, while only half of the VS patients without pursuit movements emerged from VS. Similarly, Ansell and Keenan (1989) found that subjects who demonstrated late improvement performed significantly better on tests of visual pursuit completed on admission to rehabilitation when compared to those who did not improve. A third study conducted by Shiel and associates (2000), found that acutely brain-injured patients who demonstrated visual pursuit on hospital admission were more likely to demonstrate social interaction and communicative behaviour later in their recovery course than those without evidence of pursuit. In light of these data, the Aspen Workgroup incorporated visual pursuit into the diagnostic criteria for MCS, recognising that this behaviour is not pathognomonic of MCS.

The 1997 study by Giacino and Kalmar also indicated that patients in MCS have a longer course of recovery and less disability on the DRS at one year post-injury relative to patients in VS. Patient groups were further subdivided by aetiology of injury (TBI vs. non-TBI) to control for the variance in outcome related to cause of injury. Results indicated that the MCS group continued to improve beyond the six month mark and went on to attain significantly better outcomes at 12 months post-injury. The difference in outcome between the groups was most significant in the traumatic MCS group which, on average, had moderate disability after one year. These studies suggest that the diagnosis of MCS appears to be associated with a reasonably favourable prognosis for recovery of function when it is diagnosed early in patients with traumatic brain injury. Clinical experience suggests that MCS may also represent a permanent outcome, although temporal cut-offs beyond which further recovery is unexpected have not yet been established empirically.

NEW DIRECTIONS FOR RESEARCH

The pace of research on disorders of consciousness has increased over the last 5 years. Advances in neuroimaging technologies have begun to elucidate the pathophysiology of VS and MCS allowing more accurate outcome prediction. Positron emission tomography (PET) studies reveal striking differences in the nature and extent of residual metabolic activity in patients diagnosed with VS and MCS (Laureys, Owen, & Schiff, 2004; Laureys et al., in press; Schiff et al., 2002). PET findings also indicate that patients in MCS, but not VS, retain function in association cortices which are believed to be responsible for mediating self and environmental awareness (Boly et al., 2004). Functional magnetic resonance imaging (fMRI) protocols designed to interrogate the integrity of sensorimotor, language and visual processing systems in patients with little to no behavioural evidence of spared function in these areas suggest that cortico-cortical connections in these networks are largely intact (Schiff et al., in press). Magnetic resonance spectroscopy and diffusion tensor imaging have been added to the cache of prognostic tools that can be exploited to increase prognostic specificity (Ashwal & Holshauser, 1997; Tong et al., 2004). Subtle forms of diffuse axonal injury, punctuate haemorrhages and hypoxic-ishaemic lesions, which contribute to morbidity but are difficult to detect on conventional MRI, show greater conspicuity when these techniques are employed.

Insights from this new generation of neuroimaging methods are expected to provide a road map for the development of novel treatment interventions. As these procedures bolster our ability to characterise the functional substrate underlying the severely limited response repertoire of patients in VS and MCS, individually-tailored neuromodulation strategies aimed at facilitating still-viable but downregulated network activity will become available. Such interventions offer the promise of restorating function during both the acute and chronic phases of recovery. Unlike the "coma stimulation" programmes of the 1980s, in this era of evidence-based medicine, treatments designed to speed recovery and improve quality of life following catastrophic brain injury will be carefully scrutinised before being accepted into mainstream rehabilitation by clinicians, payers and consumers.

CONCLUSION

Accurate differential diagnosis is an essential first step in the clinical management of patients with disorders of consciousness. In response to concerns about diagnostic and prognostic inaccuracy, consensus-based criteria have been developed to differentiate VS and MCS. The extent to which these guidelines have penetrated clinical care appears to vary by discipline and geographic location. Although the impact of these guidelines has not yet been formally assessed, their intent is to minimise the risk of misdiagnosis, inaccurate prognosis and inappropriate treatment decisions.

The development of novel neuroimaging procedures has significantly advanced our understanding of the pathophysiology of VS and MCS. The integration of structural and functional neuroimaging data with carefully-derived clinical findings obtained at the bedside is expected to increase diagnostic accuracy, improve outcome prediction and inform case-specific treatment interventions.

REFERENCES

American Academy of Neurology (1995). Practice parameter: Assessment and management of persons in the persistent vegetative state. *Neurology, 45,* 1015–1018.

American Congress of Rehabilitation Medicine (1995). Recommendations for use of nomenclature pertinent to persons with severe alterations in consciousness. *Archives of Physical Medicine and Rehabilitation, 76,* 205–209.

Andrews, K., Murphy, L., Munday, R., & Littlewood, C. (1996). Misdiagnosis of the vegetative state: Retrospective study in a rehabilitation unit. *British Medical Journal, 313,* 13–16.

Ansell, B. J., & Kennan, J. E. (1989). The Western Neuro Sensory Stimulation Profile: A tool for assessing slow-to-recover head-injured patients. *Archives of Physical Medicine and Rehabilitation, 70,* 104–108.

Arts, W. F., Van Dongen, H. R., Van Hof-Van Duin, J., & Lammens, E. (1985). Unexpected improvement after prolonged post-traumatic vegetative state. *Journal of Neurosurgery, Neurology and Psychiatry, 48,* 1300–1303.

Ashwal, S., & Holshouser, B. A. (1997). New neuroimaging techniques and their potential role in patients with acute brain injury. *Journal of Head Trauma Rehabilitation, 12*(4), 13–35.

Boly, M., Faymonville, M. E., Peigneux, P., Lambermont, B., Damas, P., Del Fiore, G., Degueldre, C., Franck, G., Luxen, A., Lamy, M., Moonen, G., Maquet, P., & Laureys, S. (2004). Auditory processing in severely brain injured patients. *Archives of Neurology, 61,* 233–238.

Childs, N. L., & Mercer, W. N. (1996). Late improvement in consciousness after post-traumatic vegetative state. *New England Journal of Medicine, 334*, 24–25.

Childs, N. L., Mercer, W. N., & Childs, H. W. (1993). Accuracy of diagnosis of persistent vegetative state. *Neurology, 43*(8), 1465–1467.

Giacino, J. T., Ashwal, S. A., Childs, N., Cranford, R., Jennett, B., Katz, D. I., Kelly, J., Rosenberg, J., Whyte, J., Zafonte, R., & Zasler, N. (2002). The minimally conscious state: Definition and diagnostic criteria. *Neurology, 58*, 349–353.

Giacino, J. T., & Kalmar, K. (1997). The vegetative and minimally conscious states: A comparison of clinical features and functional outcome. *Journal of Head Trauma Rehabilitation, 12*, 36–51.

Giacino, J. T., Kalmar, K., & Whyte, J. (2004). The JFK Coma Recovery Scale—Revised: Measurement characteristics and diagnostic utility. *Archives of Physical Medicine and Rehabilitation, 85*(12), 2020–2029.

Giacino, J. T., Zasler, N. D., Katz, D. I., Kelly, J. P., Rosenberg, J. H., & Filley, C. M. (1997). Development of practice guidelines for assessment and management of the vegetative and minimally consciousness states. *Journal of Head Trauma Rehabilitation, 12*(4), 79–89.

Haig, A. J., & Ruess, J. M. (1990). Recovery from vegetative state of six months duration associated with Sinemet (levadopa/carbidopa). *Archives of Physical Medicine and Rehabilitation, 71*, 1081–1083.

Howsepian, A. A. (1996). The 1994 Multi-Society Task Force consensus statement on the persistent vegetative state: A critical analysis. *Issues in Law and Medicine, 12*(1), 3–29.

Jennett, B., & Plum, F. (1972). Persistent vegetative state after brain damage: A syndrome in search of a name. *Lancet, 1*, 734–737.

Laureys, S., Owen, A., & Schiff, N. D. (2004). Brain function in coma, vegetative state, and related disorders. *Lancet Neurology, 3*, 537–546.

Laureys, S., Perrin, F., Faymonville, M. E., Schnakers, C., Boly, M., Bartsch, V., Majerus, S., Moonen, G., & Maquet, P. (in press). Cerebral processing in the minimally conscious state. *Neurology, 63*, 916–918.

Multi-Society Task Force on PVS (1994). Medical aspects of the persistent vegetative state. *New England Journal of Medicine, 330*, 1499–1508, 1572–1579.

Plum, F., & Posner, J. (1980). *The diagnosis of stupor and coma* (3rd ed.). Philadelphia: FA Davis.

Rappaport, M., Hall, K. M., Hopkins, K., Belleza, T., & Cope, D. N. (1982). Disability Rating Scale for severe head trauma: Coma to community. *Archives of Physical Medicine and Rehabilitation, 63*, 118–123.

Schiff, N. D., Ribary, U., Moreno, D. R., Beattie, B., Kronberg, E., Blasberg, R., Giacino, J., McCagg, C., Finns, J. J., Llinas, R., & Plum, F. (2002). Residual cerebral activity and behavioural fragments can remain in the persistently vegetative brain. *Brain, 125*, 1210–1234.

Schiff, N. D., Rodriguez-Moreno, D., Kamal, A., Him, K. H. S., Giacino, J. T., Plum, F., & Hirsch, J. (in press). Functional MRI reveals large scale network activation in minimally conscious patients. *Neurology.*

Shiel, A., Horn, S. A., Wilson, B. A., Watson, M. J., Campbell, M. J., & McLellan, D. L. (2000). The Wessex Head Injury Matrix (WHIM) main scale: A preliminary report on a scale to assess and monitor patient recovery after severe head injury. *Clinical Rehabilitation, 14*(4), 408–416.

Tong, K. A., Ashwal, S., Holshouser, B. A., Nickerson, J. P., Wall, C. J., Shutter, L. A., Osterdock, R. J., Haacke, E. M., & Kido, D. (2004). Diffuse axonal injury in children: Clinical correlation with hemorrhagic lesions. *Annals of Neurology, 56*(1), 36–50.

Tresch, D. D., Sims, F. H., Duthie, E. H., Goldstein, M. D., & Lane, P. S. (1991). Clinical characteristics of patients in the persistent vegetative state. *Archives of Physical Medicine and Rehabilitation, 151*, 930–932.

NEUROPSYCHOLOGICAL REHABILITATION
2005, 15 (3/4), 175–183

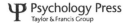

The vegetative state and the Royal College of Physicians guidance

David Bates

*Department of Neurology, Royal Victoria Infirmary,
Newcastle upon Tyne, UK*

The Royal College of Physicians of the UK, together with the Colleges of Edinburgh and Glasgow, have produced guidance on the diagnosis and management of people in the vegetative state (report of a working party of the Royal College of Physicians, 2003). Such guidance is important when the single criterion for awareness in an individual is the perception of that awareness by a potentially fallible observer. The current guidance is reviewed and comparisons made with existing arrangements in other countries. Consideration is given to the possibility of future improvements in diagnosis with the advent of imaging and metabolic assessments of brain function and the need to define the required qualifications and training for those "experts" who are currently involved in the diagnosis of the vegetative state.

INTRODUCTION

The improvement of resuscitative techniques in medicine during the middle of the 20th century saved many lives but also created the possibility of re-establishing normal cardiac activity after parts of the brain had been irretrievably injured. When the brain stem is so damaged the syndrome of brain stem death, which leads, inevitably to brain death, is recognised, the criteria defined and the management accepted throughout the world. In some patients, however, resuscitation may enable recovery of the brain stem in the absence of cortical function, either due to diffuse complete damage to the cortex or disruption of the pathways connecting the cortex to deeper structures.

Correspondence should be addressed to: Dr David Bates, Department of Neurology, Royal Victoria Infirmary, Queen Victoria Road, Newcastle upon Tyne, NE1 4LP. Email: david.bates@ncl.ac.uk

© 2005 Psychology Press Ltd
http://www.tandf.co.uk/journals/pp/09602011.html   DOI:10.1080/09602010443000399

The term "persistent vegetative state" was coined more than 30 years ago (Jennett & Plum, 1972) and has gradually come to replace the earlier descriptions of apallic syndrome, total dementia, akinetic mutism, and coma vigile.

More recently confusion has arisen over the nomenclature because the phrase "persistent vegetative state" has been replaced by the acronym PVS in which the first letter has sometimes been taken to mean "permanent". It is therefore recommended that the term "vegetative state" be used and the length of that state be separately identified to avoid the implication that a persistent vegetative state is necessarily permanent (Jennett, 1997).

It is difficult to establish the frequency with which the vegetative state occurs. Many people, as they recover from coma, pass through a transient vegetative state but it can persist until death. Assessments from studies of head injury around the world indicate a variable proportion of patients admitted with severe head injury who enter a persistent vegetative state, some authors suggesting as few as 1%, others as many as 6% or 7% (Braakman, Jennett, & Minderhoud, 1988). It is certain that as time passes fewer patients remain in the vegetative state and the prevalence of the chronic condition within the population lies probably between 20–120 people per million (Multi-Society Task Force on the Persistent Vegetative State, 1994). Approximately half of the patients so recorded enter the vegetative state following head injury, the others as the result of acute cardio-pulmonary arrest, anaesthetic accidents, stroke, cerebral haemorrhage, infection or as the terminal effect of a degenerative neurological condition (Levy et al., 1981).

In 1992, the Bland case in the English High Court raised public awareness of the condition, and since it was subsequently suggested that "every case should come to court" it was feared that there would be a huge number of cases brought before the High Court (McLean, 2001). In practice there have been less than 40 such cases during the 12 years since the index case and the Scottish, American and Dutch Court rulings that cases should only come to court when there was a dispute between relevant parties seems both acceptable and reasonable.

THE NEED FOR GUIDANCE

The relative infrequency of the condition, and the even greater infrequency of the requirement for formal reporting to a court, means that few people have sufficient expertise in the identification and assessment of the vegetative state. The variability of causation involving trauma, vascular disease, infection and degenerative disease, together with crossing the age range from paediatric to geriatric means that many different physicians and surgeons may see patients in this condition. Against this background the Royal Colleges in the UK thought it appropriate to review the topic and provide guidelines so that physicians and surgeons working in accident and emergency departments, intensive care units, medical, surgical, neurological, paediatric or geriatric units or in long-term care and rehabilitation should understand the requirements for the diagnosis and the system for documenting observations, informing the relatives of patients, and making formal decisions.

The guidelines define the terms "wakefulness" and "awareness", explain the condition of the vegetative state and recognise that the vegetative state may be termed "persistent" when it continues for more than four weeks. They also state that if a prediction of "permanence" be made, implying that awareness will never recover, it is not made with absolute certainty but based on reasonable, current evidence in relation to prognosis.

CRITERIA FOR DIAGNOSIS

Preconditions

The guidelines require important pre-conditions, which are usually easy to establish; there should be an identified cause of the condition which is recognised to be capable of resulting in the vegetative state; the persisting effects of sedative, anaesthetic or neuromuscular blocking drugs must be excluded as the continuing cause of reduced conscious level; metabolic disturbances must be corrected as far as possible, although it is recognised that metabolic changes do occur during the course of prolonged intensive care treatment and in any chronic, immobilising condition; any structural cause that is causative and potentially correctable must be excluded or reversed.

Clinical features

The clinical criteria required for diagnosis are that there must be no evidence of awareness of self or environment at any time; no response to visual, auditory, tactile or noxious stimuli of a kind suggesting volition or conscious purpose; no evidence of language comprehension or meaningful expression. In addition, it is recognised that there are typically cycles of eye closure and eye opening and that hypothalamic and brain stem function are usually sufficiently preserved to ensure the maintenance of respiration and circulation.

Examples

The guidelines outline a series of clinical features that have been documented previously in people who are in the vegetative state and which are therefore compatible with that diagnosis, a series of features that are compatible but unusual, and several clinical features that make the diagnosis untenable. Included among the latter are evidence of discriminative perception, purposeful actions, and communication. The examples given are of a smile in response to the arrival of a friend or relative, an attempt to reach out for an object or the appropriate use of language, all of which would indicate the presence of a "functioning mind" and exclude the diagnosis.

Among those unusual features compatible with the diagnosis it is recognised that some people in a vegetative state have been described to fixate a target and even follow a moving target, show isolated fragments of behaviour including the utterance of a single inappropriate word or have focal seizures. These features should always prompt careful reassessment but are not inconsistent with the decision that the individual is not aware of self or environment at any time.

Appendix

The guidance includes appendices that provide a check-list for the diagnosis of the vegetative state and the decision that the state shall be regarded as permanent, and several vignettes in which the clinical history of individuals is used to define whether they are unresponsive and unaware and reasons given for those decisions. Such descriptions of response have been found useful in earlier guidance documents (British Medical Association, 1993; International Working Party Report on the Vegetative State, 1996).

MANAGEMENT

Care

The guidelines suggest that medical care with high quality nursing is always obligatory and that as part of this care medical and nursing staff must keep relatives and carers well-informed throughout the course of the condition. It is stressed that the initial diagnosis and the subsequent monitoring must be made carefully, recognition being given to the fact that the vegetative state has previously been diagnosed in error (Andrews, Murphy, Munday, & Littlewood, 1996; Childs, Mercer, & Childs, 1993). It is recommended that the patient be examined by two doctors, both of whom have experience in assessing disorders of consciousness, although it is not defined whether they shall be neurologists, doctors involved in rehabilitation, or from other specialities. It is of course likely that they will be specialists involved in the longer-term care of individuals since, although the vegetative state may be diagnosed acutely in the intensive care unit, high dependency or general ward within a few days or weeks of the ictus, the important longer-term assessment is likely to occur months after the event and at a time when the individual is in a long-stay unit, undergoing rehabilitation, or at home.

Assessment

The guidance stresses that the doctors making the assessment must take into account information from the medical staff, other clinical staff, including neuropsychologists, occupational therapists and physiotherapists, and particularly from nurses, carers and relatives who are likely to spend most time with the patient. The two doctors making the assessment should make their assessments separately, consider the results of investigations which have been undertaken and preferably examine the patient on more than one occasion and in more than one position. It is recommended that nursing staff and relatives are present during the assessment.

Permanent vegetative state

The guidelines stress that there is no urgency in making the diagnosis of permanence in the vegetative state. If there is any uncertainty the diagnosis should not be made and the patient should be reassessed. It may, for example, be reasonable to suggest the withdrawal of some potentially sedating agent before reassessing the patient, or to take more information from nurses and carers.

Formal procedure

It is accepted in the guidelines that when a diagnosis of the permanent vegetative state is made, having established the cause of the syndrome, confirming the clinical state and with the passage of time, then recovery cannot reasonably be expected and further therapy is futile. The continuation of artificial feeding and hydration merely prolongs an insentient life for the patient and a hopeless vigil entailing major emotional costs for relatives and carers. When this decision is made the clinical team should review the evidence formally, discuss it sensitively with relatives who should then be given time to consider the implications including the possibility of the withdrawal of artificial means of administering nutrition and hydration.

It is noted that, at present, in England and Wales the courts require that the decision to withdraw nutrition and hydration should be referred to them before any action is taken (British Medical Association, 2001; General Medical Council, 2002). In Scotland the court does not have such requirement and there is great variation around the world, North America and much of northern Europe holding a view similar to that in Scotland while much of southern Europe has laws and recommendations like those in England and Wales. The guidelines, nonetheless, suggest that even within Scotland it would be appropriate for a doctor to seek the authority of the Court of Session to guarantee that the Lord Advocate would not initiate a criminal prosecution.

Other therapies

The guidance also considers the possibility of withdrawing other life-sustaining medication, including insulin or dialysis and advises that these be referred to the courts. The guidance, however, suggests that the decision not to intervene with cardio-pulmonary resuscitation, antibiotics, dialysis or insulin can be taken clinically in the best interests of the patient and after full discussion with those concerned, although this information may now be out of date in light of the recent Bourke case in the UK.

Relatives/carers/friends

Perhaps the most important aspect of the guidance from the Royal Colleges is a five page appendix which is intended for relatives, carers and friends of the person in the vegetative state. It is a lay version of the information about the state, its causation, assessment, prognosis and management which has been written by, and for, patient organisations.

THE SITUATION ELSEWHERE

The American Medical Association and the Multi-Society Task Force in the USA have been major driving forces in the decisions about management of people in the vegetative state. It is widely accepted that although there is a high mortality in adults during the first year in the vegetative state, those who survive for a year may live on for several more years and although only anecdotal information is available in the longer term there are reports of people surviving for decades. In the wake of the Karen Ann Quillin case in 1976 there were many court applications to limit ventilation, surgery, chemotherapy and tube feeding and in 1983 the President's Commission for the Study of Ethical Problems in Medicine declared that the withdrawal of tube feeding from vegetative patients not expected to recover, was good clinical practice (President's Commission, 1983).

By the late 1980s the courts in America stated that it was "no longer necessary or desirable for these cases to be brought to court unless there was dispute between relevant parties" and in 1990 the US Supreme Court reaffirmed that artificial nutrition and hydration are medical treatments that can be withdrawn. This decision has received support from the American Academy of Neurology, (1989) the American Medical Association (1990) and the American Neurological Association (1993). It has also received support from the British Medical Association (1993), The Netherlands Health Council (Health Council of The Netherlands, 1994), and the New Zealand Medical Association (1994) and in 1989 the World Medical Association approved treatment withdrawal once "permanence" was established (World Medical Association, 1989).

Similar views followed in 1992 in Belgium and in 1994 in The Netherlands, and most of these centres allowed withdrawal of tube feeding without reference to the courts 6 months after anoxic damage, or 12 months after traumatic brain damage. The original Royal College of Physicians guidance in 1996

(Royal College of Physicians, 1996) adopted identical views and similar practice is extant in Norway, Sweden, Denmark, and Japan.

The continuing requirement that every case should come to court in the UK is unique and studies of physicians' opinion in the UK and Belgium indicate that only a minority of physicians would like to see every case go to court. Most would prefer legalisation to allow physicians and families to make decisions according to agreed guidelines or guidance. There is wide international consensus that prolonging the survival of patients in a vegetative state is not in the patient's best interests and the physician therefore has no moral or legal obligation to continue life-sustaining treatment or to intervene to treat life-threatening complications (Grubb et al., 1996; Payne, Taylor, Stocking, & Sack, 1996). There is, however disagreement, in Mediterranean and Eastern European countries it is thought morally and legally necessary to continue active treatment indefinitely and there is no true uniformity in practice.

DIFFICULTIES IN DIAGNOSIS

The major driving force for the Royal College of Physicians guidance is the recognition that there are problems in making an assessment of awareness which is inevitably subjective. The initial College guidelines were probably too stringent in requiring certain reflex anomalies to be demonstrated and they were not in the spirit of the original paper from Jennett and Plum (1972). The more modern guidelines try to explain, as others have done, by the use of patient vignettes, those things that are acceptable and those that are not acceptable as part of the diagnosis. The major problem lies in distinguishing the vegetative state from the minimally conscious state.

Emphasis is firmly placed on loss of awareness as the single cardinal feature and patients who do not meet this criterion are considered to be "minimally conscious". There are no universally recognised systems for assessing the vegetative state as distinct from the minimally conscious state and features such as spontaneous limb movement, head movement, exploration of body parts, quasi-purposeful movements, grunting, grinding teeth, frowning, groaning, grimacing and brief visual tracking present difficulties because they are poorly defined and the assessor has to make a purely subjective judgement to interpret whether the behaviour is a significant response, which is reproducible and indicative of awareness.

Techniques have been developed to improve and standardise clinical evaluations such as the Sensory Modality Assessment Rehabilitation Tool (SMART) but they are time taking and not yet validated (Gill-Thwaites, 1997). It is widely recognised that nurses, occupational therapists, psychologists and physiotherapists who spend considerable time as part of a multidisciplinary team with the vegetative patient are well positioned to make frequent and meaningful observations. The Wessex Head Injury Matrix (WHIM; Shiel et al., 2000) has been validated in part, and may be an additional method to assess such patients. There are also other and newer, although less well-validated, behavioural assessments.

The question which arises is whether neuro-imaging or neurophysiological techniques might, in future, provide better information about brain activity. In this special issue the value of neurophysiological techniques are considered and the suggestion made that there may be sub-types of the vegetative state identifiable neurophysiologically which may have clinical correlates. In a recent formal review of the value of imaging techniques it is recognised that they are methodologically complex, need more careful quantative analysis and interpretation and have nothing to add to clinical examination at present (Laureys, Owen, & Schiff, 2004). Longitudinal studies, such as described elsewhere in this special issue, when related to clinical responses, may assist in defining the clinical state. Neuro-imaging techniques are very important in clinical research, they will extend our understanding of the underlying mechanisms of consciousness and coma but they are not yet useful in determining the presence of awareness (Shiel et al., 2004).

REFERENCES

American Academy of Neurology (1989). Position of the American Academy of Neurology on certain aspects of the care and management of the persistent vegetative state patient. *Neurology, 39*, 125–126.

American Medical Association. Council on Scientific Affairs and Council on Ethical and Judicial Affairs (1990). Persistent vegetative state and the decision to withdraw or withhold life support. *Journal of the American Medical Association, 263*, 426–430.

American Neurological Association Committee on Ethical Affairs (1993). Persistent vegetative state. *Annals of Neurology, 33*, 386–390.

Andrews, K., Murphy, L., Munday, R., Littlewood, C. (1996). Misdiagnosis of the vegetative state. *British Medical Journal, 313*, 13–16.

Braakman, R., Jennett, W. B., & Minderhoud, J. M. (1988). Prognosis of the posttraumatic vegetative state. *Acta Neurochir (Wien), 95*(1–2), 49–52.

British Medical Association (1993). *Guidelines on treatment decisions for patients in the persistent vegetative state—Annual report* (Appendix 7). London: BMA.

British Medical Association (2001) *Withholding and withdrawing life-prolonging medical treatment: Guidance for decision making* (2nd ed.). London: BMJ Books.

Childs, N., Mercer, W. N., & Childs, H. W. (1993). Accuracy of diagnosis of the persistent vegetative state. *Neurology, 43*, 1465–1467.

General Medical Council (2002). *Withholding and withdrawing life-prolonging treatment: Good practice in decision making.* London: GMC.

Gill-Thwaites, H. (1997). The Sensory Modality Assessment Rehabilitation Technique—A tool for assessment and treatment of patients with severe brain injury in the vegetative state. *Brain Injury, 11*, 723–734.

Grubb, A., Walsh, P., Lambe, N., Murrells, T., & Robinson, S. (1996). Survey of British clinician's views on management of patients in persistent vegetative state. *Lancet, 348*, 35–40.

Health Council of The Netherlands (1994). *Committee on Vegetative State. Patients in a vegetative state.* The Hague, The Netherlands: Health Council of The Netherlands.

International Working Party (1996). *Report on the vegetative state.* London: Royal Hospital for Neuro-Disability.

Jennett, B. (1997). A quarter century of the vegetative state: An international perspective. *Journal of Head Trauma Rehabilitation, 12,* 1–12.

Jennett, B., & Plum, F. (1972). Persistent vegetative state after brain damage. *Lancet, 1* (April, 7753), 734–737.

Laureys, S., Owen, A. M., & Schiff, N. D. (2004). Brain function in coma, vegetative state, and related disorders. *Lancet, 3,* 537–546.

Levy, D. E., Bates, D., Caronna, J. J., Cartlidge, N. E., Knill-Jones, R. P., Lapinski, R. H., Singer, B. H., Shaw, D. A., & Plum, F. (1981). Prognosis in non-traumatic coma. *Annals of Internal Medicine, 94*(3), 293–301.

McLean, S. (2001). Permanent vegetative state and the law. *Journal of Neurology, Neurosurgery, and Psychiatry, 71*(Suppl 1), i26–i27.

Multi-Society Task Force on the Persistent Vegetative State (1994). Medical aspects of a persistent vegetative state. *New England Journal of Medicine, 330,* 499–508, 572–579.

New Zealand Medical Association Public Issues Advisory Committee (1994). *Policy paper: Persistent vegetative state.* Wellington, New Zealand: New Zealand Medical Association.

Payne, K., Taylor, R. M., Stocking, C., & Sack, G. A. (1996). Physicians attitudes about the care of patients in the persistent vegetative state: A national survey. *Annals of Internal Medicine, 125,* 104–110.

President's Commission for the Study of Ethical Problems in Medicine (1983). *Deciding to forgo life-sustaining treatment.* Washington DC: US Government Printing Office.

Royal College of Physicians (1996). *The permanent vegetative state* [A Working Party report]. London: Royal College of Physicians.

Royal College of Physicians (2003). *The vegetative state: Guidance on diagnosis and management* [Report of a Working Party]. London: Royal College of Physicians.

Shiel, A., Gelling, L., Wilson, B., Coleman, M., & Pickard, J. D. (2004). Difficulties in diagnosing the vegetative state. *British Journal of Neurosurgery, 18,* 5–7.

Shiel, A., Horn, S. A., Wilson, B. A., Watson, M. J., Campbell, M. J., & McLenlan, D. L. (2000). The Wessex Head Injury Matrix (WHIM) main scale: Preliminary report on a scale to assess and monitor patient recovery after severe head injury. *Clinical Rehabilitation, 14,* 408–416.

World Medical Association (1989). *Statement on persistent vegetative state.* Ferney-Voltaire, France: World Medical Association.

NEUROPSYCHOLOGICAL REHABILITATION
2005, 15 (3/4), 184–189

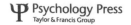
Ψ Psychology Press
Taylor & Francis Group

Incidence and prevalence of the vegetative and minimally conscious states

J. Graham Beaumont and Pamela M. Kenealy

Royal Hospital for Neuro-disability, London and School of Human and Life Sciences, Roehampton University, London, UK

The methodological difficulties of obtaining accurate epidemiological data for vegetative state (VS) and minimally conscious state (MCS) are considered, and prompt the conclusion that published data are of uncertain validity, partly due to variation in the criteria for diagnosis. On the basis of these data, incidence of VS continuing for at least six months arises at a rate of between 5 and 25 per million population (PMP). The prevalence of VS in adults in the US is between 40 and 168 PMP, and may be lower in the UK, but precise figures are not available. The incidence and prevalence of MCS have yet to be established.

INTRODUCTION

To establish valid epidemiological data depends critically on two principal factors: Clear, precise and universally accepted criteria for the diagnosis of a disorder, stable over time; and adequate systems for the collection of epidemiological data. Neither exists for vegetative state (VS) or for minimally conscious state (MCS). As a consequence, the available information concerning incidence and prevalence remains a rather unsatisfactory estimate.

Neither VS nor MCS are formal diagnoses under either DSM-IV-TR (American Psychiatric Association, 2000) or ICD-10 (World Health Organization, 1992) and as a consequence official national statistics are not available for these conditions. While clear criteria have evolved for VS over the period

Correspondence should be sent to Professor J. Graham Beaumont, Department of Clinical Psychology, Royal Hospital for Neuro-disability, West Hill, Putney, London SW15 3SW, UK. Tel: 020 8780 4500 x 5013, Fax: 020 8780 4501. Email: gbeaumont@rhn.org.uk

© 2005 Psychology Press Ltd
http://www.tandf.co.uk/journals/pp/09602011.html   DOI:10.1080/09602010443000489

since it was initially described by Jennett and Plum (1972), there are as yet no internationally agreed criteria for diagnosis, and there has been change over time. The position with regard to MCS, as a more recently formalised diagnosis (Giacino, Ashwal, Childs, Cranford, Jennett, Katz, et al., 2002), is naturally even less clear. Within these significant limitations, the current state of knowledge will be reviewed.

INCIDENCE OF VS

The most influential criteria for the diagnosis of VS have been the findings of the Multi-Society Task Force on PVS (1994), generally referred to as the "Task Force", although the UK Royal College of Physicians (1996) working party report and the International Working Party (1996) have also been influential. It remains to be seen whether the more recent report of the Royal College of Physicians (2003) effectively supersedes these earlier criteria.

The difficulty for establishing incidence has lain not so much in the criteria for diagnosis of VS as a general condition, but in the period before which it should be regarded as *permanent, persistent*, or *persisting*. For example, a continuing difficulty has been that the Task Force regarded VS as permanent after one year (for traumatic causes; although after three months for non-traumatic aetiology), while the Royal College of Physicians (1996) as after six months. As VS may be a relatively brief transitory state between coma and consciousness in the early period following insult, it is only in the continuing state of impaired consciousness and awareness that these differing diagnostic criteria are of considerable importance. The Royal College of Physicians (2003) guidance suggests that VS be regarded as *persistent* after four weeks, and that a later stage it may be considered *permanent* although on clinical rather than temporal considerations. These anomalies risk increasing the confusion concerning the diagnosis, and many believe that these terms would be better abandoned, and the diagnosis qualified by cause and duration from onset.

It has also been accepted that misdiagnosis occurs with unacceptable frequency in relation to VS (Andrews, Murphy, Munday, & Littlewood, 1996; Childs, Mercer, & Childs, 1993; Tresch et al., 1991); and the cause is generally thought to be an inadequate frequency, duration and range of observations of each patient with a disorder of consciousness. Andrews and colleagues, for example, identified a misdiagnosis rate as high as 42% in their study. Strens, Mazibrada, Duncan, and Greenwood (2004) have also illustrated the role of medication in misdiagnosis. Approaches to data collection have also proved unreliable. In Japan, Higashi (1995) attempted to collect epidemiological data by postal survey, but subsequently found only 57% of those reported to be in VS, actually were upon examination. The disparate placements of patients continuing in VS, from a variety of care institutions to being at home, also hinders the collection of relevant data.

There are also considerable national variations in reported rates for VS. As one of the major causes of VS is traumatic brain injury (accounting for up to half of vegetative survivors), this is unsurprising as rates of severe head injury differ markedly between countries. In the US severe brain injury occurs at a rate of about 200 per million population (PMP) giving, after 15% mortality, a general rate of 170 PMP (Giacino & Zasler, 1995), although it is accepted that the incidence in the UK is roughly half of this rate. The potential pool of those at risk for VS therefore appears to differ markedly as a result of social and economic factors which may include the risk of traumatic injury (especially the incidence of motor vehicle accidents) and access to emergency medicine. Differences in emergency room practice, among countries and across time, also have an impact on those with extremely severe trauma who may survive in a continuing VS (Sazbon & Dolce, 2002).

Bearing in mind all these considerations, the most authoritative and complete recent review of incidence has been provided by Jennett (2002a, b). Full details are available in these publications, but Jennett essentially finds that for the countries where adequate data are available, the estimated annual incidence (PMP) for VS from all acute causes (so excluding congenital and progressive degenerative causes) at various periods post-incident is: UK, 14 at 1 month, 8 at 3 months, and 5 at 6 months; USA, 46 at 1 month, 27 at 3 months, and 17 at 6 months; France, 67 at 1 month, 40 at 3 months and 25 at 6 months.

Sazbon and Dolce (2002) have reported data from Israel over 23 years; Israel is a special case as all patients in VS at one month are transferred to a single specialist hospital. Between 1975 and 1983 there were an average of 16.3 admissions per year, while from 1983 to 1998 the annual rate rose to 30 cases. This results in incidence figures of 4–5 PMP.

PREVALENCE OF VS

The determination of prevalence is confounded by all the above factors which affect the estimation of incidence. In particular, changing medical practice over time has an important influence on survival and therefore prevalence. An additional minor factor is the varying legal position in different countries with respect to the withdrawal of artificial nutrition and hydration leading to the termination of life in VS.

Again, Jennett's recent work (2002a, 2002b) is the most thorough and useful source of information concerning prevalence. Prevalence is a simple function of incidence and survival, but in VS is complicated by the fact that with an increasing period of survival in VS (as opposed to death or recovery) the likely period of further survival increases. The Task Force demonstrated that mean survival of those in VS at one month post-incident was 2–5 years, but for those surviving in VS at one year, if young, the mean survival was 10.5 years (although given the positively skewed distribution, the median statistic of 5.2 years may be more appropriate). For those in VS at 4 years, the mean survival was a mean 12.2 *further* years (median 7 further years). Prevalence estimates on the basis of extensive data have only been calculated for the US and vary between 40 and 168 PMP for adults, and 16 and 40 PMP for children. Jennett's comment that "the wide range of these estimates emphasises the uncertainty that remains about the size of the problem" (2002b, p. 36) seems entirely apposite.

Additional data have become available since Jennett's survey for Austria (Stepan, Haidinger, & Binder, 2004) which gives a prevalence of 19 PMP; and for Denmark (Engberg & Teasdale, 2004) which indicates a point prevalence for VS at 5 years post-incident of 1.3 PMP. A survey in Northern Ireland has been reported by Wilson, Harpur, Watson, and Morrow (2002) with 23 PMP in VS or a minimally responsive state.

Long survivors, and late recoveries, have been of particular interest in VS and while these concepts are essentially distinct, they are often confused in the limited available literature. It is also the case that reports of extraordinary survival have appeared more frequently in the media than in the scientific literature. Late discovery of earlier recoveries is a natural confounding factor in these data. Jennett (2002a, 2002b) is again the source of an authoritative review of well-documented cases and, while the Task Force accepted occasional survivals of 20 or more years, the longest well-documented survival identified by Jennett was 84 months in VS (Dyer, 1997). The disparity between this information based on single cases, and the estimated survival predictions reported above will be noted; but currently cannot be resolved.

MCS

The existence of states which do not fully qualify as VS but which share many critical features has long been recognised, and often conceived of as emergence from VS. Such a state is not uncommonly transitional in the period before a more adequate level of consciousness and responsivity is gained, although it should also be recognised that MCS may be an initial condition in its own right without a prior period in VS, or following a deterioration in the level of consciousness.

Such states have been recently placed on a more formal basis as MCS by Giacino and colleagues (Giacino et al., 2002) as either developing out of VS or coma, or else resulting from congenital nervous system disorders. They are often transient, but may exist as a continuing outcome and are characterised by inconsistent but clearly discernible behavioural evidence of consciousness. They are distinguished from VS and coma by the presence of specific behavioural phenomena which are absent in these conditions: The evidence of some degree of awareness, a definite response to noxious stimuli, and some verbal or purposeful motor behaviour even where this may be inconsistent (as indicated, for example, by the Sensory Modality Assessment Rehabilitation Technique, SMART; Gill-Thwaites & Munday, 1999; see also Koren, Gil, & Sazbon, 2002, for a review of other assessment instruments). MCS has now been accepted within the diagnostic classification proposed by the Royal College of Physicians (2003), replacing earlier alternative terms such as "minimally responsive" or "low awareness" state.

It is difficult to judge how patients now regarded as in MCS were previously classified with respect to incidence and prevalence. It seems likely that those with very minimal responsiveness were classified with VS, while those with clearer evidence of response to their environment were not. Giacino and colleagues accurately state that estimates of the incidence and prevalence of severe disorders of consciousness are unavailable, although their own estimate of adult and paediatric prevalence of MCS in the US is 48–96 PMP.

CONCLUSION

Epidemiological data concerning VS are indifferent in quality, and subject to a variety of sources of error. Calculation of incidence depends heavily upon the period post-incident at which VS is considered, and there are considerable national variations, but incidence of VS continuing for at least six months arises at a rate of between 5 and 25 PMP according to published data. In the US, the prevalence of VS in adults is reported to be between 40 and 168 PMP, although the figure may be lower in the UK and other European countries; accurate figures are not available at the present time. The incidence and prevalence of MCS have yet to be established.

REFERENCES

American Psychiatric Association (2000). *Diagnostic and statistical manual of mental disorders* (4th ed., text revision). Washington, DC: American Psychiatric Association.

Andrews, K., Murphy, L., Munday, R., & Littlewood, C. (1996). Misdiagnosis of the vegetative state: Retrospective study in a rehabilitation unit. *British Medical Journal, 313*, 13–16.

Childs, N. L., Mercer, W. N., & Childs, H. W. (1993). Accuracy of diagnosis of persistent vegetative state. *Neurology, 43*, 1465–1467.

Dyer, C. (1997). Hillsborough survivor emerges from the permanent vegetative state. *British Medical Journal, 314*, 996.

Engberg, A. W., & Teasdale, T. W. (2004). A population-based study of survival and discharge status for survivors after head injury. *Acta Neurologica Scandinavica, 110*, 281–290.

Giacino, J. T., & Zasler, N. D. (1995). Outcome after severe traumatic brain injury: Coma, the vegetative state and the minimally responsive state. *Journal of Head Trauma Rehabilitation, 10*, 40–56.

Giacino, J. T., Ashwal, S., Childs, N., Cranford, R., Jennett, B., Katz, D. I., et al. (2002). The minimally conscious state: Definition and diagnostic criteria. *Neurology, 58*, 349–353.

Gill-Thwaites, H., & Munday, R. (1999) The Sensory Modality Assessment and Rehabilitation Technique (SMART): A comprehensive and integrated assessment and treatment protocol for the vegetative state and minimally responsive patient. *Neuropsychological Rehabilitation, 9*, 305–320.

Higashi, K. (1995). Epidemiology of catastrophic brain injury. In H. S. Levin & A. L. Benton (Eds.), *Catastrophic brain injury* (pp. 15–35). Oxford: Oxford University Press.

International Working Party (1996). *Report on the vegetative state.* London: Royal Hospital for Neuro-disability.

Jennett, B. (2002a). The vegetative state. *Journal of Neurology, Neurosurgery and Psychiatry, 73*, 355–357.

Jennett, B. (2002b). *The vegetative state: Medical facts, ethical and legal dilemmas.* Cambridge: Cambridge University Press.

Jennett, B., & Plum, F. (1972). Persistent vegetative state after brain damage. *Lancet, 1* (April, 7753), 734–737.

Koren, C., Gil, M., & Sazbon, L. (2002). Assessment of the vegetative state. In G. Dolce & L. Sazbon (Eds.), *The post-traumatic vegetative state* (pp. 46–59). Stuttgart: Thieme.

Multi-Society Task Force on PVS (1994). Medical aspects of the vegetative state, (in two parts). *New England Journal of Medicine, 330*, 1499–1508, 1572–1579.

Royal College of Physicians (1996). *The permanent vegetative state: A working party report.* London: Royal College of Physicians.

Royal College of Physicians. (2003). *The vegetative state: Guidance on diagnosis and management.* London: Royal College of Physicians.

Sazbon, L., & Dolce, G. (2002). Preliminary concepts. In G. Dolce & L. Sazbon (Eds.), *The post-traumatic vegetative state* (pp. 3–10). Stuttgart: Thieme.

Stepan, C., Haidinger, G., & Binder, H. (2004). Prevalence of persistent vegetative state/apallic syndrome in Vienna. *European Journal of Neurology, 11*, 461–466.

Strens, L. H., Mazibrada, G., Duncan, J. S., & Greenwood, R. (2004). Misdiagnosing the vegetative state after severe brain injury: The influence of medication. *Brain Injury, 18*, 213–218.

Tresch, D. D., Sims, F. H., Duthie, E. H., Goldstein, M. D., & Lane, P. S. (1991). Clinical characteristics of patients in the persistent vegetative state. *Archives of Internal Medicine, 151*, 930–932.

Wilson, F. C., Harpur, J., Watson, T., & Morrow, J. I. (2002). Vegetative state and minimally responsive patients: Regional survey, long-term case outcomes and service recommendations. *Neurorehabilitation, 17*, 231–236.

World Health Organisation (1992). *The ICD-10 Classification of mental and behavioural disorders: Clinical descriptions and diagnostic guidelines.* Geneva: World Health Organisation.

NEUROPSYCHOLOGICAL REHABILITATION
2005, 15 (3/4), 190–197

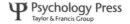

Recovery of consciousness and life expectancy of children in a vegetative state

Stephen Ashwal

Department of Pediatrics, Loma Linda University School of Medicine, Loma Linda, CA, USA

The vegetative state does occur in children and is most commonly due to acquired traumatic and non-traumatic injuries. However, neurometabolic and degenerative diseases, as well as certain developmental brain malformations such as anencephaly, can also cause this condition. There are limited data available in children concerning recovery of consciousness and function from the vegetative state as well as life expectancy. This review concentrates on these issues and is based primarily on the data published in the Multi-Society Task Force Report on PVS which was published in 1994 as well as other epidemiological studies. Children in a vegetative state do have a poor prognosis for recovery of consciousness and function and do have a shortened life expectancy. Further research is needed to better understand what variables might contribute to recovery and what therapies might be of benefit.

INTRODUCTION

Very limited data are available regarding recovery from the vegetative state (VS) and the life expectancy of children with this condition. In 1994, the Multi-Society Task Force (MSTF) on the persistent vegetative state published data extracted from the world's literature regarding these two issues (MSTF, 1994) and since then several epidemiological studies have been published that have further examined these issues (Ashwal, Eyman, & Call, 1994; Strauss, Shavelle, & Ashwal, 1999; Strauss, Ashwal, Day, & Shavelle, 2000).

Correspondence should be addressed to Stephen Ashwal MD, Department of Pediatrics, Loma Linda University School of Medicine, 11175 Campus Street, Loma Linda, CA 92350. Tel: 909 558-8242, Fax: 909 558-0479, Email: sashwal@ahs.llumc.edu

http://www.tandf.co.uk/journals/pp/09602011.html   DOI:10.1080/09602010443000281

TABLE 1
Worldwide prevalence of children aged less than 15 years in a vegetative state

Region	Total Population (<15 years)	Average number of VS patients	Low estimate of number of VS patients	High estimate of number of VS patients
World	1,894,200,000	92,816	11,365	151,536
Continents				
North America	67,830,000	3,324	407	5,426
Latin America	172,800,000	8,467	1,037	13,824
Europe	123,590,000	6,056	742	9,887
Asia	1,149,000,000	56,301	6,894	91,920
Africa	361,620,000	17,719	2,170	28,930
Selected Countries				
Belgium	1,872,000	92	11	150
China	283,514,000	13,892	1,701	22,681
Denmark	1,026,000	50	6	82
Finland	936,000	46	6	75
France	11,362,000	557	68	909
Germany	12,390,000	607	74	991
Greece	1,540,000	75	9	123
Iceland	69,000	3	0	6
India	384,696,000	18,850	2,308	30,776
Ireland	840,000	41	5	67
Israel	1,876,000	92	11	150
Italy	8,008,000	392	48	641
Japan	17,850,000	875	107	1,428
Netherlands	3,078,000	151	18	246
Norway	920,000	45	6	74
Portugal	1,664,000	82	10	133
Russia	26,190,000	1,283	157	2,095
Spain	6,195,000	304	37	496
Sweden	1,620,000	79	10	130
Switzerland	1,241,000	61	7	99
United Kingdom	11,248,000	551	67	900
United States	61,215,000	3,000	367	4,897

Population data obtained from http://www.prb.org/datafind/datafinder.htm. Prevalence rates are based on previously published data as summarised in Ashwal et al., 1994. These prevalence data were then used to calculate an average prevalence rate and this rate was used for the population of children <15 years of age for each region or country listed in the table. Overall, the average prevalence of VS patients was 49 per million with the low estimate being 6 per million and the high estimate being 80 per million.

EPIDEMIOLOGY

It is difficult to obtain accurate data regarding the prevalence of VS among children. Based on previously published estimates from many countries and available worldwide population data, it is possible to estimate the number of children in a VS (Table 1). The estimated number of children aged under 15 years worldwide in a VS is approximately 93,000 (range 11,365–151,536).

As the neurological insults occurring in children are different from adults, the risk for developing as well as recovering from VS also differs (Ashwal et al., 1994). Acute traumatic and non-traumatic injuries to the nervous system in children accounts for approximately 30% of cases. Perinatal insults (17.7%), chromosomal disorders or congenital malformations (13.0%), and infections (10.3%) occur less frequently (Ashwal et al., 1994). As clinical experience suggests, in a number of patients (28%), no specific cause can be determined. The aetiology of VS in children can be classified into three broad groups of disorders including (1) acute traumatic and non-traumatic brain injuries; (2) metabolic and degenerative disorders affecting the nervous system; and (3) developmental malformations. Children who are in VS due to acquired brain injury, particularly if it is traumatic, have the best chance for recovery of consciousness and function whereas children in whom the aetiology is due to a metabolic or degenerative disease are unlikely to recover consciousness and may have a shorter life expectancy (MSTF, 1994). In children in whom the VS is due to a cerebral malformation, the chances of recovery of consciousness remain small, but long-term studies of such individuals have not been reported.

RECOVERY

As described in the MSTF report, recovery from VS can be considered in terms of recovery of consciousness and recovery of function (MSTF, 1994).

Acute traumatic and non-traumatic injuries in children

Traumatic injuries. Recovery of awareness from post-traumatic VS appears to be somewhat better in children compared to adults. The MSTF on PVS has collected data (Table 2) on the potential for recovery from VS after severe traumatic brain injury in adults and children. Of 106 children in VS one month after severe head injury, 24% regained awareness by 3 months. At 1 year, 29% remained in VS, 9% had died, and 62% had recovered consciousness. Late recoveries after 12 months were not reported although a study by Kriel and co-investigators found that two of 40 children with traumatic brain injury began to recover after 1 year in VS (Kriel, Krach, & Jones-Saete, 1993). One patient had limited language function and was described as "able to express wants and needs". The other child had no language but was socially responsive and smiled in response to a voice or face. It is not clear whether this patient actually regained consciousness. In this study, eight of nine patients in VS for less than 3 months recovered to a severe disability; the remaining

TABLE 2
Incidence of recovery of consciousness and function in children in VS one month
after traumatic and non-traumatic brain injury

	Outcome at 3, 6, and 12 months as a percentage of children diagnosed VS 1 month after insult			Functional recovery of those patients who recovered consciousness by 12 months	
	3 months (%)	6 months (%)	12 months (%)	Recovery	(%)
Traumatic (n = 106)					
Dead	4	9	9	Severe disability	35
VS	72	40	29	Moderate disability	16
Recovered consciousness	24	51	62	Good recovery	11
Total	100%	100%	100%		62%
Non-traumatic (n = 45)					
Dead	20	22	22	Severe disability	7
VS	69	67	65	Moderate disability	0
Recovered consciousness	11	13	13	Good recovery	6
Total	100%	100%	100%		13%

This table was adapted from the Multi-Society Task Force on PVS (1994).

patient was moderately disabled. In the 15 patients in VS for 3–6 months, 12 recovered to a severe disability and three to a moderate disability and in those five patients in VS for 6–12 months three were severely and two moderately disabled. No good recoveries were reported in this series of 40 children who were in post-traumatic VS for 3 months. This data can be compared to the MSTF report where it was observed that of the 62% of children who did recover consciousness from post-traumatic VS, recovery of function (based on the use of the Glasgow Outcome Scale score) were: good recovery (11%), recovery to a moderate disability (16%), and recovery to a severe disability (35%).

Only one other study has provided data on recovery after TBI in children who were in VS one month after injury (Heindl & Laub, 1996). At 19 months post-injury, 84% of children (total $n = 82$) had recovered consciousness and 16% of these children became independent in daily activities. Less than 5% of children recovered consciousness beyond nine months of injury.

Non-traumatic injuries.   Children in non-traumatic VS have a much poorer potential for recovery of consciousness and function at 12 months post-injury than from traumatic VS (MSTF, 1994). Data collected by the MSTF on PVS showed that only 11% of children regained awareness by 3 months after injury (MSTF, 1994). At 1 year most children remained in VS (65%) or died (22%); only 13% showed recovery and this was usually to a severe disability.

Good or moderate functional recovery is extremely unlikely but may occur in children in VS due to a non-traumatic brain insult. In most of the patients who show recovery, awareness can usually be detected within 3 months of injury. Kriel et al. also reported in their recent studies that three of 13 children in post-anoxic VS for longer than 12 months (i.e., 370, 480, and 840 days) showed recovery of consciousness (Kriel et al., 1993). These patients recovered to a severe disability and in some of these children it was unclear whether this reflected recovery of consciousness or a patterned subcortical behavioural response.

Additional data from another study on post-hypoxic VS ($n = 55$) found that only 55% recovered consciousness by 19 months and only 4% became independent (Heindl & Laub, 1996). Less than 5% recovered beyond 9 months after injury. In this study children in VS due to hypoxic ischaemia also had a higher incidence of seizures and complications such as pneumonia, gastrointestinal complications and heterotopic calcifications.

Degenerative and metabolic disorders

Children in VS due to degenerative or metabolic diseases have virtually no possibility of recovering because these diseases are progressive or reach a clinical plateau in their terminal stages. In some children who are not vegetative but severely disabled an intercurrent illness may cause them to appear vegetative. As the illness improves the child may recover to his/her previous state of limited cognition.

Developmental malformations

Infants and children with congenital brain malformations severe enough to cause developmental VS are unlikely to acquire awareness. Anencephaly is the only malformation in which the prognosis for no recovery can be made at birth (Medical Task Force on Anencephaly, 1990). Other malformations diagnosed at birth may result in a vegetative outcome and if confirmed by clinical examination at 3–6 months of age, the prognosis for any improvement is extraordinarily small. The majority of infants with such malformations who recover consciousness have extremely limited awareness and minimal functional capacities.

Probability for recovery

The MSTF on PVS (1994) has estimated the probability for recovery of consciousness and function from traumatic and non-traumatic VS in adults and children who were vegetative one month after an acute injury (Table 3). Calculations of the probability for recovery were based on data from the

TABLE 3

Probabilities for recovery of consciousness and function at 12 months in children in PVS after traumatic and non-traumatic brain injury

	Outcome probabilities at 12 months	
	Traumatic PVS (n = 106)	Non-traumatic PVS (n = 45)
Patients in PVS for 3 months		
Dead (%)	14	3
PVS (%)	30	94
Severe (%)	24	3
Mod/Good (%)	32	0
Patients in PVS for 6 months		
Dead (%)	14	0
PVS (%)	54	97
Severe (%)	21	3
Mod/Good (%)	11	0

Modified from the Multi-Society Task Force on PVS (1994). Severe = recovery to a severe disability; Mod/Good = recovery to a moderate disability or to a good recovery.

previous sections, which provided the actual frequencies of recovery. Outcome probabilities at 12 months were determined for patients who remained vegetative at 3 and 6 months. Functional recovery was determined for two possible outcomes: (1) good recovery or recovery to a moderate disability and (2) recovery to a severe disability. Based on these probabilities (MSTF, 1994), the following statements can be made:

1. After 3 months, children in post-traumatic VS have a 56% chance of recovering consciousness in contrast to only 3% in children in non-traumatic VS. Of those children who recover, the probability for recovering to a severe disability is 24% and of making a moderate or good recovery 32%.

2. After 6 months, children in post-traumatic VS have a 31% chance of recovering consciousness in contrast to only 3% of children in non-traumatic VS. However, the chance of making a moderate or good recovery is now much less (i.e., 11%); recovery to a severe disability is more likely (21%).

3. VS is also likely to be permanent 12 months after traumatic brain injury and 3 months after non-traumatic injury in children. The chance for recovery after this time period seems to be exceedingly rare and almost always to a severe disability.

Life expectancy

Both adults and children in VS have shortened life expectancies despite preservation of brain stem and autonomic functions. In adults, long-term studies have shown that about 82% of patients will die within 3 years and about 10% of adults who are in VS will survive 5–10 years and only 4% beyond that time (MSTF, 1994).

As noted in Table 2, 91% of children in VS one month after traumatic brain injury were alive at one year; of those children in VS from non-traumatic injury, 78% survived. A large population-based study examining 847 children and adults considered to be in VS found approximately the same duration of survival for older children but a much shortened median life expectancy in children aged under 1 year (Ashwal et al., 1994). The life expectancy of infants and children in VS appeared to be an age-dependent phenomenon. For example, the median survival time of children less than 1 year of age was 2.6 years in contrast to children aged 2–6 years where it was 5.2 years. There is also likely to be some relation between certain aetiologies of the VS and survival times. For the data available it appears that children in VS from non-traumatic injury (8.6 years) and chromosomal disorders (8.2 years) have a longer life expectancy than children in whom the VS is due to perinatal disorders (4.1 years), traumatic brain injury (3.0 years), or infection (2.6 years). This does not appear to be due to any interdependency between age and aetiology. The reasons for these limited differences remain unclear. One possible explanation is that the shortened life expectancies observed in the perinatal or infection groups may be due to a greater degree of permanent brain stem or hypothalamic injury which causes greater immobility, an increased risk for aspiration, and an overall poorer nutritional status which renders these patients more susceptible to infection or cardiorespiratory arrest.

Life expectancy does not appear to be affected by the residential location of a child in VS. There were no differences reported in life expectancy in those children living at home (4.5 years) compared to those living in an institution (5.2 years); life expectancy of children living in a skilled nursing facility or private hospital setting was somewhat shortened (3.2 years). Although there is no definite reason to explain these limited differences in life expectancy, our experience suggests that the associated medical problems of VS patients are similar irrespective of facility. In cases where there are more serious acute or chronic medical problems, additional home nursing care is frequently provided to families or the incidence of hospital readmissions is increased; if patients are in institutions or skilled nursing facilities their care levels are upgraded to meet their specific needs.

Additional data have been reported concerning life expectancy of children in a permanent vegetative state (Strauss et al., 1999) as well as comparing life expectancy of children in VS to those in a minimally conscious state (MCS)

(Strauss et al., 2000). Both studies were from a similar population as the above-cited paper (i.e., Ashwal et al., 1994) that was based on data from patients who were residents of California and in whom an annual Client Development Evaluation report was completed. The first report was based on data from 1,021 VS patients and two major findings emerged. The first was that of a secular trend towards higher life expectancy in more recently diagnosed VS patients (Strauss et al., 1999). Life expectancy was 3.6 years in VS patients diagnosed in 1980 compared to 7.2 years for those diagnosed in 1990. Also life expectancy was longer in patients who were in VS for 4 years (life expectancy of 12.2 years) compared to those who were in VS for 1 year (10.5 years). In the second study (Strauss et al., 2000), no differences were found in the percentage of patients surviving for 8 years between those patients in VS (63%) and those in an immobile MCS (65%) or a mobile MCS (81%). These findings suggested that the presence or absence of consciousness might not be a critical factor determining life expectancy.

There are no data concerning extraordinary long survival (i.e., greater than 15 years) for children in VS. Rare cases of prolonged survival for periods up to 10–20 years were reported in the survey of child neurologists (Ashwal, Bale, Coulter, Eiben, Garg, Hill et al., 1992). The MSTF on PVS (1994) has estimated that the probability of an individual patient having prolonged survival is less than 1 in 15,000 to 75,000.

REFERENCES

Ashwal, S., Eyman, R. K., & Call, T. L. (1994). Life expectancy of children in a persistent vegetative state. *Pediatric Neurology, 10*, 27–33.

Ashwal, S., Bale, J. F., Coulter, D. L., Eiben, R., Garg, B. P., Hill, A., et al. (1992). The persistent vegetative state in children: Report of the Child Neurology Society Ethics Committee. *Annals of Neurology, 32*, 570–576.

Heindl, U. T., & Laub, M. C. (1996). Outcome of persistent vegetative state following hypoxic or traumatic brain injury in children and adolescents. *Neuropediatrics, 27*, 94–100.

Kriel, R. L., Krach, L. E., & Jones-Saete, C. (1993). Outcome of children with prolonged unconsciousness and vegetative states. *Pediatric Neurology, 9*, 362–368.

Strauss, D. J., Ashwal, S., Day, S. M., & Shavelle, R. M. (2000). Life expectancy of children in vegetative and minimally conscious states. *Pediatric Neurology, 23*, 312–319.

Strauss, D. J., Shavelle, R. M., & Ashwal, S. (1999). Life expectancy and median survival time in the permanent vegetative state. *Pediatric Neurology, 21*, 626–631.

Multi-Society Task Force Report on PVS (1994). Medical aspects of the persistent vegetative state. *New England Journal of Medicine, 330*, 1499–1508, 1572–1579.

Medical Task Force on Anencephaly (1990). The infant with anencephaly. *New England Journal of Medicine, 322*, 669–674.

NEUROPSYCHOLOGICAL REHABILITATION
2005, 15 (3/4), 198–213

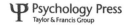

Neuropathology of the vegetative state after head injury

D. I. Graham, J. H. Adams, L. S. Murray, and B. Jennett

University of Glasgow, UK

A detailed neuropathological study of patients identified clinically after head injury as either severely disabled (SD, $n = 30$) or vegetative (VS, $n = 35$) has been carried out to determine the nature and frequency of the various pathologies that form the basis of these clinical states. Patients who were SD were older (SD median 49.5 yrs vs. VS median 38 yrs, $p = .04$), more likely to have a lucid interval (SD 31% vs. VS 9%, $p = .03$), and to have had an acute intracranial haematoma (SD 70% vs. VS 26%, $p < .001$). SD patients less often had severe, Grades (2 or 3) of traumatic diffuse axonal injury (SD 30% vs. VS 71%, $p = .001$) and less often had thalamic damage (SD 37% vs. VS 80%, $p < .001$). Similar features of both focal and diffuse damage were present in some SD and VS cases with both groups having considerable damage to white matter and to the thalamus. It is concluded that the principal structural basis of both SD and VS is diffuse traumatic axonal injury (DAI) with widespread damage to white matter and changes in the thalami. However, both ischaemic brain damage and the vascular complications of raised intracranial pressure contributed to the clinical signs and symptoms.

INTRODUCTION

A survey of head injuries by the European Brain Injury Consortium provided outcome data on 94% of patients assessed by the Glasgow Outcome Scale (GOS) 6 months after injury: 31% had died, 3% were vegetative, 16% severely disabled, 20% moderately disabled, and 31% had made a good

Correspondence should be sent to Professor David I. Graham, Academic Unit of Neuropathology, Institute of Neurological Sciences, Southern General Hospital, 1345 Govan Road, Glasgow G51 4TF. Tel: 0141 201 2113, Fax: 0141 201 2998.
Email: d.graham@clinmed.gla.ac.uk

recovery (Murray et al., 1999). The structural basis of both the vegetative state after an acute brain insult including trauma (Adams et al., 1999; Adams, Graham, & Jennett, 2000) and severe disability after traumatic brain injury (Jennett, Adams, Murray, & Graham, 2001) have been studied. The objectives of this study were to revisit the neuropathology of these previously reported cases in order to consider what light it sheds on the mechanism underlying these two types of disability.

MATERIALS AND METHODS

With the co-operation of the relevant legal authorities and the forensic pathologists in the West of Scotland, a comprehensive database of brain damage in fatal head injuries has been established in the Institute of Neurological Sciences, Glasgow. The database now comprises a consecutive series of more than 1,500 patients with fatal blunt head injuries occurring over a 30 year period who underwent post mortem examination after which the brain was suspended in 10% formal saline for 3–4 weeks before being dissected. The cerebral hemispheres were cut in the coronal plane and the cerebellar hemispheres at right angles to the folia, and the brainstem horizontally. Comprehensive histological studies, including immunohistochemistry, were undertaken (Adams et al., 1980).

Some features were recorded as being present or absent, e.g., raised intracranial pressure (Adams & Graham, 1976), whereas others were quantified and graded. The severity of ischaemic brain damage was graded: It was classified as severe when the lesions were diffuse or multifocal, or took the form of infarcts within specific arterial territories, and moderate when ischaemic damage was limited to arterial boundary zones, singly or in combination with subtotal infarction in the distribution of arterial territories (Graham et al., 1989). Surface contusions were assessed semi-quantitatively using the total contusion index (TCI). This takes into account the depth and extent of the contusions in various parts of the brain: 0 means that there were no contusions; a contusion index of less than 9 is indicative of minimal contusions; one of more than 37 is indicative of severe contusions (Adams et al., 1985). Diffuse traumatic axonal injury (DAI) was graded. In this series most examples were of the more severe Grades 2 and 3. In Grade 3 there are focal lesions in the corpus callosum and in the dorsolateral sector(s) of the rostral brainstem and in Grade 2 there is a focal lesion only in the corpus callosum. In Grade 1 there is again axonal damage diffusely throughout the white matter but there are no focal lesions in the corpus callosum or the brainstem (Adams et al., 1989). Only traumatic haematomas considered to be sufficiently large to act as significant intracranial expanding lesions (more than 35 ml) were recorded. The great majority of the haematomas so recorded had been evacuated before death. Changes in the thalamus and ventricular system were assessed semi-quantitatively.

The outcome on the GOS (Jennett & Bond, 1975) was determined following review of the hospital case notes by one of the researchers (BJ). In a retrospective review it was inevitable that there were some cases in which the outcome could not be assessed with confidence and these were not included. Patients were deemed vegetative if they had periods of spontaneous eye opening but had no evidence of awareness and were tube fed, thus meeting the initial criteria of Jennett and Plum (1972), most recently updated by the Royal College of Physicians (2003). Severely disabled patients had persisting disability, either mental or physical but usually both, that made them dependent on at least one other person for some of their activities every day.

The clinical records were also assessed with particular reference to any deterioration in the level of consciousness after a lucid interval. The lucid interval was defined as being total if the patient had been able to talk rationally after injury, and partial if talking had been confused and disorientated (Reilly, Graham, Adams, & Jennett, 1975). All cases survived for at least four weeks after having been managed by the Department of Neurosurgery in the Institute of Neurological Sciences.

Statistical analysis

For features reported with median values the groups were compared using a Mann-Whitney test; for those reported with percentages a Chi-squared test of association was used. All analyses were carried out using the statistical package Minitab Release 12.21.

RESULTS

The data will be presented in two groups: severely disabled (SD, $n = 30$) and vegetative (VS, $n = 35$). The principal clinical features of the SD and VS patients are given in Tables 1 and 2 and summarised in Table 3, and the focal and diffuse neuropathological features in Tables 4 and 5, respectively.

The basic clinical and neuropathological information (Tables 1 and 3) is similar in the two groups of cases. The exceptions are that in contrast to VS patients, the SD were older, tended to live for a shorter time and were more likely to have had a lucid interval recorded some time after injury.

In Table 4 it can be seen that compared with the VS there is a higher incidence in the SD group of fracture of the skull, contusions as assessed by the TCI, and a significantly higher number of intracranial haematomas (70% vs.

26%), most of which had been evacuated surgically. The features of raised intracranial pressure were less common in the SD group in spite of the greater frequency of intracranial haematomas. Lesions in the brainstem were seen in approximately equal numbers in SD and VS.

The diffuse neuropathological features are shown in Table 5, which highlights the significantly increased frequency of DAI in VS patients compared with SD (80% vs. 50%). This difference was even more striking for the severe Grades (2 and 3) of DAI (VS 71% vs. SD 30%). In contrast there was no evidence of a difference in the frequency of ischaemic brain damage or hydrocephalus between the two groups.

In summary there was more focal pathology in the SD than in the VS patients (Tables 4 and 5). However, further analysis shows that although there were "pure" examples of either focal or diffuse changes, many of the cases in both outcome categories had a mixture of both focal and diffuse changes.

Review of the abnormalities in the thalamus (Table 6) highlights the significantly increased frequency of these in VS cases (80%) compared with SD (37%). All but one of the 24 VS patients who survived for more than three months had thalamic damage (96%). In patients who survived for more that three months it was possible to identify histologically the nature of, and therefore the most likely cause of, the changes in the thalamus. For example, transneuronal changes reflect disconnection and therefore would likely be a consequence of DAI; diffuse ischaemic damage would be secondary to global hypoxia; and focal ischaemia would likely be a consequence of the vascular complications of raised intracranial pressure. However, in some cases there were features that suggested more than one mechanism. For example in SD patients the more severe grades of DAI alone and the combination of this with thalamic damage without ischaemic damage were less common than in VS (10% vs. 20%, and 10% vs. 34%). Thalamic damage with ischaemic damage but without DAI was similar in the SD and VS patients (20% vs. 26%). However, the most striking difference was that 15 (50%) of the SD cases had neither Grade 2 or 3 DAI, and no thalamic damage and 10 of these did not have any ischaemic damage. These combinations did not occur in a single one of the VS cases.

There were 15 (50%) SD and 7 (20%) VS patients in whom it was not possible to identify any DAI. The brain damage found in these patients is set out in Table 7. The frequency of an intracranial haematoma alone or with ischaemic damage, and of the associated vascular complications of raised intracranial pressure are apparent particularly in the SD cases in which a haematoma was present in all of this subset of cases (100%) whereas in the VS patients a haematoma was a contributing factor in 5 (71%): In the other two cases of VS ischaemic damage in association with raised intracranial pressure was a feature. In one SD case the only lesion was Grade 1 DAI.

TABLE 1

Principal clinical and neuropathological features of severely disabled cases

Case No	Age (yrs)	Sex	Cause	Survival	Lucid	Skull fracture	Brain weight	ICH	ICP+	TCI	DAI	IBD	Abnormalities in				
													Neocx	SCWM	Thalamus	Brain-stem	Hydrocephalus
1	29	M	RTA	1m	No	No	NK	No	Yes	5	2m	No	No	D	No	No	–
2	23	M	Assault	1m	No	No	1480	No	No	0	2m	+	No	D	F	No	–
3	76	M	Fall	5w	P	Yes	1200	ICH	No	18	1	No	No	No	No	No	–
4	17	M	RTA	6w	No	Yes	1620	No	Yes	1	3Mm	No	No	D	D	No	–
5	61	M	RTA	7w	No	Yes	1755	ICHe	Yes	28	No	+	BZ	F	No	L	++
6	70	F	Fall	7w	No	No	1200	SDHe	No	8	No	+	No	No	F	No	++
7	17	M	Assault	2m	T	Yes	1420	ICH	Yes	48	No	No	No	No	No	L	++
8	64	M	Fall	2m	P	Yes	1240	SDHe	Yes	13	1	No	No	No	No	No	–
9	51	M	RTA	2m	No	Yes	NK	SDHe	No	6	1	No	No	No	F	No	++
10	72	M	RTA	2m	T	No	1270	SDHe	No	1	No	++	BZ	No	No	No	–
11	26	F	RTA	10w	No	Yes	1450	SDHe	Yes	30	1	No	No	D	No	No	++
12	55	M	RTA	3m	No	No	1280	No	No	16	3Mm	+	F	No	No	No	++
13	60	M	RTA	3m	P	No	1260	ICHe	Yes	3	No	No	No	No	No	No	++
14	74	F	RTA	3m	P	No	1150	SDHe	Yes	12	No	+	No	No	F	No	++
15	79	M	NK	4m	No	No	1370	SDHe	No	0	No	+	F	No	No	No	++
16	39	M	RTA	4m	No	Yes	1520	SDHe	Yes	17	No	+	AT	Yes	No	No	++
17	55	M	RTA	4m	No	Yes	NK	ICHe	Yes	35	2m	No	No	D	No	No	++

Case	Age	Sex	Cause	Survival	Lucid	ICP+	Brain weight (g)	Haematoma	Evac.	TCI	DAI	IBD	Neocx	SCWM	Thalamus	Brainstem	Hydrocephalus
18	65	M	NK	4.5m	No	Yes	1440	No	No	0	1	No	No	No	No	No	+
19	17	M	Assault	5m	T	No	1400	EDHe	Yes	2	No	+	F	No	F	No	−
20	60	M	RTA	5m	No	No	1380	No	Yes	14	3M	No	No	D	T	No	+++
21	39	M	Assault	6m	No	No	1600	No	No	0	2m	No	No	D	No	No	−
22	48	F	RTA	7m	No	No	1230	No	No	0	3M	No	No	D	T	No	+
23	48	F	RTA	8m	No	Yes	1250	EDHe	Yes	11	No	+	BZ	No	No	L	++
24	67	M	Fall	8m	No	Yes	1390	SDHe	Yes	13	No	++	AT	F	D	No	++
25	31	M	RTA	1y6m	No	Yes	1020	ICHe	No	48	No	No	No	No	No	No	++
26	48	M	Assault	3y	No	Yes	1120	ICHe	No	21	No	No	No	No	No	No	+
27	29	M	Assault	7y	No	Yes	1450	SDHe	Yes	3	No	+	AT	F	F	M	++
28	53	M	Fall	8y	P	No	1240	SDHe	Yes	32	1	No	No	No	No	No	++
29	28	M	Assault	8y	T	No	1140	SDHe	Yes	0	No	++	AT	F	F	No	++
30	43	M	RTA	14.5y	NK	No	1250	No	No	1	3M	+	F	D	T	No	+++

RTA = road traffic accident; Lucid: T = totally lucid immediately after injury, P = partially lucid; SDH = subdural haematoma, EDH = extradural haematoma, ICH = intracerebral haematoma, e = evacuated; ICP+ = raised intracranial pressure; TCI = total contusion index; DAI = diffuse axonal injury: 1, 2 & 3 indicate Grade, m = focal lesions seen only microscopically, M = seen macroscopically, the other only microscopically; IBD = ischaemic brain damage in cerebral cortex: + = moderate, ++ = severe; Neocx = Neocortex: BZ = IBD in arterial boundary zones, AT = in arterial territories, D = diffuse damage, F = focal, C = contusions (for severity, see TCI); SCWM = subcortical white matter: D = diffuse damage, F = focal damage in relation to ischaemic damage; Thalamus: F = focal damage, T = transneuronal damage, D = diffuse ischaemic damage; Brainstem: M = focal damage in mid-line, L = lateral damage; Hydrocephalus: + = slight enlargement of the ventricular system, ++ = moderate, +++ = severe; M = male, F = female; NK = not known; g = grams; Survival: w = week(s); m = month(s); y = year(s)

TABLE 2
Principal clinical and neuropathological features of patients

Case No	Age (yrs)	Sex	Cause	Survival	Lucid	Skull fracture	Brain weight (g)	Intracranial haematoma	ICP+	TCI	DAI	IBD	Neocx	SCWM	Thalamus	Brain-stem	Hydrocephalus
1	57	M	RTA	5w	No	Yes	1450	ICH	Yes	19	No	+	C	No	D	No	–
2	36	M	RTA	6w	No	Yes	1540	No	No	4	3Mm	No	C	D	No	No	–
3	9	M	RTA	7w	No	No	1430	No	Yes	0	3m	No	No	D	No	No	+
4	18	M	RTA	7w	No	Yes	1490	No	Yes	3	3Mm	No	C	D	No	No	–
5	32	M	RTA	7w	No	No	1500	No	No	3	3Mm	No	C	D	No	No	++
6	38	M	Fall	8w	P	No	1250	SDHe	Yes	7	1	No	C	D	F	M	–
7	59	M	Assault	8w	No	No	1370	No	No	4	3M	No	C	D	T	No	–
8	47	M	Assault	8w	No	No	1390	No	No	6	3M	No	C	D	No	No	+
9	43	M	Fall	10w	No	Yes	1350	No	Yes	14	No	+	C:BZ	D	F	No	+
10	24	M	RTA	10w	No	Yes	1520	SDHe	Yes	16	1	++	C:BZ	D	D	No	++
11	29	M	Fall	12w	NK	No	1650	No	No	0	3M	No	No	D	No	No	–
12	15	F	Fall	3m	NK	No	1160	No	No	4	3M	No	C	D	T	No	–
13	65	M	RTA	3m	No	Yes	1440	No	Yes	15	1	+	C:BZ	D	D	M	+++
14	18	M	RTA	3m	No	Yes	1160	No	Yes	19	3m	+	C:F	D	T	No	+
15	27	M	RTA	4m	No	Yes	1430	SDHe	No	6	2m	++	C	D	D	No	–
16	31	M	RTA	6m	No	No	1300	No	Yes	6	3Mm	No	C	D	T	No	++
17	42	M	Assault	9m	No	No	1270	No	Yes	0	3Mm	No	No	D	T	No	++
18	58	M	RTA	9m	No	No	1550	No	Yes	0	3m	No	No	D	T	No	++
19	56	M	RTA	9m	No	No	1190	No	Yes	4	3M	No	C	D	T	No	++

20	75	F	Assault	11m	No	No	1260	No	No	0	2M	No	No	D	T	No	++
21	50	M	Assault	1y	No	No	1260	SDHe	Yes	4	No	+	C:BZ	F	D	M	++
22	49	M	Assault	1y	T	No	1070	SDHe	Yes	9	No	++	C:AT	F	F	L	++
23	34	F	RTA	1y6m	No	No	1070	No	Yes	21	3Mm	+	C:D	D	D	No	++
24	64	M	Assault	1y6m	No	Yes	1150	No	Yes	3	2M	No	C	D	T	No	++
25	27	M	NK	1y6m	No	No	1130	No	No	0	3Mm	No	No	D	No	No	++
26	18	M	Assault	2y	No	No	1200	No	Yes	6	3Mm	No	C	D	T	No	++
27	44	M	NK	2y2m	No	Yes	1300	No	Yes	6	3Mm	No	C	D	T	No	++
28	61	M	NK	2y3m	No	No	1350	ICH	Yes	6	No	++	C:D	No	D	No	++
29	52	M	RTA	2y4m	No	No	NK	No	Yes	0	3Mm	+	AT	D:F	D	T	M	++
30	7	M	RTA	2y5m	No	Yes	NK	No	No	3	3M	No	C	D	D	T	No	++
31	56	M	Assault	3y	No	No	1260	No	No	0	3M	No	No	D	D	T	No	++
32	15	M	RTA	3y	No	No	1140	No	Yes	20	3M	++	C:D	No	D	D	No	+++
33	8	M	Fall	4y	T	Yes	670	EDHe	Yes	4	No	++	C:D	No	D	D	No	+++
34	20	M	RTA	6y	No	No	1020	No	Yes	3	3Mm	+	C:BZ	D	D	D	No	++
35	42	M	Fall	8y6m	No	No	1220	SDHe	Yes	14	3M	+	C:BZ	D	D	D	No	+++

RTA = road traffic accident; Lucid: T = totally lucid immediately after injury, P = partially lucid; SDH = subdural haematoma, EDH = extradural haematoma, ICH = intracerebral haematoma, e = evacuated; ICP+ = raised intracranial pressure; TCI = total contusion index; DAI = diffuse axonal injury: 1, 2 & 3 indicate Grade, m = focal lesions seen only microscopically, M = seen macroscopically, the other only microscopically; IBD = ischaemic brain damage in cerebral cortex: + = moderate, ++ = severe; Neocx = Neocortex: BZ = IBD in arterial boundary zones, AT = in arterial territories, D = diffuse damage, F = focal, C = contusions (for severity, see TCI); SCWM = subcortical white matter: D = diffuse damage, F = focal damage in relation to ischaemic damage; Thalamus: F = focal damage, T = transneuronal damage, D = diffuse ischaemic damage; Brainstem: M = focal damage in mid-line, L = lateral damage; Hydrocephalus: + = slight enlargement of the ventricular system, ++ = moderate, +++ = severe; M = male, F = female; NK = not known; g = grams; Survival: w = week(s); m = month(s); y = year(s)

Reproduced with permission from Adams et al. (2001). The neuropathology of the Vegetative State after acute brain insult. *Brain, 123*, 1327–1388

TABLE 3
Summary of clinical features of the severely disabled and the vegetative state after head injury

	Severely disabled n = 30	Vegetative state n = 35	p-value
Gender	25 male/5 female	33 male/2 female	
Age: Median (range) years	49.5 (17–79)	38.0 (7–75)	.04
Cause of injury			
Road traffic accident	16/28 (57%)	17/32 (53%)	.95 ($\chi^2 = 0.11$, 2df)
Assault	7 (25%)	9 (28%)	
Fall	5 (18%)	6 (19%)	
Survival: Median (range) months	4 (1–174)	9 (1–102)	.24
Survival > 3 months	19 (63%)	24 (69%)	.66 ($\chi^2 = 0.20$, 1df)
Lucid interval	9/29 (31%)	3/33 (9%)	.03 ($\chi^2 = 4.8$, 1df)

TABLE 4
Focal neuropathological features of the severely disabled and the vegetative state after head injury

	Severely disabled n = 30	Vegetative state n = 35	p-value
Skull fracture	15 (50%)	12 (34%)	.20 ($\chi^2 = 1.64$, 1df)
Intracranial haematoma	21 (70%)	9 (26%)	<.001 ($\chi^2 = 12.7$, 1df)
Subdural	12 (all e)	6 (all e)	
Intracranial	7 (5 e)	2 (not e)	
Extradural	2 (2 e)	1 (e)	
Total contusion index Median (range)	9.5 (0–48)	4 (0–21)	.23
Raised intracranial pressure	17 (57%)	25 (71%)	.22 ($\chi^2 = 1.54$, 1df)
Lesions in the brainstem	4	5	

e = evacuated

TABLE 5
Diffuse neuropathological features of the severely disabled and the vegetative state after head injury

	Severely disabled n = 30	Vegetative state n = 35	p-value
DAI	15 (50%)	28 (80%)	.01 ($\chi^2 = 6.5$, 1df)
DAI Grade 2 or 3	9 (30%)	25 (71%)	.001 ($\chi^2 = 11.1$, 1df)
Ischaemic damage	14 (47%)	15 (43%)	.10 ($\chi^2 = 0.76$, 1df)
Mild	11	9	
Moderate	3	6	
Severe	0	0	
Hydrocephalus	22 (73%)	27 (77%)	.72 ($\chi^2 = 0.13$, 1df)

DAI = Traumatic diffuse axonal injury

TABLE 6
Frequency and nature of abnormalities in the thalamus

	Severely disabled n = 30	Vegetative state n = 35	p-value
Frequency of any abnormality	11 (37%)	28 (80%)	<.001 (χ^2 = 12.6, 1df)
Type of abnormality			
Transneuronal	3 (10%)	13 (37%)	
Diffuse ischaemic	2 (7%)	12 (34%)	
Focal ischaemic	6 (20%)	3 (9%)	

TABLE 7
Principal features of the severely disabled and the vegetative state after head injury in patients without traumatic diffuse axonal injury

	Severely disabled n = 15	Vegetative state n = 17
Intracranial haematoma	2	0
Intracranial haematoma with raised ICP	2	0
Intracranial haematoma with IBD	3	0
Intracranial haematoma with IBD and raised ICP	8	5
IBD and raised ICP	0	2

ICP = Intracranial pressure; IBD = Ischaemic brain damage

DISCUSSION

Like most post mortem series it is necessary to reflect on the inclusion/ exclusion criteria for selection as an indication of the extent to which these cases are representative of the whole population under study. The two main inclusion criteria for this study were that a full autopsy had been undertaken, and that hospital records were available and had recorded sufficient clinical details to allow the assessment of the criteria necessary for GOS. The first criterion was met by analysing the 1,500+ database of fatal blunt head injury for those cases surviving at least four weeks after head injury, and had undergone a full autopsy including comprehensive neuropathological examination. The second criterion was more difficult to meet as the review of the hospital records was retrospective and data were often not recorded in sufficient detail to allow cases to be included. Further, as these cases had been accrued by the department over a 40+ year period it should be remembered that the diagnostic criteria are relatively new and are in fact still evolving (Jennett & Plum, 1972; Multi-Society Task Force on PVS, 1994; Giacino et al., 1997; Jennett, 2002; Royal College of Physicians, 2003).

There have been several reports of SD and the VS after acute insults to the brain (Adams, Brierely, Connor, & Treip, 1966; Brierley, Graham, Adams, & Simpson, 1971; Cole & Cowie, 1987; Dougherty, Rawlinson, Levy, & Plum, 1981; French, 1952; Ingvar, Brun, Johansson, & Samuelsson, 1978; Relkin, Petito, & Plum, 1990). Many emphasised the vulnerability of the brain to ischaemic damage. The structural basis of the VS due to trauma and other causes was reviewed by Kinney and Samuels (1994) who concluded that end-stage non-traumatic neurological disease often has the features of SD or VS and that there are different causes in children and adults. Nevertheless, after reviewing the literature Kinney and Samuels (1994) concluded that VS may be associated with three main patterns of brain damage (1) widespread destruction of the cortical ribbon, (2) widespread damage to white matter tracts, and (3) damage to the thalamus. Examples of each of these three patterns were found in the current series of cases. More recent reviews of VS include Adams et al. (2000) and Jennett et al. (2001).

The first pattern of extensive damage to the neocortical ribbon (and sub-cortical grey matter) was a particular feature of 14 (47%) cases of SD and 15 (43%) of the VS cases. In some of these it appeared to be the principal underlying structural abnormality. Such cases have been reported previously (Adams et al., 1966; Cole & Cowie, 1987; Dougherty et al., 1981; Kinney & Samuels, 1994) and are brought about by a period of cardiac arrest or pro-longed profound hypotension. Essentially similar patterns of brain damage may occur as a result of other types of hypoxic injury such as status epilepti-cus, carbon monoxide poisoning and asphyxia (Adams et al., 2000; Graham & Lantos, 2002).

The second pattern described by Kinney and Samuels (1994) was that of widespread damage to white matter. The importance of this pattern was first recognised by Strich (1956) who in a series of cases with "severe post-traumatic dementia" described widespread Wallerian-type degeneration throughout the neuraxis. Alternative hypotheses about the cause of this type of brain damage included hypoxia, ischaemia, brain swelling and damage to the brainstem secondary to a high intracranial pressure (Jellinger, 1977; Jellinger & Seitelberger, 1970; Peters & Rothemund, 1977). These have now been discounted as the primary cause of the damage, which is attributed to diffuse (traumatic) axonal injury (Adams et al., 1989), although hypoxia, swelling, etc., may contribute to the overall amount of brain damage. The fact that DAI was present in 15 (50%) of SD and 28 (80%) of VS indi-cates the major contribution that damage to myelinated axons makes to the categories of SD and VS after head injury.

The third pattern of brain damage described by Kinney and Samuels (1994) is the least common in our experience, and was found as both diffuse and focal involvement of the thalamus in both SD (8, 27%) and VS (15, 43%). The former pattern occurred as a consequence of global ischaemia (cardiac arrest) and the latter most likely secondary to raised intracranial pressure. Bilateral damage to the thalamus has also been reported (Jellinger, 1994; Kinney et al., 1994).

Brain damage due to head injury is frequently classified as focal or diffuse (Graham, Gennarelli, & McIntosh, 2002). Focal damage includes contusions on the surface of the brain and intracranial haematomas. Diffuse brain damage is fundamentally different and comprises diffuse traumatic axonal injury (DAI), hypoxic/ischaemic brain damage, and diffuse brain swelling. Whereas, the focal lesions may cause secondary brain damage—including haemorrhage and infarction in the brainstem, the diffuse types of lesions cause coma not by compression of the brainstem but by diffuse injury to the cerebral hemispheres, and/or the brainstem (Gennarelli, 1983). The most common mechanical input to the head is dynamic loading—either impact or impulsive—the duration of which is a critical factor in determining the type of head injury produced. Epidemiological studies have shown that, in general, impact loading is most likely due to a fall which is associated with focal lesions whereas impulsive loading is most likely due to a road traffic accident which results in diffuse lesions (Graham et al., 1995). In many cases there is both impact and impulsive loading that result in focal and diffuse pathologies.

It might have been anticipated that the neuropathology in SD would have been similar to those in VS but less severe given the similarity of causes of the injury. However, in 15/30 cases of SD neither Grade 2 or 3 nor thalamic damage was seen, a combination that was not found in any case of VS. The lesions underlying the SD cases appear to have been an aggregate of focal damage (contusions, intracranial haematoma, and vascular complications of raised intracranial pressure including secondary damage to the brainstem). Six SD cases had Grade 1 DAI, one of which had no other identifiable lesions indicating that the diffuse damage to white matter in DAI alone may be sufficiently extensive to result in SD. Some SD cases, however, had lesions similar to those in the VS cases; 30% had Grade 2 or 3 DAI and about one-third had thalamic lesions.

It has been recognised for some 10 years that there is a potential for a degree of recovery in VS particularly after trauma (Multi-Society Task Force, 1994). This is hypothesised to be in large measure due to the nature and the amount of damage to the thalamus. For example, there is evidence that hypoxic damage is likely to cause irreversible ischaemic neuronal necrosis whereas traumatic axonal injury may result in partial atrophy but without cell loss as a result of transneuronal change after disconnection. Given the frequency of DAI in both SD (15, 50%) and VS (28, 80%) and ischaemic damage in SD (14, 47%) and VS (15, 43%) it seems likely that either or both or usually a combination contribute to the pattern of thalamic damage in each patient.

Increased attention is now being given not only to the pattern of damage in the brain after head injury but also to the type and amount and its distribution, particularly as it is well known that different causes produce a differential response in different parts of the brain. For example, after cardiac arrest the CA1 and CA4 sections of the hippocampus are more at risk than CA2 and CA3 (Auer & Sutherland, 2002), and the anterior and dorso-medial nuclei of the thalamus are most at risk of damage (Brierley et al., 1971; Cole & Cowie, 1987; Dougherty et al., 1981; French, 1952), whereas in DAI there is particular involvement of the lateral and ventral nuclei (Adams et al., 2000). These classical descriptions have remained true and, as suggested by Kinney and Samuels (1994), need to be supplemented by quantitative data. By stereological techniques quantitative data have now been obtained for the hippocampus after head injury with confirmation of the pattern of severity but at different rates of involvement (Maxwell et al., 2003). Recent studies using similar techniques have confirmed that the various nuclei of the thalami also respond differently ranging from cell loss to cell atrophy in association with reactive changes in microglia, macrophages, and astrocytes (Maxwell, personal communication).

That not all of the cellular changes occur acutely—and presumably a consequence of hypoxia/ischaemia, has been suggested by experimental laboratory evidence (Bramlett, Dietrich, Green, & Busto, 1997; Dixon et al., 1999; McIntosh et al., 1998; Pierce, Smith, Trojanowski, & McIntosh, 1998; Smith et al., 1997) in which the volume of cortical contusion and the ventricles become larger, and delayed changes develop in the thalami (Chen, Pickard, & Harris, 2003) with increasing survival. These delayed changes with a more protracted time course may be due to programmed cell death (Rink et al., 1995) which has now been identified in the white matter of patients surviving after DAI for between 4 weeks and 2 years, 5 months (Wilson et al., 2004). Commensurate with these cellular changes is a reduction in the bulk of the central white matter with hydrocephalus ex vacuo and an increase in the consistency of the tissue due to astrocytosis. Whether these changes are passive, reflecting processes with a long natural history from the time of injury, or whether they are active and might be due to withdrawal of trophic factors after axon loss, or to continuing microglial/macrophage activation with continuing death of oligodendrocytes, is not clear (Wilson et al., 2004).

It is concluded from this review there are both similarities and differences in the structural basis of SD and VS. These clinical categories of the GOS may variously be due to extensive damage to the cortex, to white matter, or to subcortical grey matter and in particular the thalami. In fact this study has confirmed the importance of structural damage to the thalami especially when occurring in association with damage to white matter as the structural basis of the GOS.

REFERENCES

Adams, J. H., Brierley, J. B., Connor, R. C., & Treip, C. S. (1966). The effects of systemic hypotension upon the human brain. Clinical and neuropathological report the two cases. *Lancet*, *89*, 235–268.

Adams, J. H., Doyle, D., Ford, I., Gennarelli, T. A., Graham, D. I., & McLellan, D. R. (1989). Diffuse axonal injury in head injury: Definition, diagnosis and grading. *Histopathology*, *15*, 49–59.

Adams, J. H., Doyle, D., Graham, D. I., Lawrence, A. E., McLellan, D. R., Gennarelli, T. A., Pastuszko, M., & Sakamoto, T. (1985). The contusion index: A reappraisal in human and experimental non-missile head injury. *Neuropathology and Applied Neurobiology*, *11*, 299–308.

Adams, J. H., & Graham, D. I. (1976). The relationship between ventricular fluid pressure and the neuropathology of raised intracranial pressure. *Neuropathology and Applied Neurobiology*, *2*, 323–332.

Adams, J. H., Graham, D. I., & Jennett, B. (2000). The neuropathology of the vegetative state after acute brain insult. *Brain*, *123*, 1327–1338.

Adams, J. H., Graham, D. I., Scott, G., Parker, L. S., & Doyle, D. (1980). Brain damage in fatal non-missile head injury. *Journal of Clinical Pathology*, *33*, 1132–1145.

Adams, J., Jennett, B., McLellan, D. R., Murray, L. S., & Graham, D. I. (1999). The neuropathology of the vegetative state after head injury. *Journal of Clinical Pathology*, *52*, 804–806.

Auer, R. M., & Sutherland, G. R. (2002). Hypoxia and related conditions. In D. I. Graham & P. L. Lantos (Eds.), *Greenfield's neuropathology* (7th ed., pp. 233–280). London: Arnold.

Bramlett, H. M., Dietrich, W. D., Green, E. J., & Busto, R. (1997). Chronic histopathological consequences of fluid percussion brain injury in rats: Effects of post-traumatic hypothermia. *Acta Neuropathology*, *93*, 190–199.

Brierley, J. B., Graham, D. I., Adams, J. H., & Simpson, J. A. (1971). Neocortical death after cardiac arrest: A clinical, neurophysiological and neuropathological report of two cases. *Lancet*, *2*, 560–565.

Chen, S., Pickard, J. D., & Harris, N. G. (2003). Time course of cellular pathology after controlled cortical impact injury. *Experimental Neurology*, *182*, 87–102.

Cole, G., & Cowie, V. A. (1987). Long survival after cardiac arrest: Case report and neuropathological findings. *Clinical Neuropathology*, *6*, 104–109.

Dixon, C. E., Kochanek, P. M., Yan, H. Q., Schiding, J. K., Griffith, R. G., Baum, E., Marion, D. W., & DeKosky, S. T. (1999). One-year study of spatial memory performance, brain morphology, and cholinergic markers after moderate controlled cortical impact in rats. *Journal of Neurotrauma*, *16*, 109–122.

Dougherty, J. H. Jr., Rawlinson, D. H., Levy, D. E., & Plum, F. (1981). Hypoxic-ischaemic brain injury and the vegetative state: Clinical and neuropathologic correlation. *Neurology*, *31*, 991–997.

French, J. D. (1952). Brain lesions associated with prolonged unconsciousness. *Acta Neurology and Psychiatry*, *68*, 727–740.

Gennarelli, T. A. (1983). Head injury in man and experimental animals—clinical aspects. *Acta Neurochirurgica Supplement*, *32*, 1–13.

Giacino, J. T., Zasler, N. D., Katz, D. I., Kelly, J. P., & Rosenberg, J. H. (1997). Development of practice guidelines for assessment and management of the vegetative and minimally conscious status. *Journal of Head Trauma Rehabilitation*, *12*, 79–89.

Graham, D. I., Adams, J. H., Nicoll, J. A. R., Maxwell, W. L., & Gennarelli, T. A. (1995). The nature, distribution and causes of traumatic brain injury. *Brain Pathology*, *5*, 1–13.

Graham, D. I., Ford, I., Adams, J. H., Doyle, D., Teasdale, G. M., & Lawrence, A. E. (1989). Ischaemic brain damage is still common in fatal non-missile head injury. *Journal of Neurology, Neurosurgery and Psychiatry, 52*, 346–350.

Graham, D. I., Gennarelli, T. A., & McIntosh, T. K. (2002). Trauma. In D. I. Graham & P. L. Lantos (eds.), *Greenfield's neuropathology* (pp. 823–898). London: Edward Arnold.

Graham, D. I., & Lantos, P. L. (Eds.). (2002). *Greenfields neuropathology* (7th ed.). London: Edward Arnold.

Ingvar, D. H., Brun, A., Johansson, L., & Samuelsson, S. M. (1978). Survival after severe cerebral anoxia with destruction of the cerebral cortex: The apallic syndrome. *Annals of New York Academy of Science, 315*, 184–214.

Jellinger, K. (1977). Pathology and pathogenesis of apallic syndrome following closed head injuries. In O. G. Dalle, F. Gerstenbrand, C. H. Lucking, F. Peters, & U. H. Peters (eds.), *The apallic syndrome* (pp. 88–103). Berlin: Spinger-Verlag.

Jellinger, K. A. (1994). The brain of Karen Ann Quinlan (Letter). *New England Journal of Medicine, 331*, 1378–1379.

Jellinger, K., & Seitelberger, F. (1970). Protracted post-traumatic encephalopathy: Pathology pathogenesis and clinical implications. *Journal of Neurology and Science, 10*, 51–94.

Jennett, B. (2002). *The vegetative state*. Cambridge: Cambridge University Press.

Jennett, B., Adams, J. H., Murray, L. S., & Graham, D. I. (2001). Neuropathology in vegetative and severely disabled patients after head injury. *Neurology, 56*, 486–490.

Jennett, B., & Bond, M. (1975). Assessment of outcome after severe brain damage. *Lancet, 1*, 480–484.

Jennett, B., & Plum, F. (1972). Persistent vegetative state after brain damage. A syndrome in search of a name. *Lancet, 1*, 734–737.

Kinney, H. C., Korein, J., Panigraphy, A., Dikkes, P., & Goode, R. (1994). Neuropathological findings in the brain of Karen Ann Quinlan. The role of the thalamus in the persistent vegetative state. *New England Journal of Medicine, 330*, 1469–1475.

Kinney, H. C., & Samuels, M. A. (1994). Neuropathology of the persistent vegetative state. A review. *Journal of Neuropathology and Experimental Neurology, 53*, 548–558.

McIntosh, T. K., Saatman, K. E., Raghupathi, R., Graham, D. I., Smith, D. H., Lee, V. M., & Trojanowski, J. Q. (1998). The molecular and cellular sequelae of experimental traumatic brain injury: Pathogenic mechanisms. *Neuropathology and Applied Neurobiology, 24*, 251–267.

Maxwell, W. L., Dhillon, K., Harper, L., Espin, L., McIntosh, T. K., Smith, D. H., & Graham, D. I. (2003). There is differential loss of pyramidal cells from the human hippocampus with survival after blunt head injury. *Journal of Neuropathology and Experimental Neurology, 62*, 272–279.

Multi-Society Task Force on PVS (1994). Medical aspects of the persistent vegetative state. *New England Journal of Medicine, 330*, 1572–1579.

Murray, G. D., Teasdale, G. M., Braakman, R., Cohadon, F., Dearden, M., Iannotti, F., Karimi, A., Lapierre, F., Maas, A., Ohman, J., Persson, L., Servadei, F., Stocchetti, N., Trojanowski, T., & Unterberg, A. (1999). The European brain injury consortium survey of head injuries. *Acta Neurochirurgica (Wein), 19*, 223–236.

Peters, G., & Rothemund, E. (1977). Neuropathology of the traumatic apallic syndrome. In O. G. Dalle, F. Gerstenbrand, C. H. Lucking, F. Peters, & U. H. Peters (eds.), *The apallic syndrome* (pp. 78–87). Berlin: Springer-Verlag.

Pierce, J. E., Smith, D. H., Trojanowski, J. Q., & McIntosh, T. K. (1998). Enduring cognitive, neurobehavioural and histopathological changes persist for up to one year following severe experimental brain injury in rats. *Neuroscience, 87*, 359–369.

Reilly, P. L., Graham, D. I., Adams, J. H., & Jennett, B. (1975). Patients with head injury who talk and die. *Lancet, 2*, 375–377.

Relkin, N. R., Petito, C. K., & Plum, F. (1990). Coma and the vegetative state associated with thalamic injury after cardiac arrest. (Abstract). *Annals of Neurology, 28,* 221–222.

Rink, A., Fung, K. M., Trojanowski, J. Q., Lee, V. M., Neugebauer, E., & McIntosh, T. K. (1995). Evidence of apoptotic cell death after experimental traumatic brain injury in the rat. *Annals of Journal of Pathology, 147,* 1575–1583.

Royal College of Physicians (2003). The vegetative state. *Clinical Medicine, 3,* 249–254.

Smith, D. H., Chen, X-H, Pierce, J. E. S., Wolf, J. A., Trojanowski, J. Q., Graham, D. I., & McIntosh, T. K. (1997). Progressive atrophy and neuronal death for one year following brain trauma in the rat. *Journal of Neurotrauma, 14,* 715–727.

Strich, S. J. (1956). Diffuse degeneration of the cerebral white matter in severe dementia following head injury. *Journal of Neurology, Neurosurgery and Psychiatry, 19,* 163–185.

Wilson, S., Raghupathi, R., Saatman, K. E., MacKinnon, M. A., McIntosh, T. K., & Graham, D. I. (2004). Continued *in situ* DNA fragmentation of microglia/microphages in white matter weeks and months after traumatic brain injury. *Journal of Neurotrauma, 21,* 239–250.

NEUROPSYCHOLOGICAL REHABILITATION
2005, 15 (3/4), 214–223

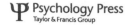
Psychology Press
Taylor & Francis Group

The neurological assessment of patients in vegetative and minimally conscious states

Roger A. Barker

Department of Neurology and Cambridge Centre for Brain Repair,
Addenbrooke's NHS Trust, Cambridge

Patients with serious central nervous system (CNS) injuries can enter a chronic state in which there is impaired awareness, but the presence of preserved basic vegetative functions. Such cases present formidable challenges to the medical practitioner in terms of clinical assessment and thus management. This paper presents the neurological approach to such patients highlighting the clinical clues that need to be sought to decide whether the patient is in a persistent vegetative or minimally conscious state (i.e., showing any responsiveness to external stimuli), or alternatively suffering from a locked-in syndrome. This neurological clinical formulation is then assimilated with other tests and assessments from a range of medical specialities, and by so doing helps confirm the clinical impression. This multidisciplinary approach is vital in the assessment of such patients and ideally should also include neurophysiological and functional imaging paradigms.

INTRODUCTION

The assessment of patients who have experienced significant cerebral trauma with altered consciousness and awareness poses a major problem to the examining clinician, as the normal neurological examination is not possible for obvious reasons. In the acute stage the loss of consciousness, wakefulness and awareness is termed coma, and the comatosed patient does not vocalise,

Correpondence should be addressed to: Dr Roger Barker, Department of Neurology and Cambridge Centre for Brain Repair, Addenbrooke's NHS Trust, Hills Road, Cambridge CB2 2PY. Tel: 01223 331160, Fax: 01223 331184. Email: rab46@hermes.cam.ac.uk

I would like to thank Alasdair Coles for his insightful comments.

http://www.tandf.co.uk/journals/pp/09602011.html   DOI:10.1080/09602010443000344

open either eyes or follow commands (Zeman, 2001). However, patients who survive this phase may go on into a vegetative state (VS), characterised by a loss of awareness but the presence of basic vegetative functions such as breathing and sleep–wake cycles. If this latter stage then persists for at least a month then the patient is said to have a persistent vegetative state, and if it persists for over one year following trauma or six months from a non-traumatic aetiology then it is termed a permanent vegetative state (Zeman, 2003). In such conditions there is typically diffuse and extensive damage involving the thalamus, cortex and white matter connections and the prognosis is poor.

The assessment of such patients in the acute phase is often done in the context of intensive care units and the use of various monitoring devices such as EEG, evoked potentials, intracranial pressure measurements and such like. In the chronic phase the assessments are done in the context of rehabilitation wards and, while involving imaging and neurophysiology (Laureys, Owen, & Schiff, 2004), relies heavily on a multi-disciplinary approach including the neurological examination. This examination serves several important functions. At its most basic, the question arises as to whether the patient that is conscious, is also aware, as the original description of the VS by Jennett and Plum (1974) described the condition as one of 'wakefulness without awareness'.

In this paper I have laid out my neurological approach to such a patient, which I have found to be helpful and reliable especially when taken in the context of other assessment modalities from a range of other medical practitioners. In particular the history and examination of the patient is designed to answer the following three questions:

1. Are there any focal deficits, which help localise the main site of injury and which may be complicating the interpretation of the patient's responses/behaviour?

2. Is the patient in a persistent vegetative or minimally conscious state? The latter being defined as the presence of reproducible but inconsistent evidence of awareness; i.e., showing definite if limited responsiveness to external stimuli?

3. And, most importantly, is the patient suffering from a locked-in syndrome?

A summary of these three questions is given in Table 1, which is taken from a recent short review by Zeman (Zeman, 2003; Royal College of Physicians, 2003).

However, the neurological assessment is only part of a much wider multi-disciplinary approach, each component of which brings vital information to

TABLE 1
The major features of states of impaired consciousness (modified from Zeman, 2003;
Royal College of Physicians, 2003)

Condition	VS	Minimally conscious state	Locked in syndrome
Awareness	Absent	Present	Present
Sleep–wake cycle	Present	Present	Present
Response to noxious stimuli	±	Present	Present in eyes only
Motor function	No purposeful movements	Some consistent or inconsistent verbal or purposeful motor responses	Volitional vertical eye movements or eyeblink preserved
Respiratory function	Preserved	Preserved	Preserved
Prognosis	Poor	Variable	Depends on aetiology but full recovery is unlikely
EEG	Normally slow wave activity	Unknown	Typically normal

the final clinical diagnosis. These assessments should ideally be conducted over time (i.e., repeated assessments) and involve neuropsychologists, physiotherapists, occupational therapists, speech and language therapists as well as the family and nursing staff. In this review though, a summary is given of the contribution of the neurologist to the diagnosis and management of patients in this state, an assessment that typically is conducted months after the original insult.

HISTORY

As with all medical issues a good account of the original insult and subsequent course is extremely helpful in the initial assessment of such patients.

Type of insult. Head injury, subarachnoid haemorrhage, cardiac or respiratory arrest, etc. This is important not only in helping with the localisation of the likely deficit, but also the period required for assessment to determine whether the patient has entered into a permanent VS. For example, if the patient collapsed with a basilar thrombosis, then there is a much higher probability of the patient developing a locked-in syndrome with localised pontine pathology as opposed to the patient who sustained a prolonged cardiac arrest in which diffuse cerebral damage is more likely with the development of a VS.

Site of injury. To some extent this relates to the type of injury, but in particular it is important to know whether the speech or pontine areas were preferentially targeted as this may give a false impression of the level of impairment. Furthermore cortical damage may evoke seizures and thus it is critical to ensure that all patients are not in some form of complex partial status, as this will clearly adversely affect the level of consciousness. If the lesion is located in the pons, a locked-in syndrome can occur, as there is disruption of the corticobulbar and corticospinal tracts, depriving the patient of speech or useful limb movement. However, the somatosensory pathways are often intact, as are the ascending brainstem activation pathways and the midbrain nuclei involved with eye movements (Leon-Carrion, van Eeckhout, & Dominguez-Morales Medl, 2002). Therefore, in any patient with such a lesion, evidence for a locked-in (or de-efferented state) must be sought.

Time since injury. The timing of the injury relative to the time of assessment is important, as the closer the two are to each other, the greater the need for reassessment at later time points. This is especially true with young patients and traumatic brain injury.

Age of patient. The level of plasticity within the CNS changes with age, becoming less in older patients. Thus younger patients may be expected to do better and so require more active reassessments compared to older patients.

Time of day and previous activities in that day. Patients with major CNS damage are not unlike normal people in getting tired, and so any assessment should ideally be done when patients are at their most alert. Thus assessing patients after they have just returned from physiotherapy, for example, can give a false impression of their true capability.

Medication. It is critical to get an up-to-date list of the medications that the patient is taking. It is easy for such patients to end up being put on a wide range of drugs, many of which are sedative. Thus anti-epileptic and anti-spastic drugs are commonly used, most of which are sedative, especially in the context of a damaged CNS. It is therefore extremely difficult to make any objective assessment if patients are on high doses of such drugs, and careful consideration should be given to slowly reducing these with a view to further assessment.

Nursing staff and relatives. It is extremely helpful to get an account of what the patient seems to be able to do by talking to the relatives that have been visiting the patient regularly, as well as the normal nursing staff. Obviously such accounts can be misleading, as relatives, for example, may over-interpret spontaneous actions as being more specific and responsive in their intent. Nevertheless, such accounts give some impression of what might be the level of awareness of the patient. Thus it is useful to find out whether patients:

- seem to follow objects/people with their eyes when they enter the room or approach the bed;
- are able to make any vocalisations, and if so, are these reliably in response to given stimuli;
- show a change in arousal when a person close to them is in the room;
- ever move their limbs towards specific stimuli—for example, suction catheters, electrodes for EEG, etc.;
- evidence of a normal circadian rhythm of wakefulness.

Obviously spontaneous flexor movements can give the impression of being targeted to stimuli, but any such movements do need to be critically evaluated (see below).

Finally, an account as to how these responses have changed over time, in particular, are these behaviours becoming more frequent? And, if they have suddenly stopped, is there some other reason for this, such as an infection?

EXAMINATION

General

The examination in the first instance relies on observation. It can be extremely educational to simply observe what patients are capable of doing on their own or in response to nursing care or relatives talking and interacting with them. So for example, does the patient spontaneously move any limb? Do any of the limbs move with turning of the patient, suction, etc., and if so is it flexor or extensor? Does the patient make any noise? Does the patient move his or her eyes spontaneously, if so is this towards specific stimuli? Does the patient have contractures?

Most patients, by this stage of the assessment for their PV or minimally conscious state, are spontaneously breathing with a normal pattern of respiration. Clearly, if there is disordered respiration, e.g., Cheyne–Stokes breathing, this implies significant brainstem or cardiovascular damage/instability and carries with it a correspondingly poor prognosis.

Finally it is important to ensure that patients are in the optimal position for assessment, and that they have not just been subject to a physically or mentally demanding exercise/therapy as this will adversely affect their conscious level and abilities.

Overall level of consciousness

The easiest way to assess the overall responsiveness of the patient, is using the Glasgow Coma Scale score (see Table 2) (Teasdale & Jennett, 1974). However, this tool is relatively insensitive and not especially informative in patients with VS or a MCS, as a result other assessment tools are employed such as the Sensory Modality Assessment Rehabilitation Technique (SMART) or Wessex Head Injury Matrix (WHIM) (Gill-Thwaites, 1997; Shiel et al., 2000).

Cranial nerves

Pupils. The size and responsiveness of pupils can be very helpful especially in the acute stage in the comatosed patient (Plum & Posner, 1980). However, it is of limited value in the chronic state as patients will have been imaged and the site and extent of damage known and thus pupillary size and reactivity to light can be easily predicted. However, it can be helpful in localising the site of major injury in brainstem events (e.g., pons with pin-point pupils) as well as ensuring that patients are not being over-sedated with opiate-like drugs, for example.

TABLE 2
Glasgow Coma Scale (after Teasdale & Jennett, 1974)

E: EYE OPENING
1 None
2 To pain
3 To sound and speech
4 Spontaneously

M: MOTOR FUNCTION
1 None
2 Extends to pain
3 Flexes to pain
4 Withdraws to pain
5 Localises to pain
6 Normal and follows commands

V: VERBAL RESPONSE
1 None
2 Incomprehensible
3 Inappropriate words
4 Confused
5 Orientated

Eye movements.   This can be very helpful. In the first instance it is useful to see the extent of spontaneous eye movements, and whether there is any nystagmus or tendency to gaze to one side implying a significant lateralised cerebral insult. It is then useful to see the extent of eye movements using oculocephalic movements, and finally the response to commands to follow a moving target such as a hand or torch. It is also useful to walk around the bed and see whether the patient's eyes track you as you move around.

Other cranial nerves.   This is of limited value in such patients. However, it is useful to see whether there is a major abnormality, in particular any lower brainstem signs which may point towards a predominant brainstem lesion, and thus the possibility of a locked-in syndrome. Furthermore one may be able to gauge the hemisphere most affected by looking for unilateral upper motor neuron facial palsies. Finally, the response to suction may be helpful, and in anyone with spontaneous facial movements it is important to exclude any ongoing partial epileptic activity. However, I do not tend to assess vestibular function using caloric tests, as this is generally only helpful in patients being assessed for brain death, or in the acute stages of coma.

Limb examination

Observation.   It is worth assessing whether there is either any asymmetry in the postures of the two sides, or contractures. It is also worth looking for scars from surgery, either previous to or as a result of the initial cerebral insult, as this may explain some of the limb abnormalities (O'Connor, 2004). Wasting is generally only seen in the context of global wasting as a result of debilitating illness, but its presence in a focal region suggests a lower motor neuron lesion consistent with either a segmental spinal cord lesion, root avulsion, or peripheral nerve damage/entrapment.

Tone.   This is generally increased in all limbs and may be so great that the limb cannot be bent. This may reflect hypertonicity or contractures and the easiest way to distinguish the two is to assess the patient when asleep, when spasticity should be reduced and contractures sustained. However, knowing when the patient is asleep may be difficult.

Power.   This is hard to assess, as patients cannot follow commands. However, gently raising and dropping limbs can give an impression of how much movement may be possible in the limb.

Reflexes and plantar responses.   These are usually not helpful as the reflexes are either increased or absent from hypertonicity and the plantars are extensor in nearly all cases.

Response to painful stimuli.   The pressing of the nailbed or sternum, while looking cruel, is necessary to see what movement can be elicited by powerful noxious sensory stimuli. This response is recorded in the GCS, and is helpful in allowing one to assess the extent of cerebral injury.

Finally it is worth while checking that the patient does not have an infection, by looking at the urine, listening to the chest and looking at the site of the Percutaneous Endoscopic Gastrostomy (PEG). If any of these areas look infected, it is worth while culturing the affected site, treating with antibiotics and reassessing the patient at a later date, as all infections will deleteriously affect the neurological status of the patient.

FORMULATION

At the conclusion of the history and examination, one should be able to ascertain:

- The nature, extent and anatomical sequelae of the initial insult to the CNS.

- The natural history of the patient's condition from that time, in particular any sign of improvement.

- The normal responsiveness and behaviour of the patient, especially to powerful sensory stimuli and specific simple commands.

- The diagnosis as being one of VS, a minimally conscious state or a locked in syndrome.

At this stage further investigation can be helpful, especially in cases where one is concerned about the possibility that the patient may be in a locked-in state. In these cases asking *simple* questions with yes or no responses should be sought—the response being limited to eye blinking or eyebrow/eye movements (e.g., vertical eye movements). Thus the questioning must be done slowly and carefully. If it is rushed, then the patient may appear not to be responding appropriately and consistently, which may mislead the examiner.

However, the use of other investigative tools can often be very helpful in arriving at a diagnosis of a locked-in syndrome, especially the use of evoked potentials, EEG, and functional activation imaging studies (see Table 1 and other papers in this special issue).

TREATMENT

Once a diagnosis has been made, appropriate treatment should be considered, although most patients by this stage are normally in well-established units with appropriate support and therapy. However, particular attention should be paid to:

- The provision of constant interactions and vocal encouragement.

- Physiotherapy to avoid contractures.

- Modification of drug therapies to ensure that the patient is not over-sedated.

- Instigation of anti-epileptic therapies if epilepsy is proven or strongly suspected.

- Antibiotic therapy, if appropriate, for a proven infection (changes in the temperature of a patient is not uncommon in these states, due to the nature of the lesion, and so other evidence for an infection is normally needed outside of a pyrexia).

- Exploration of communication is needed if it is suspected that the patient is in a locked-in state.

- Consideration of transfer to a specialist rehabilitation unit is strongly recommended as these units have all the expertise to assess and manage these patients most effectively.

CONCLUSION

Overall, the assessment of patients once they have entered into a persistent vegetative or minimally conscious state, is difficult and rudimentary compared to the normal neurological examination. However, a detailed history coupled to a targeted neurological examination can provide the information necessary to localise the major pathological site, and the likely state of the patient. In particular, the anxiety of missing a patient with a locked-in state is a real, if rare, event and thus must be actively sought in patients with predominant brainstem, especially pontine, lesions. In such cases, additional assessments using neurophysiological and functional imaging are helpful.

However, even in such cases, sometimes, repeated assessments are needed to clarify the diagnosis—a diagnosis which has important management implications especially due to the public and media interest in cases of VS given that such patients have been the subject of court decisions on withdrawal of treatment (Anon, 1993). It is therefore imperative that in all such cases, a multidisciplinary approach is adopted for investigation, assessment and treatment.

REFERENCES

Anon (1993). Tony Bland awaits final hearing. *British Medical Journal, 306*, 11–12.

Gill-Thwaites, H. (1997). The Sensory Modality Assessment Rehabilitation Technique: A tool for assessment and treatment of patients with severe brain injury in a vegetative state. *Brain Injury, 11*, 723–734.

Jennett, B., & Plum, F. (1972). Persistent vegetative state after brain damage. *Lancet, 1* (April 1, 7753), 734–737.

Laureys, S., Owen, A. M., & Schiff, N. D. (2004). Brain function in coma, vegetative state and related disorders. *Lancet Neurology, 3*, 537–546.

Leon-Carrion, J., van Eeckhout, P., & Dominguez-Morales Medl, R. (2002). The locked in syndrome: A syndrome looking for a therapy. *Brain Injury, 16*, 555–569.

O'Connor, R. (2004). Musculoskeletal complications of neurological conditions. *Advances in Clinical Neuroscience & Rehabilitation, 4*, 27–29.

Plum, F., & Posner, J. B. (1980). *Diagnosis of stupor and coma* (3rd ed.). Philadelphia, PA: Davis.

Royal College of Physicians (2003). The vegetative state: Guidance on diagnosis and management. *Clinical Medicine, 3*(3), 249–254.

Shiel, A., Horn, S. A., Wilson, B. A., Watson, M. J., Campbell, M. J., & McLellan, D. L. (2000). The Wessex Head Injury Matrix (WHIM) main scale: A preliminary report on a scale to assess and monitor patient recovery after severe head injury. *Clinical Rehabilitation, 14*, 408–416.

Teasdale, G., & Jennett, B. (1974). Assessment of coma and impaired consciousness. *Lancet, 2*, 81–84.

Zeman, A. (2003). What is consciousness and what does it mean for the persistent vegetative state? *Advances in Clinical Neuroscience & Rehabilitation, 3*(3), 12–14.

Zeman, A. (2001). Consciousness. *Brain, 124*, 1263–1289.

NEUROPSYCHOLOGICAL REHABILITATION
2005, 15 (3/4), 224–236

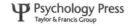

Hydrocephalus, ventriculomegaly and the vegetative state: A review

John D. Pickard, Martin R. Coleman, and Marek Czosnyka

University of Cambridge, Addenbrooke's Hospital, Cambridge, UK

The revised guidelines from the Royal College of Physicians make it clear that structural problems such as hydrocephalus should be excluded before the diagnosis of vegetative state (VS) can be made. Ventriculomegaly is common after severe head injury but the distinction between atrophy and potentially treatable hydrocephalus cannot be made on the basis of conventional computerised tomographic (CT) or magnetic resonance (MR) scanning alone—physiological measurements of intracranial pressure (ICP) and cerebrospinal fluid (CSF) outflow resistance may be helpful. These techniques are reviewed together with the limited literature available that documents the effect of CSF diversion on outcome in "vegetative" patients.

INTRODUCTION

It is essential, as part of the process to confirm the diagnosis of vegetative state (VS), to exclude conditions—of which hydrocephalus is one—that might retard or prevent recovery (Royal College of Physicians, 2003). Unfortunately, the detection of hydrocephalus that might respond to treatment is not straightforward. We here discuss the pathophysiological basis of hydrocephalus, its distinction from ventriculomegaly and describe a method to detect hydrocephalus in vegetative and minimally conscious patients.

Correspondence should be sent to Professor John Pickard, University of Cambridge, Academic Neurosurgery Unit, Box 167, Addenbrooke's Hospital, Cambridge, CB2 2QQ. Tel: +44 (0)1223 336946, Fax: +44 (0)1223 216926. Email: jdp.secretary@medschl.cam.ac.uk

The authors are very grateful to Professor David Graham for his permission to reproduce Figure 1. This work was supported by the Smith's Charity, UK and an MRC Programme Grant (number G9439390 ID56833).

---

http://www.tandf.co.uk/journals/pp/09602011.html   DOI:10.1080/09602010443000614

HYDROCEPHALUS IN NON-COMATOSE AND NON-VEGETATIVE PATIENTS

Hydrocephalus is defined as the accumulation of excess cerebrospinal fluid (CSF) within the head, often but not always associated with dilatation of the ventricles, due to an abnormality of secretion, circulation or absorption of CSF. True hydrocephalus should be distinguished from ventriculomegaly secondary to cerebral atrophy or "hydrocephalus ex vacuo". CSF hypersecretion is rare but it has been described in choroidal villous hypertrophy in childhood (Fujimoto, Matsushita, Plese, & Marino, 2004). The great majority of cases of hydrocephalus are the result of blockage within or at the outlets of the ventricular system (obstructive) or within the basal cisterns/subarachnoid space or arachnoid granulations (communicating).

True hydrocephalus may present with the symptoms and signs of raised intracranial pressure (ICP): headache, nausea, vomiting, transient visual obscurations with papilloedema, and "false" localising signs such as a VIth nerve palsy. The conscious level will deteriorate if raised ICP is left untreated. Alternatively, patients may present much more insidiously with so-called normal pressure hydrocephalus (NPH). NPH was first formally described by Hakim and Adams in 1965 and consists of a clinical triad of gait disturbance (magnet gait), "dementia", and urinary incontinence with ventricular dilatation and apparently normal CSF pressure as recorded briefly through a lumbar puncture needle. However, overnight ICP monitoring may reveal increased CSF pressure with an increased frequency and amplitude of vasogenic waves of ICP. Typically, the resistance to CSF absorption is increased (*vide infra*). NPH may be idiopathic or may follow meningitis, subarachnoid haemorrhage or trauma among other conditions, often many years later. Characteristically it is a condition of late middle age and the elderly, particularly in its idiopathic form. Patients with aqueduct stenosis may remain asymptomatic for many years but in older life may present with NPH. NPH is important because it is potentially reversible by CSF shunting or, in some of the patients in the subgroup with late presentation of aqueduct stenosis, by IIIrd ventriculostomy. The gait disturbance is often improved by shunting as are many of the problems of higher mental function except for the frontal dysexecutive component (Iddon et al., 1999). Patients with a chronically depressed level of consciousness may take many months to improve after a shunt so that test removal of some CSF is not a reliable predictor of outcome following a shunt (*vide infra*).

Although considered to be a disorder of the CSF circulation, there is evidence, particularly in idiopathic NPH, to suggest that the cerebral vasculature may play a role in its pathogenesis through effects on the biomechanical properties of the cerebral mantle. Indeed, it is appropriate to refer to the patients presenting with the Hakim triad as complex dementia as there is often considerable overlap in the same patient between NPH, cerebrovascular disease (Earnest, Fahn, Karp, & Rowland, 1974), and Alzheimer's (Silverberg et al., 2003). The challenge for the clinician is to identify those patients with a remediable hydrocephalic component that will respond to shunting. Some patients may respond for a few years to a shunt, but then other processes including Alzheimer's and cerebrovascular disease may supervene—for example, when systemic hypertension is not adequately controlled.

HYDROCEPHALUS IN VEGETATIVE PATIENTS

It is important in the context of possible VS to emphasise that post-traumatic hydrocephalus is less likely to present as obviously raised intracranial pressure but more insidiously as failure to improve—the natural history following a head injury is usually to continue to improve (Cohadon, 2000; Dolce & Sazbon, 2002; Jennett, 2002; Jennett & Plum, 1972). When patients do not improve after brain injury, the question should always be asked: why not? Some patients with large skull defects due to decompressive craniotomy may develop the "syndrome of the trephined" particularly if they become dehydrated and are sat up for prolonged periods of time. Such patients may improve after cranioplasty (insertion of an acrylic, titanium or bone plate to fill in the skull defect). Other patients with borderline hydrocephalus may deteriorate after a cranioplasty and require a shunt vide infra.

INCIDENCE OF "HYDROCEPHALUS" IN VS PATIENTS

Ventriculomegaly is commonly seen at post-mortem in patients who have died in VS (Figure 1). The Glasgow study recorded an incidence of "hydrocephalus" of 77% but not all ventriculomegaly is true hydrocephalus (Jennett, Adams, Murray, & Graham, 2001). No mass lesions causing obstructive hydrocephalus were described in the Glasgow study. It is important to appreciate the limitations of neuropathology in defining true communicating hydrocephalus. The only pathological substrates that may accompany communicating hydrocephalus would be obliteration of the subarachnoid space, basal cisterns or arachnoid granulations and possibly selective periventricular white matter loss. It would be unusual to examine the extracerebral structures in the preserved brain. Hence the figure of 77% for "hydrocephalus" probably represents both hydrocephalus ex vacuo as well as true hydrocephalus. This supposition is born out by the incidence of both diffuse axonal injury and thalamic abnormalities of 80% (Jennett et al., 2001). In the VS cohort, there was reduction in the area of

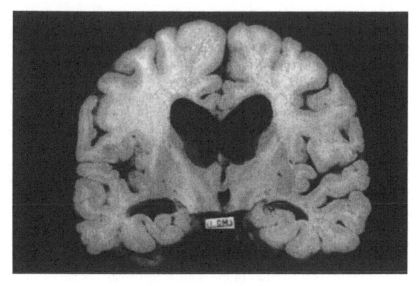

Figure 1. Coronal section of the brain of a VS patient

the dorsomedial and ventroposterior thalamic nuclei with a reduction in the number but not size of the thalamic neurones.

BRAIN SCANNING IN VS PATIENTS

Air and isotope studies revealed post-traumatic ventriculomegaly many years ago (Dandy & Blackfan, 1914; Granholm & Svendgaard, 1972; Gurdjian & Fisher, 1966; Hawkins, Lloyd, Fletcher, & Hanka. 1976; Lewin, 1968). The air studies probably overestimated the degree of ventriculomegaly, perhaps because of post-traumatic changes in the biomechanical properties of the cerebral mantle. CT scanning has been reported to show ventricular dilatation in some 25–51% of patients in VS although the definition of ventriculomegaly has differed between reports (Beyerl & Black, 1984; French & Dublin, 1977; Gudeman et al., 1981; Katz, Brander, & Sahgal, 1989; Kishore et al., 1978; Koo & LaRoque, 1977; Levin, Meyers, & Grossman, 1981; Merino-de Villasante & Taveras, 1976; Meyers, Levin, Eisenberg, & Guinto, 1983; Paoletti, Pezzotta, & Spanu, 1983). Shunt-responsive hydrocephalus occurs in fewer patients (0.7% Cardoso & Galbraith, 1985; 3.9% Groswasser, Cohen, Reider-Groswasser, & Stern. 1988; 20% Marmarou et al., 1996). The phenomenon certainly occurs in childhood (Silver & Chinarian, 1997). Careful longitudinal studies have revealed that hydrocephalus may be preceded by transient subdural collections of CSF (Licata et al., 2001; Yoshimoto, Wakai, & Hamano, 1998). Studies of patients with normal pressure hydrocephalus have demonstrated that there is no reliable way of using CT scanning to distinguish between shunt-responders and non-responders. A favourable response to shunting might be expected in NPH patients where there is no superficial cortical atrophy, the IIIrd ventricle is enlarged, and there is periventricular hypodensity suggestive of oedema due to CSF extravasation and reversal of drainage of interstitial fluid. However, there are many exceptions and periventricular changes in chronic hydrocephalus are more likely to represent periventricular gliosis and infarcted white matter rather than the oedema of acute obstructive hydrocephalus. MR scanning is more sensitive in detecting such changes. Progressive ventriculomegaly on successive CT scans does not differentiate hydrocephalus from atrophy. Figures 2 and 3 illustrate the MR scans of patients from the Cambridge Coma Study Group cohort (N = 20; 10 VS and 10 MCS; 16 male, average age = 43 years, range 19–67) who were investigated between 3 weeks and 122 months post-insult. The bicaudate ratio—the width of the lateral ventricles at the level of the caudate nuclei relative to the internal diameter of the skull at that level—of the patients in VS was 0.26 (range 0.17–0.40) and in the minimally conscious was 0.24 (range 0.10–0.30). In other words, the ventricles were dilated in many of the patients in both groups. There are no specific features about such MR scans that are diagnostic of either VS or MCS: the same scan appearances may be seen in patients who are fully conscious and present with other problems or might be asymptomatic, particularly in the elderly.

When air, isotope or contrast is injected into the lumbar theca, it normally passes into the cortical subarachnoid space. In communicating hydrocephalus, such tracers do not enter the cortical subarachnoid space ("convexity block") but pass retrogradely into the ventricles ("ventricular reflux"). Unfortunately, such findings do not help to predict reliably whether the individual patient will respond to a shunt.

PHYSIOLOGICAL STUDIES OF THE CSF CIRCULATION

In patients who have failed to progress or regressed clinically and who have ventriculomegaly on CT or MR scanning, consideration should be given to assessing their intracranial pressure and CSF dynamics. In patients in VS or MCS, it is very difficult to detect subtle changes in their neurological condition. Single measurements of CSF pressure through a lumbar puncture needle and fluid column manometer will miss most of the important information (Czosnyka & Pickard, 2004, for review). Considerable controversy surrounds which investigations provide the most reliable prediction of outcome following shunting. Prolonged external drainage of CSF has many advocates as does measurement of the resistance to CSF absorption (R_{csf}).

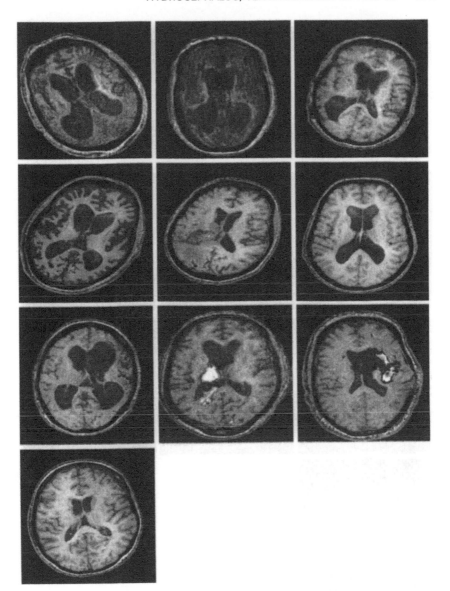

Figure 2. Montage of MR scans for 10 VS patients

The CSF infusion test depends upon Davson's equation, which describes the relationships between CSF pressure, production and absorption:

$$Pcsf = (If \times Rout) + Psss$$

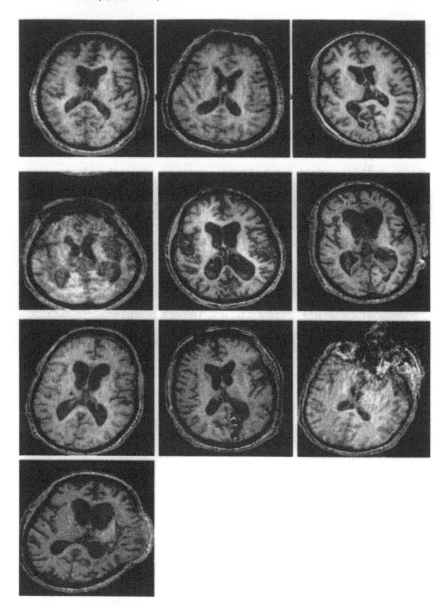

Figure 3. Montage of MR scans for 10 MCS patents

where *Rout* is the resistance to CSF outflow, *If* is the CSF formation rate, and *Psss* is the sagittal sinus pressure.

The infusion study may be performed via the lumbar CSF space or via a pre-implanted ventricular access device. In both cases two needles are inserted (22 g spinal needles for lumbar tests; 25 g butterfly needles for ventricular studies). One needle is connected to a pressure transducer via a stiff saline-filled tube and the other to an infusion pump mounted on a purpose-built trolley containing a pressure amplifier (and IBM-compatible personal computer running software for data analysis — www.neurosurg.cam.ac.uk/icmplus/). After 10 minutes of baseline measurement, the infusion of normal saline at a rate of 1.5 ml/min or 1 ml/min (if the baseline pressure was higher than 15 mmHg) is started and continued until a steady state ICP plateau is achieved. If the ICP increases to 40 mmHg, the infusion is stopped. Following cessation of the saline infusion, ICP is recorded until it decreases to steady baseline levels (Figure 4). All compensatory parameters are calculated using computer-supported methods based on physiological models of the CSF circulation. Baseline ICP and R_{csf} characterise the static properties of the CSF circulation. Using similar physiological tests, Marmarou and colleagues have distinguished five subgroups among patients after severe head injury:

- Normal ventricular size and normal ICP (41.3 %).

- Normal ventricular size but raised ICP ("benign intracranial hypertension"—type profile—14.7%).

- Ventriculomegaly, normal ICP and Rout (atrophy group—24%).

- Ventriculomegaly, normal ICP but raised Rout (NPH group—9.3%).

- Ventriculomegaly, elevated ICP with or without raised Rout (high pressure hydrocephalus group—10.7%).

Care should be taken with the interpretation of Rout following a decompressive craniectomy: Rout may be apparently normal but a cranioplasty may precipitate acute neurological deterioration if ventriculomegaly is present (Figure 5, Czosnyka et al., 2000).

TIMING OF INVESTIGATIONS AND COUNSELLING OF THE FAMILY

Many patients who fail to progress from coma may not be scanned after the initial acute phase. The family may have adjusted to the apparently dismal prognosis. It may appear as perverse or meddlesome to suggest further invasive investigations unless the family has been forewarned as part of the earlier counselling that such tests may become appropriate later. Such conflicts may arise when care is transferred between hospitals and community facilities or when second opinions are sought. Why bother doctor? Is it not unkind? Even

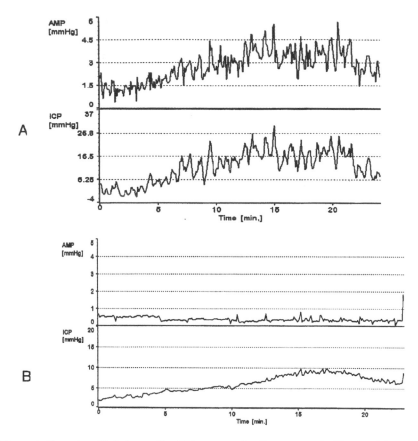

Figure 4. Examples of infusion studies. ICP—mean value (8 sec average) of intracranial pressure, and AMP—value of pulse amplitude of ICP waveform. In response to constant rate infusion ICP increases and, after finishing infusion, it decreases back to the baseline (a) normal pressure hydrocephalus, resistance to CSF outflow 14.5 mmHg/(ml/min), normal baseline ICP. There are vasogenic waves in the recording ("B" waves and amplitude of ICP is strictly proportional to mean ICP, (b) brain atrophy: normal baseline ICP, low resistance to CSF outflow 6 mmHg/(ml/min), no vasogenic waves, pulse amplitude does not change when ICP increases

if a shunt is indicated and leads to improvement in a minority of cases, does this not increase the awareness by the patients of their appalling deficits? Early counselling is essential together with understanding of the need to look for remediable hydrocephalus sooner rather than later by serial scanning accompanied by physiological tests if progressive ventriculomegaly or failure to progress is noted. Both families and the clinical staff need to be aware that any benefits of shunting may take many weeks or even months to become manifest, even in cases of known hydrocephalus who have had a shunt

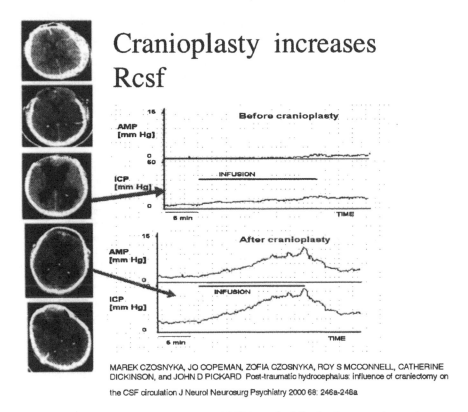

Cranioplasty increases Rcsf

MAREK CZOSNYKA, JO COPEMAN, ZOFIA CZOSNYKA, ROY S MCCONNELL, CATHERINE DICKINSON, and JOHN D PICKARD Post-traumatic hydrocephalus: influence of craniectomy on the CSF circulation J Neurol Neurosurg Psychiatry 2000 68: 246a-248a

Figure 5. Effect of cranioplasty on intracranial CSF dynamics following decompressive craniectomy for refractory intracranial hypertension after severe head injury. ICP—mean ICP; AMP—pulse amplitude of ICP waveform. First scan just after injury, shows tight brain. Second scan after bifrontal decompressive craniectomy. Third scan several months later, showing dilated ventricles and no cranioplasty. Infusion test performed at this stage revealed normal CSF circulation, with little "atrophic" features. Next scan, after cranioplasty, infusion test revealed substantial CSF circulatory deficit. Last scan, after successful shunting, ventricles decreased and patient dramatically improved clinically

blockage or intracranial haemorrhage. Paradoxically, ventricular size need not shrink after a shunt for clinical improvement to occur.

OUTCOME FOLLOWING CSF SHUNTING

Table 1 summarises the current literature, which is rather limited. It is not clear how many of these patients were vegetative or minimally conscious, nor what the timing of assessment or of shunting was. Most patients were investigated by CT or MR scanning alone with few physiological tests

TABLE 1
Outcome following CSF shunting in patients in VS or "prolonged posttraumatic coma or unawareness"

Author	Investigation	Patients	Outcome
Kalisky et al., 1895 Houston, USA	CT (ICP)	1	No change
Sazbon & Grosswasser, 1990 Tel-Aviv, Israel	CT	17	7 recovered consciousness (number of true VS patients?; timing?)
Tribl & Oder, 2000 Vienna, Austria	CT	18	6 improved, 12 no change (VS and MCS; degree of improvement?)
Licata et al., 2001 Verona, Italy	CT (MRI, RISA, ICP)	26	4 good recovery, 3 partial disability, 19 persistent coma (timing?)
Mazzini et al., 2003 Torino, Italy	MR (SPECT)	5	3 improved, 2 no change (degree of improvement?)

MR = Magnetic resonance scanning; ICP = intracranial pressure studies; CT = computerised tomography; RISA = radioiodinated serume albumen cisternography; SPECT = single photon emission computerised tomography. Tests bracketed in column 2 of the table were only conducted in a minority of patients.

being performed. The suspicion however is that a few patients in VS/MCS did improve after shunting.

SUMMARY

The revised Royal College of Physician guidelines make it clear that conditions such as hydrocephalus should be excluded before the diagnosis of VS can be made. Ventriculomegaly is common after severe head injury but the distinction between atrophy and potentially shunt-responsive hydrocephalus cannot be made on the basis of conventional CT or MR scanning alone—physiological measurements of ICP and CSF outflow resistance are required. A more systematic approach is required to this problem that should include careful early counselling of a patient's family in order not to raise undue expectations but equally not to deny a patient potential treatment.

REFERENCES

Beyerl, B., & Black, P. M. (1984). Post-traumatic hydrocephalus. *Neurosurgery, 15*, 257–261.
Cardoso, E. R., & Galbraith, S. (1985). Post-traumatic hydrocephalus—A retrospective review. *Surgical Neurology, 23*, 261–264.

Cohadon, F. (2000). *Sortir du coma*. Paris: Editions Odile Jacob.

Czosnyka, M., Copeman, J., Czosnyka, Z., McConnell, R., Dickinson, C., Pickard, J. D. (2000). Post-traumatic hydrocephalus: influence of craniectomy on the CSF circulation. *Journal of Neurology, Neurosurgery and Psychiatry, 68*, 246–248.

Czosnyka, M., Pickard, J. D. (2004). Monitoring and interpretation of intracranial pressure. *Journal Neurology, Neurosurgery and Psychiatry, 75*, 813–821.

Czosnyka, M., Whitehouse, H., Smielewski, P., Simac, S., & Pickard, J. D. (1996). Testing of cerebrospinal compensatory reserve in shunted and non-shunted patients: A guide to interpretation based on an observational study. *Journal of Neurology, Neurosurgery and Psychiatry, 60*, 549–558.

Dandy, W., & Blackfan, K. D. (1914). Internal hydrocephalus. An experimental, clinical and pathological study. *American Journal of Diseases of Children, 8*, 406–482.

Dolce, G., Sazbon, L. (2002). *The post-traumatic vegetative state*. Stuttgart: Thieme.

Earnest, M. P., Fahn, S., Karp, J. H., & Rowland, L. P. (1974). Normal pressure hydrocephalus and hypertensive cerebrovascular hypertensive disease. *Archives of Neurology, 31*, 262–266.

French, B. N., & Dublin, A. B. (1977). The value of computerised tomography in the management of 1000 consecutive head injuries. *Surgical Neurology, 7*, 171–183.

Fujimoto, Y., Matsushita, M., Plese, J. P., & Marino, R. (2004). Hydrocephalus due to diffuse villous hypertrophy of the choroid plexus. *Paediatric Neurosurgery, 40*, 32–36.

Granholm, L., Svendgaard, N. (1972). Hydrocephalus following traumatic head injuries. *Scandinavian Journal of Rehabilitation Medicine, 4*, 31–34.

Groswasser, Z., Cohen, M., Reider-Groswasser, I., & Stern, M. J. (1988). Incidence, CT findings and rehabilitation outcome of patients with communicative hydrocephalus following severe head injury. *Brain Injury, 2*, 267–272.

Gudeman, S. K., Kishore, P. R. S., Becker, D. P., Lipper, M. H., Girevendulis, A. K., Jeffries, B. F., & Butterworth, J. F., 4th. (1981). Computed tomography in the evaluation of incidence and significance of post-traumatic hydrocephalus. *Radiology, 141*, 397–402.

Gurdjian, E. S., Fisher, R. A. (1966). Post traumatic hydrocephalus in head injury. In W. F. Caveness (Ed.), *Head injury conference proceedings* (pp. 550–555). Philadelphia: Lippincott.

Hakim, S., Adams, R. D. (1965). The special clinical problem of symptomatic hydrocephalus with normal CSF pressure. *Journal of Neurological Sciences, 2*, 307–327.

Hawkins, T. D., Lloyd, A. D., Fletcher, G. K., & Hanka, R. (1976). Ventricular size following head injury: A clinico-radiological study. *Radiology, 27*, 279–289.

Iddon, J. L., Pickard, J. D., Cross, J. J., & Griffiths, P. D., Czosnyka, M., Sahakian, B. J. (1999). Specific patterns of cognitive impairment in patients with idiopathic normal pressure hydrocephalus. *Journal of Neurology, Neurosurgery and Psychiatry, 67*, 723–732.

Jennett, B. (2002). The vegetative state: medical facts, ethical and legal dilemmas. Cambridge, UK: Cambridge University Press.

Jennett, B., Adams, J. H., Murray, L. S., & Graham, D. I. (2001). Neuropathology in vegetative and severely disabled patients after head injury. *Neurology, 56*(4), 486–490.

Jennett, B., & Plum, F. (1972). Persistant vegetative state after brain damage: A syndrome in search of a name. *Lancet, 1*, 734–737.

Kalisky, Z., Morrison, D. P., Meyers, C. A., & Von Laufen, A. (1985). Medical problems encountered during rehabilitation of patients with head injury. *Archives of Physical Medicine and Rehabilitation, 66*, 25–29.

Kampfl, A., Franz, G., Aichner, F., Pfausler, B., Haring, H. P., Felber, S., Luz, G., Schocke, M., & Schmutzhard, E. (1998). The persistent vegetative state after closed head injury: Clinical and magnetic resonance imaging findings in 42 patients. *Journal of Neurosurgery, 88*, 809–816.

Katz, R. T., Brander, V., & Sahgal, V. (1989). Updates on the diagnosis and management of post-traumatic hydrocephalus. *American Journal of Physical Medicine and Rehabilitation*, *68*, 91–96.

Kishore, P. R. S., Lipper, M. H., Miller, J. D., Gyrevendulis, A. K., Becker, D. P., & Vives, F. S. (1978). Post-traumatic hydrocephalus in patients with severe head injury. *Neuroradiology*, *16*, 261–265.

Koo, A. H., & LaRoque, R. L. (1977). Evaluation of head trauma by computed Tomography. *Radiology*, *123*, 345–350.

Levin, H. S., Meyers, C. A., Grossman, R. G., & Sarwar, M. (1981). Ventricular enlargement after closed head injury. *Archives of Neurology*, *38*, 623–629.

Lewin, W. (1968). Preliminary observation on external hydrocephalus after severe head injury. *British Journal of Surgery*, *55*, 747–751.

Licata, C., Cristofori, L., Gambin, R., Vivenza, C., & Turazzi, S. (2001). Post-traumatic hydrocephalus. *Journal of Neurosurgical Science*, *45*, 141–149.

Marmarou, A., Foda, M. A., Bandoh, K., Yoshihara, M., Yamamoto, T., Tsuji, O., Zasler, N., Ward, J. D., & Young, H. F. (1996). Post-traumatic ventriculomegaly: Hydrocephalus or atrophy? A new approach for diagnosis using CSF dynamics. *Journal of Neurosurgery*, *85*, 1026–1035.

Mazzini, L., Campini, R., Angelino, E., Rognone, F., Pastore, I., & Oliveri, G. (2003). Post-traumatic hydrocephalus: A clinical, neuroradiologic and neuropsychologic assessment of long-term outcome. *Archives of Physical Medicine and Rehabilitation*, *84*, 1637–1641.

Merino-de Villasante, J., & Taveras, J. M. (1976). Computerised tomography in acute head trauma. *American Journal of Roentgenology*, *126*, 765–778.

Meyers, C. A., Levin, H. S., Eisenberg, H. M., & Guinto, F. C. (1983). Early versus late lateral ventricular enlargement following closed head injury. *Journal of Neurology, Neurosurgery and Psychiatry*, *46*, 1092–1097.

Paoletti, P., Pezzotta, S., & Spanu, G. (1983). Diagnosis and treatment of post-traumatic hydrocephalus. *Journal of Neurosurgical Science*, *27*, 171–175.

Royal College of Physicians of London (2003). The vegetative state: Guidance on diagnosis and management. *Clinical Medicine*, *3*, 249–254.

Sazbon, L., & Groswasser, Z. (1990). Outcome in 134 patients with prolonged post-traumatic unawareness. Part I: parameters determining late recovery of consciousness. *Journal of Neurosurgery*, *72*, 75–80.

Silver, B. V., & Chinarian, J. (1997). Neurologic improvement following shunt placement for post-traumatic hydrocephalus in a child. *Pediatric Rehabilitation*, *1*, 123–126.

Silverberg, G. D., Mayo, M., Saul, T., Rubenstein, E., & McGuire, D. (2003). Alzheimer's disease, normal pressure hydrocephalus and senescent changes in CSF circulatory physiology—a hypothesis. *Lancet Neurology*, *2*, 506–511.

Tribl, G., & Oder, W. (2000). Outcome after shunt implantation in severe head injury with post-traumatic hydrocephalus. *Brain Injury*, *14*, 345–354.

Yoshimoto, Y., Wakai, S., Hamano, M. (1998). External hydrocephalus after aneurysm surgery—paradoxical response to ventricular shunting. *Journal of Neurosurgery*, *88*, 485–489.

NEUROPSYCHOLOGICAL REHABILITATION
2005, 15 (3/4), 237–250

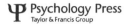

Permanent vegetative state: The legal position

Sheila A. M. McLean

School of Law, University of Glasgow, UK

Medicine's diagnostic and therapeutic capacities raise increasingly complex ethical and legal issues for consideration. This is particularly so when the patient is in a permanent vegetative state. This article reviews the current legal position in the case of adults in permanent vegetative state (pVS), with particular attention to the devices used by courts in reaching decisions about whether or not to prolong assisted nutrition and hydration. The article further considers the impact of the Human Rights Act 1998, and argues that the current legal position is significantly, if not determinatively, based on clinical judgement, even where there is some doubt about whether or not the cases actually meet the terms of the Royal College of Physicians (RCP) diagnostic guidelines. In addition, the article asks whether or not the devices used by courts to permit withdrawing assisted nutrition and hydration from patients in pVS could be categorised as assisted death, and notes the (arguable) weakness of these devices as a basis for derogation from the sanctity of life principle.

Few clinical situations are likely to generate as many profound legal, ethical and personal dilemmas as those presented by the patient in a vegetative state (VS). Although there are variations in the vegetative state, this commentary will confine itself to those diagnosed as being in a permanent vegetative state (pVS), since it is at this extreme end of human existence that clinical decisions become most acutely problematic. Moreover, this discussion will concern itself only with adults diagnosed as being in a pVS.

DIAGNOSIS AND CLINICAL MANAGEMENT

The Royal College of Physicians (2003) has issued guidelines on the diagnosis and management of the VS, which provide a template for those

Correspondence should be addressed to Professor Sheila A. M. McLean, International Bar Association Professor of Law and Ethics in Medicine, School of Law, The University, Glasgow G12 8QQ. Tel: 0141 330 5577, Fax: 0141 330 4698, Email: S.A.M.McLean@law.gla.ac.uk involved in such cases. In addition to these guidelines, a body of common law, which will be considered later, has developed around the management of patients in pVS. In terms of the RCP's guidelines, caution is urged in the diagnosis of pVS, because of its consequences; first, that "a prediction is being made that awareness will never recover", even although, as the RCP notes, "[t]his prediction cannot be made with absolute certainty"[1]. Further, the RCP guidelines caution that the diagnosis of VS should be specific and exclude other conditions, such as brainstem death and coma[2]. Moreover, the RCP insists that the diagnosis of pVS should not be made until "12 months after head injury (traumatic brain injury) and six months after other causes before the VS is judged to be 'permanent' "[3]. Diagnosis should be made by two suitably qualified doctors,[4] and with "great care"[5].

The reasons for caution and care are self-evident. The notion that human life is sacred, or has a special intrinsic worth, is widely accepted even in secular societies. As the person in pVS is alive for legal purposes, just as with any other living patient decisions about whether or not medical intervention to sustain that life should be provided have considerable significance. The consequence of this diagnosis will often result in discussion of the possibility of removing life-sustaining treatment, primarily assisted nutrition and hydration. Although in some situations, the provision of nutrition and hydration—even if this needs to be done artificially—is seen as basic care, and therefore to be provided without question, for the patient in pVS the issue has taken on a different significance.

The RCP Guidelines also make specific reference to the concept of futility, saying that when "recovery cannot reasonably be expected", then "further therapy is futile. It merely prolongs an insentient life and a hopeless vigil entailing major emotional costs for relatives and carers"[6]. The imposition of futile treatment is not regarded as being in the best interests of the patient. However, definitions of what is "futile" treatment vary, leading Mason, McCall Smith and Laurie (2002) to say that "the whole topic of medical futility. . . . is fraught with difficulties and contradictions"[7].

---

[1]Royal College of Physicians (2003). *The vegetative state: Guidance on diagnosis and management, Report of a Working Party of the Royal College of Physicians*, p.2, para 1.9.

[2]p. 4, para 2.5

[3]p. 5, para 2.8

[4]p. 7, para 3.3

[5]p. 7, para 3.2

[6]p. 9, para 3.5

[7]Mason, J. K., McCall Smith, R. A., & Laurie, G. T. (2002). *Law and medical ethics*, (6th Edn.), London: Butterworths, at p. 473, para 16.10

THE SANCTITY OF LIFE

Before considering the major legal cases involving patients in pVS, it is worth briefly expanding on the importance of this doctrine in legal thinking. The sanctity of human life might appear to mandate that all lives, irrespective of quality, should be maintained when possible. However, this has not been the approach adopted by the law. Lord Donaldson, for example, has said that "[t]here is without doubt a very strong presumption in favour of a course of action which will prolong life, but . . . it is not irrebuttable"[8]. Additionally, other principles (such as that of autonomy) can "trump" the State's interest in respecting the sanctity of all life. In the case of *Re T (adult: refusal of treatment)* it was said:

> The patient's interest consists of his right to self-determination—his right to live his own life as he wishes, even if it will damage his health or lead to his premature death. Society's interest is in upholding the concept that all human life is sacred and that it should be preserved if at all possible. *It is well established that in the ultimate the right of the individual is paramount.*[9] (Emphasis added)

Equally, the law makes a distinction between acts and omissions; that is, we are generally culpable in respect of our acts but not our omissions to act. A distinction is drawn between killing and letting die; thus, a doctor may not directly kill a patient, but may "let nature take its course". However, as the Court of Human Rights noted recently, this distinction may not always operate. In the case of *David Glass v UK*, the court said:

> It cannot be excluded that the acts and omissions of the authorities in the field of health care may in certain circumstances engage their responsibility under the positive limb of Article 2[10].

The doctrine may also come second to an assessment of the best interests of a given patient (sometimes apparently in combination with some concept of futility). Thus, in *Airedale NHS Trust v Bland*, which will be considered in more detail *infra*, Lord Goff said:

> The question is not whether the doctor should take a course which will kill his patient, or even take a course which has the effect of accelerating

---

[8]*Re J (a minor) (wardship: medical treatment)* [1990] 3 All ER 930 at p 938
[9]*Re T (adult: refusal of treatment)* 9 BMLR 46 (1992) at p. 59
[10]*David Glass v The United Kingdom* [2004] Lloyd's Rep Med 76 (ECHR) at p. 85

death. The question is whether the doctor should or should not continue to provide his patient with medical treatment or care which, if continued, will prolong his patient's life. . . . [T]he question is not whether it is in the best interests of the patient that he should die. The question is whether it is in the best interests of the patient that his life should be prolonged by the continuance of this form of medical treatment or care.[11]

Finally, the law accepted the theologically derived doctrine of double effect in the case of *R v Adams*[12]. Mason et al. (2002) describe this doctrine as follows:

. . . . an action which has a good objective may be performed despite the fact that the objective can only be achieved at the expense of a coincident harmful effect. . . . the action itself must be either good or morally indifferent, the good effect must not be produced by means of the ill-effect and there must be a proportionate reason for allowing the expected ill to occur.[13]

The net effect of these various legal devices is that although the sanctity of life is said to be a primary underpinning of the law, there are some circumstances in which it does not dominate decision-making or directly inform the outcome. Nonetheless, it is *prima facie* the guiding principle in all personal interactions, including those between doctor and patient, and derogations from it will not be made lightly. If it is to perform its protective function, justifications are needed for any derogation. As Lord Lowrie said in the landmark case of *Airedale NHS Trust v Bland*, it is important that "society's notions of what is the law and what is right should coincide"[14]. If the proper management of patients in pVS is on occasion to include hastening their death, then it is manifestly important that there is some consensus on the rationale(s) given to permit this, not least because, as Lord Mustill has said:

. . . . the authority of the State, through the medium of the court, is being invoked to permit one group of its citizens to terminate the life of another.[15]

---

[11][1993] 1 All ER 821, at p. 869
[12][1957] Crim LR 365.
[13]Mason, L. K., McCall Smith, R. A., & Laurie, G. T. (2002). *Law and Medical Ethics*, (6th Edn.), London, Butterworths, p. 558, para 18.77
[14]*supra*, note 7, at p. 123
[15]*supra*, note 7, per Lord Mustill at p. 131

THE CASES

The first, and arguably most significant, case for discussion is that of *Airedale NHS Trust v Bland*[16]. This case involved a young man who had been in what was then described as a persistent vegetative state (PVS) for over 3 years, following a tragic accident at a football ground. His parents and doctors were agreed that nutrition and hydration should be removed, allowing him to die. There was no prospect of recovery, the court was told, and, on the basis of a number of arguments discussed below, permission was sought, and granted, to remove the assisted feeding. This case was followed by the Scottish case of *Law Hospital v Lord Advocate*[17], where a similar conclusion was reached. No reported cases have arisen in Scotland following this judgement, perhaps because there is technically no requirement to seek court authority to discontinue assisted nutrition and hydration, unlike the situation in England and Wales[18]. However, the Lord Advocate did indicate that protection from prosecution could only be guaranteed to doctors were court authority to remove nutrition and hydration obtained[19]. As will be seen later, the precise legal position in Scotland is less than clear; it is uncertain whether such decisions fall to be considered under the common law or the terms of the Adults With Incapacity (Scotland) Act 2000.

In the case of *Re G*[20], it was held to be lawful to remove assisted feeding. In *Frenchay Healthcare NHS Trust v S*[21], it was held lawful not to reinsert a dislodged feeding tube, and in *Swindon and Marlborough NHS Trust v S*[22], it was lawful not to seek to unblock a feeding tube. The criminal law situation also seems to have been clarified in England and Wales by the case of *R v Bingley Magistrates' Court, ex parte Morrow*[23]. In this case, Morrow asked magistrates to issue a summons charging Anthony Bland's doctor with murder. The Magistrates refused, a decision which was upheld on appeal to the Queen's Bench Division, where it was said that ". . . . a declaration by a civil court should normally inhibit a future prosecution"[24].

On what grounds, therefore, have these decisions been made? If it is accepted that they are complex and sensitive, and that they require justification, it is

---

[16][1993] 1 All ER 821

[17]1996 SLT 848; 1996 SLT 869

[18]*Practice Note* [1996] 4 All ER 766

[19]For a brief discussion of the differences between Scottish and English law, see McLean, S. A. M. (2001). Permanent vegetative state and the law. *Journal of Neurology Neurosurgery and Psychiatry* 7(suppl 1): 126–127.

[20][1995] Med.L.Rev. 80

[21]17 BMLR 156 (1994) (CA)

[22][1995] Med.L.Rev. 84

[23][1995] Med.L.Rev. 86

[24][1995] Med.L.R. 86, at p. 87

worth exploring in some detail the grounds on which courts have concluded on the lawfulness of the removal of assisted nutrition and hydration.

CONSENT

It is trite to repeat that it is the consent of the patient that renders interventions lawful (McLean, 1989; Mason et al., 2002). In situations such as pVS, of course, the patient is not in a position to give such a consent. Where treatment is for the benefit of the incompetent patient, it may be given using the doctrine of necessity in England and Wales[25], and in terms of the Adults with Incapacity (Scotland) Act 2000 in Scotland. The question then is whether or not the provision of assisted nutrition and hydration would be for the benefit of (or in the best interests of) the patient. However, before considering this, there is one further issue which was given some prominence in the *Bland* case. Viewed from the opposite perspective it could be argued that it is unlawful to treat a patient who has not consented to it. Thus, it could be argued that invasive treatment of a patient who has not consented to it, where treatment offers no hope of benefit, might in fact amount to an assault. Some of the judges in the *Bland* case directly addressed this and concluded that such treatment could indeed amount to an assault.

Additionally, the adult patient may have left an advance statement of wishes. The RCP recognises the importance of any such statement in its guidelines, stating:

> Where a patient has made a valid and applicable advance directive indicating their refusal of continuing treatment, this must be respected. If not, efforts should be made to establish what the patient's views and preferences might have been, to help to make a decision in his or her best interests.[26]

The critical matter, therefore, is that—where possible—the decision about what a patient him or herself would have wanted to happen (an indication of the likelihood of their having consented to further invasive treatment) should rest on any discoverable wishes expressed by the patient, rather than the choice being presumed by others. The significance of advance statements was recently reiterated in the case of *R (Burke) v General Medical Council*[27],

---

[25]This is likely to be impacted when the draft Mental Capacity Bill becomes law, broadly equating the legal position in England and Wales with that which now exists in Scotland

[26]p. 8, para 3.8

[27][2004] EWHC 1879 (Admin)

where they were described (where "valid and relevant to the treatment in question") as being "in principle determinative"[28].

BEST INTERESTS

It has already been indicated that one way of addressing the problems posed by the patient in pVS is to ask whether or not it is in his/her interests that treatment should be continued. The application of this test is not uncontroversial, however. Lord Mustill, for example, claimed in the *Bland* case that Anthony Bland's condition meant that he had no interests at all; a position with which not everyone would agree, but which would make the application of a "best" interests test impossible. Mason et al. also question Lord Goff's view, referred to *supra*. They ask: what is the difference between saying it is not in the patient's best interests to die and saying that it is not in the patient's best interests to provide the means to allow him/her to live? Taking this question seriously, it can be argued that application of the best interests test to pVS patients seems to imply (however indirectly) that death can be preferable to life. Accepting this (as some may well do) could open the door to a reconsideration of other areas of the law, such as physician assisted death, and this the courts are traditionally reluctant to do, as is the medical profession by and large. To avoid such a potentially uncomfortable conclusion, therefore, the question is re-phrased by the courts. As Lord Goff said:

> In circumstances such as these, it may be difficult to say that it is in his best interests that the treatment should be ended. But, if the question is asked, as in my opinion it should be, whether it is in his best interests that treatment which has the effect of artificially prolonging his life should be continued, that question can sensibly be answered to the effect that it is not in his best interests to do so.[29]

In Scotland, the Adults with Incapacity (Scotland) Act 2000 provides for the means by which treatment can be administered to adults who are incapable of consenting to it. However, the Act specifically did not address the failure to provide treatment, and its relevance in the case of the pVS patient is currently unclear. Much will depend on how the concepts of "benefit" or "futility" within the Act are construed. The Code of Practice for the Act says:

> All interventions under the Act (including some omissions) must comply with the general principles that all interventions must benefit the adult,

---

[28]at para 169
[29]at p. 115

and that any intervention must be the least restrictive option in relation to the freedom of the adult. Clearly, an intervention under Part 5 of the Act which adversely affects the well-being of an adult or causes harm or even death to that adult cannot be described as bringing a benefit to that adult. Section 47 of the Act only allows intervention to "safeguard or promote the physical or mental health of the adult". This does not impose a duty to provide futile treatment or treatment where the burden to the patient outweighs the clinical benefit.[30]

To complicate further the clinician's decision, it is also clear that the notion of "best interests" is not solely (or even primarily) a medical concept, arguably irrespective of prognosis. In cases not involving patients in pVS, this has been made clear by the courts; that is, "best interests" are wider than purely medical "best interests". Indeed, in *Frenchay Healthcare NHS Trust v S*, Sir Thomas Bingham MR said:

> It is, I think, important that there should not be a belief that what the doctor says is the patient's best interest *is* the patient's best interest. For my part I would certainly reserve to the court the ultimate power and duty to review the doctor's decision in the light of all the facts.[31]

MEDICAL TREATMENT?

One further consideration raised in the *Bland* case related to whether or not assisted nutrition and hydration could properly be categorised as medical treatment. If it were basic care, there would virtually never be a lawful basis for withholding or withdrawing assistance; however, if this can be categorised as medical treatment then the decision as to its provision rests with what a "responsible body of medical opinion"[32] would have done in the circumstances. Unsurprisingly, perhaps, there was considerable disquiet at the prospect that "basic" requirements of life should be categorised as "medical". However, in *Airedale NHS Trust v Bland*, Lord Goff seemed unconcerned by the implications of this, stating:

> There is overwhelming evidence that, in the medical profession, artificial feeding is regarded as a form of medical treatment; and, even if it is

---

[30]*Code of Practice for Persons Authorised to Carry Out Medical Treatment or Research under Part 5 of the Act*, SE/2002/73 (April 2002), Scottish Executive, para 2.62

[31]at p. 164

[32]The so-called *Bolam Test*, derived from the case of *Bolam v Friern Hospital Management Committee* [1957] 2 All ER 118

not strictly medical treatment, it must form part of the medical care of the patient.[33]

Answering the question in this way leaves the discretion to the clinical team (assuming that other conditions are met, of course).

HUMAN RIGHTS

It was widely expected that the coming into force of the Human Rights Act 1998, which incorporated the European Convention on Human Rights into UK law, would have a considerable effect on medical judgements; perhaps most acutely decisions at the end of life. For patients in pVS, given that they are legally alive, it might have been thought that Article 2 (the Right to Life) would guarantee them protection from decisions admittedly designed to end their life. Naturally, had this been the case, it would have posed considerable problems for clinical staff and relatives, but it would also have satisfied those who believe that withdrawing nutrition and hydration is indistinguishable from killing.

The legal position in the UK seems, however, to have been settled by the judgement in the case of *NHS Trust A v M, NHS Trust B v H*[34]. In this case, the diagnosis of pVS had been made by four consultants in the case of "M" and five in "H". This diagnosis was made within the terms of the then existing guidelines from the RCP. Prior to the passing of the Human Rights Act, there would almost certainly have been little reason to explore these cases in any depth as they clearly satisfied the criteria accepted in UK courts. However, argument was heard on a number of Articles of the European Convention on Human Rights. As this case seems likely to dominate future jurisprudence in this area, it is worth exploring in some detail.

The first Article of the Convention to be considered was Article 2—the right to life. It is accepted that the State's obligation to preserve the right to life is both a negative and a positive one. Thus, mechanisms should be in place which provide the best possible opportunity for citizens to enjoy their right to life and also to provide life-sustaining treatment positively to preserve life. In her judgment, Dame Elizabeth Butler-Sloss said:

Although the intention in withdrawing artificial nutrition and hydration in PVS cases is to hasten death, in my judgment the phrase "depriva-tion of life" must import a deliberate act, as opposed to an omission, by someone acting on behalf of the State, which results in death. A

---

[33]at p. 117
[34]58 BMLR 87 (2000)

responsible decision by a medical team not to provide treatment at the initial stage could not amount to intentional deprivation of life by the State. Such a decision based on clinical judgement is an omission to act. The death of the patient is the result of the illness or injury from which he suffered, and that cannot be described as a deprivation.[35]

It is not entirely clear from where she derives this opinion—that is, that there must be a deliberate act—but her conclusion reinforced in law the distinction between acts and omissions, which was heavily critiqued by Lord Mustill in the *Bland* case. In that case he said:

> The acute unease which I feel about adopting this way through the legal and ethical maze is I believe due in an important part to the sensation that however much the terminologies may differ, the ethical status of the two courses of action is for all relevant purposes indistinguishable. By dismissing this appeal I fear that your Lordships' House may only emphasise the distortions of a legal structure which is already both morally and intellectually misshapen.[36]

For Dame Elizabeth Butler-Sloss, however, the protection purportedly offered by Article 2 would only be available when the omission arises in a situation where there exists a positive duty to preserve life. Relying on the decision in *Bland* in particular, she could find no such duty in the case of the patient in pVS. Indeed, she considered that where a decision to withdraw assisted nutrition and hydration is made by a responsible body of medical opinion, and is in the patient's best interests, then it cannot be in breach of the right to life.[37]

Arguments were also raised about the possible applicability of Article 3— the right not to be subjected to inhuman and degrading treatment. This is the only Article in the Convention from which no derogation is possible. The argument, therefore, would run that it is inhuman or degrading deliberately to bring about death by starvation or dehydration. In normal circumstances, of course, it is likely that this Article would indeed apply, and failure to offer nutrition and hydration (even with medical assistance) would amount to a breach of that Article. However, Dame Elizabeth Butler-Sloss interpreted the terms of the Article as implying that the inhuman and degrading treatment must be *experienced* by the "victim". Thus, in as much as she felt Article 3 was engaged by this case, she said:

---

[35]at p. 95
[36]at p. 132
[37]at p. 97

An insensate patient suffering from permanent vegetative state has no feelings and no comprehension of the treatment accorded to him or her. Article 3 does not, in my judgment, apply to these two cases.[38]

Accordingly, her conclusion was that it was not in the best interests of the two patients concerned that they should continue to receive assisted nutrition and hydration. The expected impact of the Human Rights Act was, therefore, simply to reinforce existing law. This interpretation has, however, subsequently been subject to challenge. In the case of *R (Burke) v General Medical Council*[39], Mr Justice Munby said:

. . . . however unconscious or unaware of ill-treatment a particular incompetent. . . . may be, treatment which has the effect on those who witness it of degrading the individual may come within Article 3. Otherwise. . . . the Convention's emphasis on the protection of the vulnerable may be circumvented.[40]

As this case may well be subject to appeal, this statement of the law cannot yet be taken as ultimately authoritative, but arguably it does appear to reflect the goals of the Convention rather more closely than did Dame Elizabeth's judgment, and—if upheld—could have an impact on the management of the patient in pVS. However, Mr Justice Munby was at pains to distance himself from any suggestion that withdrawing life-prolonging treatment "which satisfies the exacting requirements of the common law. . . . and in a manner which is in all other respects compatible with the patient's rights under Article 3 and Article 8 [the right to private and family life]"[41] would breach the right to life. For Mr Justice Munby, Article 3 "embraces. . . . the right to die with dignity and the right to be protected from treatment, or from a lack of treatment, which will result in one dying in unavoidably distressing circumstances"[42]. Given that it remains moot whether or not removing nutrition and hydration would amount to a breach of Article 3, it is not yet clear just what impact this case will have on the management of patients in pVS.

SLIPPERY SLOPE?

Burke apart, the conclusion that can be drawn from the above is that the decision about whether or not to remove assisted nutrition and hydration lies

---

[38]at p. 100
[39][2004] EWHC 1879 (Admin)
[40]at para 145
[41]at para 162
[42]at para 166

firmly within the medical profession itself. Although courts will evaluate these decisions, they do so relatively uncritically. In fact, as often as not, the role of the courts is to rubber stamp a responsible medical decision. This may be a matter of little concern, so long as it is generally accepted that there are no benefits for individuals in pVS in being kept alive, and of course that the diagnosis is sound and reliable. Interestingly, however, the strict adherence to the RCP guidelines, which is theoretically demanded by the judges, has not always been required in practice.

In the case of *Re G (adult incompetent: withdrawal of treatment)*[43] the patient was a woman who had suffered severe brain damage and it was considered that there was no prospect of recovery. Although not technically satisfying the RCP guidelines, Dame Elizabeth Butler-Sloss was content to allow her to "die with dignity and in peace by the withdrawal of the artificial nutrition and hydration"[44]. In *Re D*[45], again the patient did not fully satisfy the criteria for pVS laid down by the Royal College of Physicians. However, it was held that she was for all practical purposes in pVS and therefore that it was not in her best interests to continue feeding. Describing her condition as a "living death"[46], Sir Stephen Brown P held that it was not in her interest to be kept alive, and that the time for "merciful relief has arrived"[47]. In *Re H (adult: incompetent)*[48], although again the criteria were not fully met, doctors agreed that the patient was in pVS and a similar decision was reached.

Although this apparent relaxation of the rules may be welcomed by those responsible for patient care, and indeed by grieving relatives, such decisions do begin to call into question the role of the law in these situations. It is arguable that the position in England, which requires courts to agree to the withdrawal of treatment, is more in line with the requirements of Article 6 of the Convention on Human Rights—that is, the right to a fair hearing—than is the position in Scotland, which does not strictly require court endorsement of the clinical decision. It can be argued that a fair hearing (following argument for and against the decision) is never more important than when the outcome is certain death. However, the apparent safeguards of the English position are arguably considerably weakened by the courts' reluctance to gainsay clinical decisions.

---

[43] 65 BMLR 6 (2001)
[44] at p. 8
[45] 38 BMLR 1 (1997)
[46] at p. 10
[47] *id*
[48] 38 BMLR 11 (1997) (Fam Div)

CONCLUSION

This brief discussion of the legal position of the patient in pVS has raised a number of issues, some of which bear directly on other end of life debates. For example, if it can reasonably be said that it is not in an individual's interests to be kept alive (based on the lack of quality of his or her life), on what grounds (as Lord Mustill and Lord Browne-Wilkinson asked in the *Bland* case) can it ever be right not to permit a competent adult to make such a decision for themselves, and be assisted in dying? The answer that will be given is, of course, that there is a difference between actively killing and passively allowing to die; that is there is a distinction between an act and an omission. In some cases, this will indeed be the case. However, strict law dictates that where there is a pre-existing duty of care, then an omission is as culpable as an act. Thus, courts have had to use other devices (such as best interests) to claim that where a patient is in pVS there is no duty to treat, thus legally neutralising the omission to do so. However, it could equally be argued that it is not in the interests of other groups of individuals to *be* treated, and therefore that willing doctors should be allowed to assist in their death.

This is obviously not the place for a debate on euthanasia or assisted suicide, and the courts have been very clear that what they are doing in pVS cases is not equivalent to endorsing either of these. However, even if one can accept that omitting to save a patient in full pVS is not euthanasia by any other name, the rather more controversial cases described briefly above must render one less than confident of the distinction between the two situations, not least because it appears that the terms of the RCP's guidelines are not met in some cases where decisions which result in death are taken.

In the *Bland* case, Lord Goff proposed that the best way to develop an ethically sound legal framework was to ensure "mutual understanding between the doctors and the judges"[49]. This seems in large part to have been achieved. However, in that same case, Lord Browne-Wilkinson reminded us that ". . . . behind the questions of law lie moral, ethical, medical and practical issues of fundamental importance to society"[50]. This brief evaluation of the law's response to patients in pVS exposes some of these issues, and highlights the devices used by courts to permit their death. Whether or not these are morally or ethically adequate to justify derogation from the sanctity of life principle is debatable.

---

[49]at p. 118
[50]at p. 124

REFERENCES

Mason, J. K., McCall Smith, R. A., & Laurie, G. T. (Eds.) (2002). *Law and medical ethics* (6th ed.), London: Butterworths.

McLean, S. A. M. (1989). *A patient's right to know: Information disclosure, the doctor and the law*. Aldershot, UK: Dartmouth.

Royal College of Physicians (2003). *The vegetative state: Guidance on diagnosis and management. Report of a Working Party of the Royal College of Physicians*. London: RCP.

NEUROPSYCHOLOGICAL REHABILITATION
2005, 15 (3/4), 251–256

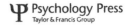
Ψ Psychology Press
Taylor & Francis Group

Forensic assessment issues in low level neurological states

Nathan D. Zasler

*CEO & Medical Director, Concussion Care Centre of Virginia, Ltd., CEO &
Medical Director, Tree of Life Services, Inc., Glen Allen, VA; Clinical Associate
Professor, Department of Physical Medicine and Rehabilitation, Virginia
Commonwealth University, Richmond, VA, USA*

Forensic assessment of persons in low-level neurological state (LLNS) is fraught
with limitations and caveats. Examiners must be aware of the nuances of forensic evaluation in the context of the conditions of examination, ethics and responsibilities that they have been charged with as an independent evaluator and
fact seeker in the context of litigation-oriented dispute resolution. This article
provides an overview of the independent medical evaluation (IME) of persons
in LLNS including ethics, contextual limitations, history gathering, corroboratory interviews and suggested examination, as well as report format, among
other important issues.

INTRODUCTION

The independent medical evaluation (IME) is a tool of dispute resolution
utilised when the disagreement between two or more parties contains one or
more key issues of a medical nature. The dispute may be narrow and specific
involving questions of causation, diagnosis, prognosis or treatment recommendations, or it may be wide ranging, involving long-range care costs or
claims of fraud and/or functional/psychiatric presentations. The role of the
IME is to review and analyse and, in some instances, update and expand the
existing evidence in order to provide guidance to the parties as to the strength
of the medical opinions of the case. The IME report, as well as the IME

Correspondence should be addressed to: Nathan Zasler, MD, Concussion Care Centre of
Virginia, 10120 West Broad Street, Suite G, Glen Allen, VA, 23060, USA. Tel: 804-346-1803,
Fax: 804-346-1956, Email: nzasler@cccv-ltd.com

---

http://www.tandf.co.uk/journals/pp/09602011.html   DOI:10.1080/09602010443000380

clinician, rates the information along a continuum from unfounded speculation through to certainty for medical knowledge in general, and for the clinical findings of a particular case. The IME report should be clear, concise and comprehensive with the understanding that either party should be able to find common ground for settlement or that the triers of fact will be assisted in making an informed determination (Ameis, Zasler, Martelli, & Bush, in press; Ameis & Zasler, 2002).

Caveats for the IME

An IME can only fulfil a contributory role if the analysis of evidence and references to facts are logical, impartial and appropriate. The examiner must fully understand and completely address all suitable questions asked without regard to the implications of any opinions, to either party, in order to assist meaningfully in dispute resolution. Clearly, in this context, there is no role for advocacy except for the truth. That is, the examining clinician should not be an advocate, either for the examinee and/or the party hiring the expert to provide medicolegal opinions (Martelli, Zasler, & Grayson, 2000). It is important to clarify the relationship of the physician to the examinee/claimant, as well as to the other parties involved in the case to negate the potential effects of conflict of interest. Unless required by legislation or pre-arranged, the examiner generally has no obligation to discuss the report with the claimant and/or any other party, other than the requesting party, given the generalised perception that there is no physician:patient relationship between an examiner and examinee and/or any other party associated with the examinee (Martelli, Zasler, & Johnson-Green, 2001).

There are various caveats that have been espoused in the independent medical literature regarding a myriad of issues including, but not necessarily limited to: conduct of the claimant and others involved in the IME process; scope and inquiry of service within the context of an IME; quality assurance issues as related to conducting IMEs including issues of impartiality and ethics of conduct; record keeping suggestions; third party observers during the evaluation and methodologies for report documentation and preparation (Zasler & Martelli, 2002).

ASSESSMENT OF LOW LEVEL NEUROLOGICAL STATES

General comments

Perhaps one of the most challenging areas of independent medical evaluations facing clinicians involved in neurological care and/or rehabilitation is the assessment of patients in LLNS. Such evaluations are challenging on numerous levels due to the complexity of the evaluation process and development of opinions, as related to this small sub-section of persons with acquired brain injury. Within the context of any discussion regarding medicolegal and forensic assessment of patients in low-level neurological states, it must be understood that, in general, examiners are only provided an opportunity for a "one-time" evaluation without access to the preferred paradigm of serial assessments. Based on current opinion within the field of neurological rehabilitation, it would certainly be preferable to advocate for, as well as allow, serial assessments, even in the context of medicolegal evaluations to provide greater levels of assurance regarding the degree of medical probability with which expert opinions are being provided (Zasler & Cantor, 2004).

Historical issues: Pre-injury, injury, and post-injury data

In the context of performing such evaluations, it is of utmost importance to obtain as complete information as possible regarding the pre-injury status of the claimant, including all pertinent information regarding past medical history, as well as psychosocial history, in conjunction with understanding the claimant's family history, the latter as it relates to genetic loading risk factors or heritable diseases, in addition to general trends of median survival time within the claimant's immediate family. Just as importantly, examining clinicians should understand details regarding the injury itself, whether traumatic or non-traumatic or some combination of both. Details regarding the initial presenting severity of the injury and/or secondary brain injury-related complications are paramount in making determinations regarding prognoses, particularly prior to "permanency" being established. Post-injury neurological recovery course and medical history certainly are pertinent in the interpretation of an individual's current status, morbidity risk factors, future needs, and general prognosis including median survival time (Zasler, 1999).

Importance of corroboratory sources

Ideally, examiners should be given opportunities to obtain information from corroboratory sources in the context of "plaintiff", as well as "defence" independent medical evaluations. This is typically not permitted, at least in the legal system used in the USA; however, this sets a precedent that may ultimately limit the scope and quality of the assessment being performed. Additionally, and in the ideal scenario, examiners should request opportunities to observe the examinee "interacting" with familiar individuals including family members, and direct care staff, among others. Again, all too often, this opportunity is prohibited by the "powers that be", within the context of both personal injury litigation and workers compensation-related litigation in the USA (Ameis & Zasler, 2002).

Basic rules of assessment to optimise examinee performance

Thorough assessment is vital for determination of an accurate neurological diagnosis. One needs to ascertain that the patient is in good general health and that there are no issues with intercurrent infection that may mask the individual's true neurological status. Attempts should be made to assure that no sedating medications or abnormal metabolic states are negatively impacting on arousal level. The examinee should be assessed in bed for determination of full integumentary status and limb range of motion, among other important physical examination points. Additionally, and as feasible, it is preferable to also examine the person in a supported seating position to optimise arousal. Efforts should be made, particularly when, in the context of most forensic assessments, there may only be one examination, to do the assessment at a time of day when the person is normally most arousable (Giacino et al., 1997). Over-stimulation and/or an environment with distractions should be avoided to optimise examinee attentional capabilities (Giacino et al., 2002; Zasler & Cantor, 2004).

Physical examination issues

As related to the physical examination of the low level neurological claimant, it is important to conduct a thorough general examination, and one not just germane to the neurological level of function of the individual in question. Specifically, appropriate evaluation of the examinee's general status including vital signs and multisystem assessment is paramount to providing a comprehensive understanding of the individual risk factors and/or complications associated with their low-level neurological state. Probably, two of the most important systems are the integument and musculoskeletal systems particularly as related to the potential negative repercussions of relative immobility.

Neurological examination should include cranial nerve assessment 1–12, deep tendon reflexes including pathological reflexes, sensory examination (including visual fields and auditory and nociceptive/tactile responsiveness), cerebellar assessment, and motor function testing, among other areas assessed. The mental status assessment of an individual in a low level neurological state relies on an in-depth, bedside, neurobehavioural assessment with a focus on evidence of responses consistent with awareness versus lack thereof, best accomplished by fastidious attention to nuances of neurobehavioural assessment, as well as use of validated assessment tools such as the Coma Recovery Scale—Revised (Zasler, 1996; Zasler & Cantor, 2004).

IME report formats and content

Within the context of providing opinions germane to the medicolegal evaluation of a person in LLNS, it is paramount to provide an in-depth delineation of all materials reviewed in the context of formulation of any and all medicole-gal opinions. Ideally, a narrative summarising the pertinent pre-injury, injury and post-injury-related history can assist in providing a foundation for the opinions being expressed in the context of the IME.

Adequate levels of sophistication are requisites for the examiner involved in the medicolegal assessment of this patient population, given the issues involved in the interpretation of examination findings in these patients; in par-ticular, as it relates to assessing cortically from subcortically mediated responses and delineating responses that are, more likely than not, consistent with con-scious behaviour. All examination findings should be thoroughly documented, both pertinent negatives and positives. Clinicians should maintain "raw notes" as verification of their findings.

Examiners should provide opinions within the context of an IME regard-ing the myriad of issues including, at a minimum, commentary regarding: (1) whether or not the claimant has reached maximal medical improvement (MMI); (2) opinions regarding apportionment and causality; (3) delineation of restrictions and risks as a consequence of the injury in question; (4) opin-ions regarding median survival time and/or life expectancy; (5) opinions regarding pain and suffering; (6) vocational and general prognoses; (7) current and future care needs; (8) general diagnostic impressions; (9) opinions regard-ing general treatment recommendations including, but not necessarily limited to, need for surgical interventions; (10) recommendations regarding discon-tinuation of drugs that may be negatively impacting on functional status; (11) opinions regarding pharmacotherapy to enhance function, as deemed clini-cally appropriate; (12) general rehabilitative treatment recommendations, among others (Ameis & Zasler, 2002; Giacino & Zasler, 1995).

CONCLUSIONS

Clearly, the knowledge base required to conduct independent medical exami-nations of individuals in low level neurological states is a "niche area" within the global field of neurological care and rehabilitation regardless of one's spe-cific medical specialty. The appropriate use of the extant scientific literature when assessing this special group of patients integrated with both clinical and medicolegal experience produces the ideal scenario for provision of thorough IMEs that are evidence based, ethical and even-handed.

REFERENCES

Ameis, A., & Zasler, N. D. (2002). The independent medical examination. *Physical Medicine and Rehabilitation Clinics of North America, 13,* 259–286.

Ameis, A., Zasler, N. D., Martelli, M. F., & Bush, S. (in press). Ethical issues in clinicolegal practice. In N. Zasler, D. Katz, & R. Zafonte (Eds.), *Brain injury medicine: Principles and practice.* New York: Demos Medical Publishers.

Giacino, J. T., Ashwal, S., Childs, N., Cranford, R., Jennett, B., Katz, D. I., Kelly, J. P., Rosenberg, J. H., White, J., Zafonte, R. D., Zasler, N. D. (2002). The minimally conscious state: Definition and diagnostic criteria. *Neurology, 58,* 349–353.

Giacino, J. T., & Zasler, N. D. (1995). Outcome after severe traumatic brain injury: Coma, vegetative state, and the minimally responsive state. *Journal of Head Trauma Rehabilitation, 10*(1), 40–56.

Giacino, J. T., Zasler, N. D., Katz, D. I., Kelly, J. P., Rosenberg, J. H., & Filley, C. M. (1997). Development of practice guidelines for assessment and management of the vegetative and minimally conscious state. *Journal of Head Trauma Rehabilitation, 12*(4), 79–89.

Martelli, M. F., Zasler, N. D., & Grayson, R. (2000). Ethical considerations in medicolegal evaluation of neurologic injury and impairments following acquired brain injury. In M. Shiffman (Ed.), *Attorney's guide to ethics in forensic science and medicine.* Springfield, IL: Charles C. Thomas.

Martelli, M. F., Zasler, N. D., & Johnson-Green, E. D. (2001). Promoting ethical and objective practice in the medicolegal arena of disability evaluation. *Physical Medicine and Rehabilitation Clinics of North America, 12*(3), 571–586.

Zasler, N. D. (1996). Vegetative state: Challenges, controversies and caveats. A physiatric perspective. In H. Stonnington & B. Uzzell (Eds.), *Recovery after traumatic brain injury.* (pp. 185–195). Proceedings from the 4th Conference, International Association for the Study of Traumatic Brain Injury, St. Louis, MO. Lawrence Erlbaum Associates.

Zasler, N. D. (1999). Physiatric assessment in traumatic brain injury. In M. Rosenthal, E. R. Griffith, J. S. Kreutzer, B. Pentaland (Eds.), *Rehabilitation of the adult and child with traumatic brain injury* (3rd ed., pp. 117–130). Philadelphia, PA: S.A. Davis.

Zasler, N. D., & Cantor, I. (2004). Medicolegal aspects of severe traumatic brain injury. *Journal of the Virginia Trial Lawyers Association. February,* 26–39.

Zasler, N. D., & Martelli, M. F. (2002). Ethics in medicolegal evaluation of neurologic disability. *Journal of Controversial Medical Claim, 9*(3), 13–19.

NEUROPSYCHOLOGICAL REHABILITATION
2005, 15 (3/4), 257–263

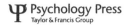

Ethics and the vegetative state

Chris Borthwick

Brunswick, Australia

Before discussing ethical issues to do with patients in permanent (or persistent) vegetative state (PVS) it is necessary to address the foundational issue of whether PVS as a concept is able to provide a robust link to situations in the real world. The high reported rates of misdiagnosis and recovery in patients diagnosed as being in PVS casts doubt upon the applicability of ethicists' thought experiments on Platonic forms to actual decision making in clinical situations. We should abandon the illusion that we can have access to logical certainty through diagnostic definition, and should instead frame our opinions and our procedures in ways that can accommodate a high element of uncertainty, and should in the light of recent studies give considerable weight to the possibility that patients, at present unable to express opinions on their care, will later become able to do so, if given proper treatment and adequate evaluation.

Ronald Dworkin, like virtually all ethicists, defines "a persistent vegetative state . . . [as one where the patients] are unconscious. . . . and the higher centers of their brains have been permanently damaged in a way that rules out any return to consciousness. They are capable of no sensation and no thought" (Dworkin, 1995).

Ethicists such as Dworkin have written largely on issues associated with the vegetative state (VS) , almost always in the form of the persistent (or permanent) vegetative state (PVS), understood in Dworkin's formulation[1].

---

[1]The nomenclature in this area is confused. Most neurologists now adopt the usage of the Royal College of Physicians (RCP) (1996) and refer only to the "vegetative state", the "continuing vegetative state", and the "permanent vegetative state". Nonetheless, almost everybody else—the press, the law, much medical literature, Hollywood, many clinicians, and the public in general—continue to use the older term "persistent vegetative state" as if it meant "permanent vegetative state". The term "post-coma unawareness", suggested by the Australian National Health and Medical Research Council (2003), would be an improvement (although in the light of Andrews' et al. (1996) findings a more accurate term might simply be "locked-in syndrome").

Correspondence should be addressed to: Chris Borthwick 74 Rose St, Brunswick, Vic 3056, Australia. Tel: (61-3) 93206824, Fax: (61-3) 9386 0761, Email: chrisb@vicnet.net.au

© 2005 Psychology Press Ltd
http://www.tandf.co.uk/journals/pp/0960201 1.html   DOI:10.1080/09602010443000308

These issues include:

1. Is a person in PVS a "person" (in a number of senses) (Gormally, 1993)?

2. Can a person in PVS have interests, or "best interests" (McLean, 2001)?

3. Should scarce medical resources be allocated to people in PVS?

4. Are nutrition and hydration for a person in PVS medical operations?

5. Is there a difference between killing a person in PVS and letting him or her die (Randall, 1997)?

6. Should people in PVS be considered to be "dead" (in a number of senses)?

These are all issues in which I have neither expertise nor interest, and I refer those who wish to survey the discussion in this area to the abundant literature reviewed in Jennet (2002).

My intention in this paper is to examine the conditions that would be necessary for those discussions to be meaningful, and to examine the evidence for the proposition that such conditions exist.

PHILOSOPHICAL INQUIRIES

Philosophers have gone to some trouble to distinguish between false statements and meaningless statements. Bertrand Russell, for example, argued that the statement "The present King of France is bald" is on the face of it not false, despite the fact that France has no king, because if the statement was false then its negation, "The present King of France has hair", would be true (Russell, 1905). Russell resolved this paradox by saying that in stating, "The present King of France is bald", we are making several separate but linked assertions—that an x exists such that x is the King of France, and that x is bald—and that the first of these, and therefore the statement as a whole, is false.

If you want a good head of hair, it is necessary to exist. However, cognitive philosophy also boasts an entire bestiary of creatures who are universally agreed not to exist but who are nonetheless employed as thought experiments to draw out the implications of different philosophical positions. The Martian lacks humanity, but has consciousness and observable behaviour; the Zombie has humanity and behaviour, but lacks consciousness (Midgely, 2004); the Robot has neither humanity nor consciousness, but has behaviour (Kirk, 1986). If we make these up into a table (Table 1), we find that there are vacant spaces for people who have humanity but neither consciousness nor

TABLE 1
Philosophical constructs

	Ordinary human	Martian	Robot	Zombie	Human in PVS	Human in LIS
Humanity	*			*	*	*
Consciousness	*	*				*
Behaviour	*	*	*	*		

behaviour, and people who have humanity and consciousness but no behaviour; and these gaps have been filled by recruiting people in PVS and locked-in syndrome (LIS).

Philosophical actors, being embodiments of defined states of being, do not pretend to be based on real-world experience, although their hypothesised behaviour may still cast light on actual phcnomcna.

ETHICAL FOUNDATIONS

Ethics, too, has its cast of didactic characters, each employed to demonstrate the implications of particular combinations of qualities. If we respect the rights of people with profound mental retardation, we should respect the rights of nonhuman primates who have demonstrated speech-related capacity (Ansotz, 1993). If we are prepared to abort a foetus a day before birth, then we should be prepared to kill a [handicapped] baby a day after birth (Kuhse & Singer, 1985). If we are forced to choose between either saving the life of a chimpanzee who wants to go on living and a human with profound brain damage who is not capable of having desires for the future because its mental capacities do not allow it to grasp that it is a mental entity existing over time, then it is entirely justifiable to choose to save the chimpanzcc (Singer, 1997).

Cells in the ethical table (Table 2) are filled roughly as follows (the assignation of subjects in each case relying on varying assumptions as to clinical observations and particular definitions of such open-ended words as "consciousness").

In the field of ethics, however, practitioners seek to make their constructs do double duty. They must both fit neatly into structures of argument and be able to be reached down from the shelf for application in actual situations. This makes it necessary to address the issue of whether the person in PVS— "a human with profound brain damage who is not capable of having desires for the future"—has existence, or whether he or she is, like the present king of France, a merely hypothetical entity.

TABLE 2
Ethical constructs

	Adult human	Ape (Koko)	Retarded adult	Human baby	Human baby (Anencephalic)	PVS	Foetus
Humanity	*		*	*	*	*	*
Consciousness	*	*	*	*			
Behaviour	*	*	*	*			
Potential	*		*			*	
Language	*	*					

It is here that the classification "vegetative state", and its extensions "permanent vegetative state" and "persistent vegetative state", become so useful. They provide ethicists with the ability to export definitional truths from the world of logic to the world of clinical reality. "By definition, patients in a persistent vegetative state are unaware of themselves or their environment. They are noncognitive, nonsentient, and incapable of conscious experience" (Multi-Society Task Force, 1994). By definition, people in a vegetative state "do not 'feel' pain in the sense of conscious discomfort of the kind that doctors would be obliged to treat" (Mitchell, Kerridge, & Lovat, 1993).

By definition, too, permanent vegetative state (or, more often, "persistent vegetative state") is permanent; a 1996 British Medical Association paper on treatment decisions for patients in persistent vegetative state, for example, said that "an enduring cause for concern . . . have [sic] been the intermittent reports of alleged 'recovery' from PVS. In the BMA's view, recoveries, where they can be verified, indicate an original misdiagnosis"(British Medical Association, 1996).

This alibi is important, because whether or not people with permanent vegetative state recover, people diagnosed as being in persistent vegetative state certainly do recover.

Historically, Jennet and Plum wanted "to identify an irrecoverable state"—irrecoverable and thus permanent. They named the syndrome "persistent vegetative state" because they did not have the data to make "permanent vegetative state" stick—as they put it, "the criteria needed to establish that prediction [of irrecoverability] reliably have still to be confirmed. Until then 'persistent' is safer than *'permanent'* or *'irreversible'* . . ." (Jennett & Plum, 1972, p. 734). The criteria that could successfully identify irreversibility, and the data that should support them, have not been developed in the 30 years since; indeed, more recent studies have cast ever-increasing doubt on the certainty of the clinician, culminating in Andrews, Murphy, Munday, and Littlewood's (1996) study in which 75% of the patients presenting with diagnoses of persistent vegetative state proved in the event to be either misdiagnosed or capable of some recovery[2]. That is to say, it is at least possible that (at most) one person in four diagnosed as having permanent (or persistent) vegetative state is permanently vegetative.

I have hypothesised elsewhere (Borthwick, in press) that clinicians have in general preferred to ignore the increasingly suspect nature of the prognosis inherent in the diagnosis of permanent (or persistent) vegetative state because they have been concerned less with issues of consciousness than with opinions about resource use (according to Jennett, 1976, physicians who care for such patients "sound . . . a death knell for those who are denied the benefits of appropriate care by [this] spendthrift attitude") and because they tend to believe severe disability to be as bad as or worse than death (Cranford, 1996, for example, commented on Andrews' results that ". . . all 17 patients who were found to be conscious were severely disabled; . . . I would speculate that most people would find this condition far more horrifying than the vegetative state itself, and some might think it an even stronger reason for stopping treatment. . . ."). The medical profession has thus been prepared to relax its standards, both in accepting a degree of error as to outcome—"Insistence on certainty beyond a reasonable point can handicap the physician dealing with treatment options in apparently hopeless cases. . . ." (Giacino et al., 2002)—and in recommending termination for a wider range of cases—"As medical knowledge about the diagnosis and prognosis of the minimally conscious state increases. . . . it may be in the best interests of some such patients to have life-sustaining treatment withdrawn (Jennett, 2002).

Both the argument from resources and the argument from disability deserve attention, but they are not arguments that relate particularly to the characteristics of the permanent (or persistent) vegetative state—permanence, lack of sensation, and absence of thought—as employed by, say, Dworkin. Unless those qualities can be regained, we are, when addressing the issues originally listed, in what might be called a King of France situation.

One argument that has been employed is that ". . . when properly diagnosed, such a condition is irreversible . . ." (Shannon & Walter, 2004)—that is, while we are in practice subject to human error, this does not affect the qualities of the Platonic ideal of the PVS patient that is the object of ethical discourse. This argument serves only to paper over the fundamental difficulty of transferring ethical prescriptions into the world of phenomena. To be told that we must treat people in properly diagnosed PVS differently from people who have been misdiagnosed as PVS is hardly helpful unless we have a way of telling them apart, while to treat them the same way rather smacks of the

---

[2]"Of the 40 patients diagnosed as being in the vegetative state, 10 (25%) remained vegetative, 13 (33%) slowly emerged from the vegetative state during the rehabilitation programme, and 17 (43%) were considered to have been misdiagnosed as vegetative."

crusader's way of distinguishing the faithful from heretics, "Kill them all. God will recognise his own".

The discussion of ethics as applied to disabilities of this nature cannot progress until we discard once and for all the notion that there is a name that, when invoked, can make our decisions simple and straightforward. These matters are not susceptible to hard-and-fast rules. It would be much easier if they were; and that is why people try to pretend that they are, or at least behave as if they thought so. Of course, you can have hard-and-fast rules if you want to, but then they will be false rules, and they will lead you wrong; because their simplicity will render them inapplicable to problems that are not simple.

The discipline of ethics should abandon the illusion that it can have access to logical certainty through diagnostic definition. Rather than relying upon abstracted but determinative ethical pronouncements we should instead frame our opinions and our procedures in ways that can accommodate a high element of uncertainty. We should in the light of Andrews et al.'s (1996) study give considerable weight to the possibility that patients at present unable to express opinions on their care will become able to do so later if given proper treatment and adequate evaluation.

REFERENCES

Andrews, K., Murphy, L., Munday, R., Littlewood, C. (1996). Misdiagnosis of the vegetative state: Retrospective study in a rehabilitation unit. *British Medical Journal, 313*, 13–16.

Ansotz, C. (1993). Profoundly intellectually disabled humans and the great apes: A comparison. In P. Cavalieri & P. Singer (Eds.), *The great ape project.* New York: St. Martins Griffin.

Borthwick, C. (in press). Permanent vegetative state: Usefulness and limits of a prognostic definition, *Neurorehabilitation.*

British Medical Association (1996). *Withholding and withdrawing life-prolonging medical treatment.* London: BMA.

Cranford, R. (1996). Misdiagnosing the persistent vegetative state. *British Medical Journal, 313*, 5–6.

Dworkin, R. (1993). *Life's dominion: An argument about abortion* (p. 187). London: Harper Collins.

Giacino, J., Ashwal, S., Childs, N., Cranford, R., & Jennett, B. (2002). The minimally conscious state: Definition and diagnostic criteria. *Neurology, 58*, 349–353.

Gormally, L. (1993). Definitions of personhood: Implications for the care of PVS patients. *Catholic Medical Quarterly, 44*(4), 7–12.

Jennett, B. (1976). Resource allocation for the severely brain damaged. *Archives of Neurology 33*, 595–597.

Jennett, B. (2002). *The vegetative state: Medical facts, ethical and legal dilemmas* (p. 144). New York: CUP.

Jennett, B., & Plum, F. (1972). Persistent vegetative state after brain damage: A syndrome in search of a name. *Lancet, 1*, 734–737.

Kirk, R. (1986). Sentience, causation and some robots. *Australasian Journal of Philosophy, 64*, 308–321.

Kuhse, H., & Singer, P. (1985). *Should the baby live?* New York: Oxford University Press.

McLean, S. (2001). Permanent vegetative state and the law. *Journal of Neurology, Neurosurgery and Psychiatry*, *71*(Suppl 1), i26–i27.

Midgley, M. (2004). Zombies can't concentrate. *Philosophy Now*, *44*, 24–25.

Mitchell, K., Kerridge, I., & Lovat, T. (1993). Medical futility, treatment withdrawal, and the persistent vegetative state. *Journal of Medical Ethics*, *19*, 71–76.

Multi-Society Task Force on PVS (1994). Medical aspects of the persistent vegetative state: Second of two parts. *New England Journal of Medicine*, *330*(22), 1572–1579.

National Health and Medical Research Council (2003). *Post-coma unresponsiveness (Vegetative State): A clinical framework for diagnosis*. Canberra: NHMRC. [http://www.health.gov.au/nhmrc/publications/synopses/hpr23syn.htm].

Randall, F. (1997). Why causing death is not necessarily equivalent to allowing to die. *Journal of Medical Ethics*, *23*, 373–376.

Royal College of Physicians. (1996). *Guidance on diagnosis and management* [Report of a working party]. London: RCP.

Russell, B. (1905). On denoting. *Mind*, *14*, 479–493.

Shannon, T., & Walter, J. (2004). Artificial nutrition and hydration: Assessing the papal statement. *National Catholic Reporter, April 16*.

Singer, P. (1997). Ethics and the limits of scientific freedom. *Monash Bioethics Review*, *16*, 2(April).

NEUROPSYCHOLOGICAL REHABILITATION
2005, 15 (3/4), 264–271

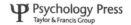

The vegetative state: Promoting greater clarity and improved treatment

Cindy Province

St Louis Center for Bioethics and Culture, Ellisville, MO, USA

The condition commonly referred to as the persistent vegetative state (PVS) or vegetative state (VS) generates tremendous confusion among health care professionals. Muddled and nihilistic views of very severe brain injury have hampered efforts to improve the diagnosis and treatment of patients thought to be in the VS. Significant obstacles to diagnostic clarity arise from multiple sources including imprecise terminology and conflation of the concepts of "behaviour" and "awareness". Failure to employ effective, uniform protocols of assessment and rehabilitation contributes to inadequate treatment of these extremely vulnerable patients. Despite diagnostic and prognostic difficulties, courts across the globe have accepted medical opinion as persuasive evidence for life-support withdrawal. A new outlook on severe brain injury is needed, with greater clarity and standardisation of assessment and care. Best practices in assessment and rehabilitation must be incorporated along with new developments in cognitive neuroscience and neuroimaging. Such a rehabilitative view will encourage intellectual curiosity towards improved quality of care for patients with severe brain injury. Attaining high levels of accuracy depends upon reaching a clearer understanding of the nature of human consciousness itself, of the condition, and of the patient's potential for full or partial recovery.

BACKGROUND

Brain injury resulting in severe impairment of consciousness presents profound medical, legal, and ethical issues. Identified in 1972, the persistent

---

Correspondence should be sent to Cindy Province, Associate Director, St. Louis Center for Bioethics and Culture, 15820 Clayton Road, Ellisville, MO, USA. Tel: (636) 798-2168. Email: cindy.province@thecbc.org

---

http://www.tandf.co.uk/journals/pp/09602011.html   DOI:10.1080/09602010443000623

vegetative state (PVS; Jennett & Plum, 1972) is emblematic of the difficulties posed by severe brain injury. Thirty years later, the minimally conscious state (MCS; Giacino et al., 2002) now presents medical professionals, the legal profession, families and society with similar problems. While much of the PVS and MCS literature has focused on undesirable aspects of life in the PVS or with severe disabilities—and in particular on proposed end-points for therapy—less attention has been directed towards the exploration of strategies for recognising and treating patients in PVS and MCS who may have the potential for recovery or significant improvement.

Since at least the mid-1990s, there has been increasing recognition that many patients with very severe brain injuries have not received optimal assessment and rehabilitative care. This recognition has been brought to the forefront by several studies that identified a disturbingly high rate of misdiagnosis among patients thought to be in the vegetative state (Andrews, Murphy, Munday, & Littlewood, 1996; Childs, Mercer, & Childs, 1993). Central to the issue of frequent misdiagnosis is the concern that specialised rehabilitative care with the intent to unmask signs of awareness and recovery potential is often not provided. Although information regarding frequent misdiagnosis and suboptimal care has been available for years, this information has been slow to percolate into general medical knowledge and the daily management of these patients, and slower still to penetrate the field of law and the overarching realm of ethics.

Although engulfed in such significant uncertainty, the VS has been the focus of several landmark legal cases that have set a precedent for patients living with such diagnoses (*Airedale NHS Trust v. Bland*, 1993; *Cruzan v. Director, Missouri Department of Health* 1990; *In the matter of Quinlan, an alleged incompetent* 1976). Withdrawal of both medical treatment and ordinary care from the patients in these cases has served as a historical galvanising point and legal "backdrop" for the right-to-die movement within the US and other countries (Cantor, 2001). Bijlani (2000) noted that, in general, courts have been willing to accept medical opinion as persuasive expert testimony when considering the withdrawal of nutrition and hydration. However, due in part to institutional medical confusion, denial, or underplaying of diagnostic and prognostic uncertainty, courts have appeared to prefer—even in the face of potential error—firm declarations of irrecoverability over less definite, but undoubtedly more honest, admissions of uncertainty. Cases such as the highly publicised Terry Schiavo case in the US, which involves a debate over alleged misdiagnosis and lack of appropriate rehabilitative care (*Schiavo v. Bush*, 2004) make clear that diagnostic accuracy, along with optimal practices in assessment and rehabilitation, are indeed a concern of life and death for many severely brain-injured patients who cannot speak for themselves and who must rely upon others to serve as advocates.

In advancing a vision for improving the care of patients with severe brain injury, Fins (2003) described a "therapeutic nihilism" that surrounds related clinical issues, as well as a "neglect syndrome" describing how the study of severe cognitive impairment has been too often ignored (p. 323). Despite growing awareness that conditions of severe brain injury have often been managed suboptimally, and despite the fact that nearly a decade has elapsed since studies began reporting significant misdiagnosis of VS (Andrews et al., 1996; Childs et al., 1993), a nearly ubiquitous, muddled (Shewmon, 2004), and/or nihilistic (Fins, 2003) view of severe brain injury persists. Families of patients thought to be in the VS may justifiably wonder why improvements in assessment and rehabilitative care have lagged so far behind recognition of these care needs. I propose that attention to the following interconnected problems is pivotal to satisfactory resolution of the issues surrounding optimal care of patients with severe brain injury:

1. Resolving definitional and diagnostic abstrusity.

2. Employment of suitable specialised assessment protocols.

3. Implementation of appropriate rehabilitative care strategies.

Care deficiencies resulting from failure to resolve these issues often constitute de facto therapeutic abandonment of these extremely vulnerable patients.

ISSUES REQUIRING RESOLUTION

Definition and diagnosis

As Shewmon (2004) noted, a lucid definition is a prerequisite for any scientific discussion or study. Such definition has, thus far, eluded professionals attempting to properly describe conditions of brain injury accompanied by profound impairments of consciousness. The initial labelling of PVS contributed to the confusion (Borthwick, 1995). As Jennett (2002), one of the two physicians who originally coined the term PVS to describe patients thought to be in a state of "wakefulness without awareness" (Jennett & Plum, 1972), declared, "The term 'vegetative state' simply describes observed behaviour, without implying specific structural pathology" (p. 355). What Jennett suggests is a taxonomic benefit is instead a serious impediment to precision in assessment, diagnosis, and care. "Awareness", per se, cannot be measured, but must be inferred from behaviour (Bernat, 2002). However, it is known that many patients who are indeed aware have great difficulty exhibiting behaviour demonstrative of their awareness (Andrews, 1997; Shiel et al., 2004). Because the definition of PVS is based upon the unknowable and immeasurable (i.e., the awareness of another individual) (Shewmon, 2004), it provides little practical guidance for the clinician.

The vague nature of the terms VS and PVS has been noted in related literature (Shewmon, 2004). However, the terms are still commonly used, albeit generically and often inappropriately, both within clinical practice and public discourse. Despite attempts to modify the term PVS (Australian Government National Health and Medical Research Council, 2003; Multi-Society Task Force on PVS, 1994), no alternative has taken hold (Andrews, 1997). This should be a concern to all professionals involved in the care of patients with severe brain injury. Negative attitudes toward these patients are inadvertently reinforced in the words we use to describe the severely disabled. In addition to its being a dehumanising label, the term VS has come to imply hopelessness with no possibility of recovery. Kilner (1992) posited that the term "vegetative state...has demeaning connotations and invites inadequate treatment" (p. 124). Recognising the difficulties inherent to attempts at naming a complex set of symptoms and dis-abilities, the health care profession is nonetheless obliged to seek, promote, and integrate accurate and precise terminology descriptive of the clinical entity. This obligation must be fulfilled without negative predetermination of the course of treatment patients will receive, and without implication that they cannot or will never recover.

From abstraction to assessment

Assessing patients for an entity that is not adequately defined presents a host of additional problems. Despite noteworthy contributions to the literature on assessment of patients with severe brain injury (Freeman, 1996; Gill-Thwaites, 1997; Whyte, Dipasquale, & Vaccaro, 1999; Wilson & Gill-Thwaites, 2000), the quality and type of assessment applied to patients thought to be in VS differs widely depending upon location, clinical setting, and other factors. In practical terms, no single standardised and uniform assessment approach has yet been adopted for pervasive use in patients with severe brain injury. In spite of apparent consensus that neuro-logical assessment should incorporate well-controlled clinical observation, augmented by advances in neuroimaging (Fins & Plum, 2004), the actual daily practice of such assessment is often haphazard at best. Poor assessment can involve unstructured, isolated, or brief observation that may not elicit the full range of behaviour (Multi-Society Task Force on PVS, 1994; Shiel et al., 2004; Zeman, 1997); cavalier or poor assessment skills; and the use of inappropriate, primitive, or nonstandardised assessment tools and methods. Additional problems include medical factors that hinder patient response such as medication effects (Strens, Mazibrada, Duncan, & Greenwood,

2004). Premature final pronouncements of a lack of patient awareness are also problematic, as are ignoring or dismissing input offered by nursing staff and family members who typically spend the longest periods of time with the patients (Shewmon, 2004; Wade & Johnston, 1999).

The inherent heterogeneity of the severely brain-injured patient population (Wilson & Gill-Thwaites, 2000) presents additional challenges for health care professionals. Heterogeneity in the patient thought to be in the VS can manifest as physical disabilities such as blindness and paralysis, which prevent engagement in activities or behaviours that could otherwise reveal patient awareness (Andrews, 1997; McMillan, 1996; Whyte et al., 1999). Multisensory approaches such as the Sensory Modality Assessment Rehabilitation Technique (SMART), a tool used to evaluate and treat patients with severe brain injury (Gill-Thwaites, 1997) show promise in the identification of awareness in patients previously thought to be "unaware", in some cases for a number of years.

Although the SMART and other assessment tools (Whyte et al., 1999) have been helpful in detecting awareness in this patient population, use of these very specifically designed instruments remains quite limited. Despite the many challenges presented by patients thought to be in the VS, immediate and extensive implementation of promising techniques, such as the SMART, can assist individual patients in demonstrating awareness and can also assist clinicians in data collection and further refinement of assessment techniques.

Rehabilitation protocol

The lack of standardised and effective rehabilitation protocols within the therapeutic environment contributes to suboptimal care of patients with severe brain injury. Rehabilitative care must be provided concurrently with ongoing assessment efforts in cases of suspected VS. Attempting to accurately assess awareness in a patient who is improperly positioned, uncomfortable, paralysed, blind, aphasic, or suffering from another of the myriad obstacles experienced by these patients, without first addressing and attempting to ameliorate these problems, can be, to say the least, a futile exercise.

Widespread, systematic use of techniques and tools such as the SMART, an instrument designed for this patient population that integrates assessment with rehabilitation, would begin the process of establishing helpful clinical benchmarks. However, neither the SMART nor any other highly specialised rehabilitation assessment tool is routinely used in severely neurologically impaired patients within the US. If sincere concern over the "best interests" of brain-injured patients exists, it makes sense that considerable effort would be made to assess and rehabilitate these patients to a point where they can make their interests and wishes known. Instances of patients thought to be in the VS who are in fact aware but have great difficulty demonstrating awareness (McMillan, 1996), provide poignant encouragement for clinicians to assist patients in overcoming physical obstacles whenever possible.

THE WAY AHEAD

The customarily grim view of severe brain injury resulting in cognitive impairment provides a disincentive for the development and implementation of rehabilitation strategies that could benefit these patients. This preconception obscures the issues surrounding care improvements (who would benefit from such improvements if all patients are deceased due to withdrawal of care in presumed "hopeless cases"?) and creates a sense of urgency for "final disposition" of these patients that would be better directed toward improvements in care. Clinicians should avoid claiming more certainty regarding diagnosis or prognosis than they can objectively discern (Bernat, 2002).

Recognition that rehabilitative care issues surrounding severe brain injury have not been optimally addressed is an important first step toward attaining greater clarity in the assessment, treatment, and rehabilitation of these patients. Fins (2003) wrote of an ideal vision for the care of brain injury: "Imagine a world where severely brain-injured patients were taken seriously. State of the art research facilities would stand next to clinical centres equipped with the latest imaging technologies to elucidate the underlying mechanisms of cognitive neurodisability" (p. 323). Sadly, the world Fins describes remains a fantasy. A paradigm shift is needed, incorporating a clearer and more progressive view of severe brain injury—a rehabilitative/ redemptive view—which would recruit and incorporate best practices in structured observation and rehabilitation techniques. It would also encourage universal adoption of rigorous, standardised assessment and rehabilitation guidelines, as well as the development of both acute and postacute centres specialising in the treatment of complex neurodisability (Fins, 2003; Gill-Thwaites, 1997). Such practices can and should be incorporated immediately. Advances in cognitive neuroscience (Fins, 2003) and neuroimaging (Kobylarz & Schiff, 2004; Owen et al., 2002) that may prove helpful in identifying predictors of recovery and in monitoring treatment effects must also be incorporated into clinical practice as they become available.

The Fins (2003) vision equates to new attitudes towards brain-injured patients and the encouragement of innovation and further research into severe brain injury. Attaining high levels of accuracy in predicting recovery potential will ultimately depend upon reaching a clearer understanding of the nature of human consciousness and of the VS condition itself. Meanwhile, improving treatment for patients with severe brain injury is both ethically and medically appropriate. Increased public awareness due to current high-profile cases, such as the Schiavo case (*Shiavo v. Bush*, 2004), helps make this an advantageous time for the neuroscience community to pursue global improvement in the care of these patients and to advocate on their behalf for funding mechanisms that will promote the development and use of advanced rehabilitative strategies and programmes.

REFERENCES

Airedale NHS Trust v. Bland (1993). 1 AL ER 821.

Andrews, K. (1997). Vegetative state: Background and ethics. *Journal of the Royal Society of Medicine, 90*, 593–596.

Andrews, K., Murphy, L., Munday R., & Littlewood C. (1996). Misdiagnosis of the vegetative state: Retrospective study in a rehabilitation unit. *British Medical Journal, 313*, 13–16.

Australian Government National Health and Medical Research Council (2003). *Post-coma unresponsiveness (vegetative state): A clinical framework for diagnosis.* Canberra: NHMRC. http://www.health.gov.au/nhmrc/publications/synopses/hpr23syn.htm

Bernat, J. L. (2002). Questions remaining about the minimally conscious state. *Neurology, 58*, 337–338.

Bijlani, A. (2000). Diagnosing permanent vegetative state. *Journal of the Royal College of Physicians of London, 34*(1), 61–62.

Borthwick, C. (1995). Persistent vegetative state: A syndrome in search of a name, or a judgement in search of a syndrome. *Monash Bioethics Review, 2*, 20–26.

Cantor, N. L. (2001). Twenty-five years after Quinlan: A review of the jurisprudence of death and dying. *Journal of Law and Medical Ethics, 29*, 182–196.

Childs, N., Mercer, W., & Childs, H. (1993). Accuracy of diagnosis of persistent vegetative state. *Neurology, 43*, 1465–1467.

Cruzan v. Director, Missouri Department of Health (1990). 110 S. Ct. 2841.

Fins, J. J. (2003). Constructing an ethical stereotaxy for severe brain injury: Balancing risks, benefits and access. *Neuroscience, 4*, 323–327.

Fins J., & Plum, F. (2004). Neurological diagnosis is more than a state of mind: Diagnostic clarity and impaired consciousness. *Archives of Neurology, 61*, 1354–1355.

Freeman, E. (1996). The coma exit chart: Assessing the patient in prolonged coma and the vegetative state. *Brain Injury, 10*, 615–624.

Giacino, J. T., Ashwal, S., Childs, N., Cranford, R., Jennett, B., Katz, D. I., et al. (2002). The minimally conscious state: Definition and diagnostic criteria. *Neurology, 58*, 349–353.

Gill-Thwaites, H. (1997). The sensory modality assessment rehabilitation technique (SMART)—A tool for assessment and treatment of patients with severe brain injury in a vegetative state. *Brain Injury, 11*(10), 723–734.

In the matter of Karen Quinlan, an alleged incompetent (1976). 70 N.J. Super 227;348 A. 2d. 801.

Jennett, B. (2002). The vegetative state. *Journal of Neurology, Neurosurgery and Psychiatry, 73*, 355–356.

Jennett, B., & Plum, F. (1972). Persistent vegetative state after brain damage: A syndrome in search of a name. *Lancet, 1*, 734–737.

Kilner, J. (1992). *Life on the line: Ethics, aging, ending patients' lives and allocating vital resources.* Grand Rapids, MI: Eerdmans.

Kobylarz, E., & Schiff, N. (2004). Functional imaging of severely brain-injured patients: Progress, challenges, and limitations. *Archives of Neurology, 61*, 1357–1360.

McMillan, T. M. (1996). Neuropsycholocial assessment after extremely severe head injury in a case of life or death. *Brain Injury, 11*(7), 483–490.

Multi-Society Task Force on PVS (1994). Medical aspects of the persistent vegetative state. *New England Journal of Medicine, 330*, 1499–1508.

Owen, A. M., Menon, D. K., Johnsrude, I. S., Bor, D., Scott, S. K., Manly, T., et al. (2002). Detecting residual function in persistent vegetative state. *Neurocase, 8*, 394–403.

Schiavo v. Bush (2004). No. 03-008212-CI-20 (Pinellas County, Florida Circuit Court, 6th Judicial District).

Shewmon, D. A. (2004). The ABC of PVS: Problems of definition. In C. A. Machato & D. A. Shewmon (Eds.), *Brain death and disorders of consciousness* (pp. 215–226). New York: Kluwer Academic/Plenum.

Shiel, A., Gelling, L., Wilson, B., Coleman, M., & Pickard, J. D. (2004). Difficulties in diagnosing the vegetative state. *British Journal of Neurosurgery, 18*(1), 5–7.

Strens, L. H., Mazibrada, G., Duncan, J. S., & Greenwood, R. (2004). Misdiagnosing the vegetative state after severe brain injury: The influence of medication. *Brain Injury, 18*(2), 213–218.

Wade, D. T., & Johnston, C. (1999) The persistent vegetative state: Practical guidance on diagnosis and management. *British Medical Journal, 319*, 841–844.

Whyte, J., Dipasquale, M. C., & Vaccaro, M. (1999). Assessment of command-following in minimally conscious brain injured patients. *Archives of Physical Medicine and Rehabilitation, 80*, 653–660.

Wilson, S. L., & Gill-Thwaites, H. (2000). Early indication of emergence from vegetative state derived from assessments with the SMART—A preliminary report. *Brain Injury, 14*(4), 319–331.

Zeman, A. (1997) Persistent vegetative state. *Lancet, 350*, 795–799.

NEUROPSYCHOLOGICAL REHABILITATION
2005, 15 (3/4), 272–275

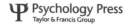

Part II: Functional imaging, electrophysiology and mechanical intervention

Foreword by John D. Pickard

Unlike brainstem death, the diagnosis of and differentiation between the vegetative, minimally conscious, and the intermittently aware may be difficult and require prolonged observation by a multidisciplinary team, experienced in the use of behavioural scales, aware of the need for appropriate seating and posture, and the need to avoid over-stimulation. Undoubtedly, objective investigations would be helpful not only to distinguish between these various states, but also to aid prognosis. Some patients do improve from one state to the next over the first few months. There is a growing interest in whether it is possible to expedite and optimise any potential for recovery. Some patients have relatively little structural damage but have severely impaired thalamo-cortical function. Uncertainties over natural history in an individual patient make trial design of interventions such as neuro-modulatory implants, stem cells and drugs very difficult.

The development of specialist investigations such as functional brain imaging and electrophysiology require that these patients, fortunately relatively very few in number, are looked after in specialist centres with the benefit of state of the art care and counselling for the families and carers. Too often in the past, such patients have been admitted to long-stay institutions where remedial causes and avoidable complications are more easily missed. Research networks are now being organised to advance our understanding of and care for these states of altered consciousness while optimising care.

Clearly patients in vegetative (VS) and minimally conscious (MCS) states cannot give informed consent to research procedures. A minority of ethics committees have difficulty engaging with this problem and consider that even assent by next of kin is insufficient. Such views contrast with the possibility of withdrawal of feeding where an individual patient obviously cannot

http://www.tandf.co.uk/journals/pp/09602011.html   DOI:10.1080/09602010443000641

give consent and may not have left an advance directive, although they may have indicated in general terms what they would wish to happen should they ever be involved in that situation. This nihilistic view towards research in these patients ignores the extensive discussions surrounding research in the cognitively impaired. For example, the Royal College of Psychiatrists report points out that it is discriminatory to deny a patient group access to research provided that it is relevant to their specific condition and the risk is minimal (Royal College of Psychiatrists, 2001). Defenceless patients must be protected but equally they should not be judged unworthy to have access to safe research, which might prove beneficial in the long term, if not to them personally. Electrophysiology and functional brain imaging are just such safe technologies and, in practice, are already beginning to provide data that is helpful in the management of the individual patient (see papers in Part II). Such benefits cannot always have been anticipated nor should such promise be used by the research team to encourage relatives to agree to research. Benefits of inclusion in research protocols include:

- State of the art care.

- Review of the diagnosis by an experienced multidisciplinary team.

- Early detection and prophylactic treatment of avoidable complications.

- Detection and treatment of contributory causes such as hydrocephalus.

- Delineation of which sensory modalities and which side for presentation should be used to communicate with the individual patient.

- More informed counselling of families and carers.

In the absence of severe hypoxia, structural brain imaging (CT or MRI) may be confirmatory of neuropathological studies in showing that patients in VS or MCS do not always have grossly atrophied brains. Ventricular dilatation, sulcal atrophy and loss of white matter are not specific to VS or MCS and may be seen in perfectly sentient people who have little or no problems with higher mental function (see papers in Part I). Measurements of cerebral metabolism by FDG-PET reveal global depression in both VS and MCS (see Beuthien-Baumann paper). There are methodological issues that need to be taken into account when interpreting such images, e.g., what is the appropriate value for the lumped constant for FDG under these pathological conditions? Recovery of metabolism in polymodal association cortex (pre-frontal, Broca, parietotemporal and precuneous) may accompany emergence from VS. Recent studies of benzodiazepine receptor density using ^{11}C-flumazenil reveal that there may be loss of neuronal integrity in patients with apparently little structural damage and that such reduction in binding potential of flumazenil may correlate at least in the more acute stages with reduction in FDG uptake (see Beuthien-Baumann paper). More long-term study is required to define whether flumazenil binding potential will differentiate between patients who will or will not emerge from VS.

Functional brain imaging studies using either PET or fMRI require preliminary behavioural and electrophysiological assessment to define which sensory pathways are reasonably intact so that an appropriate test paradigm can be designed. Great care is required with the choice of such paradigms in order to interrogate the hierarchy of responses beyond the primary sensory cortices and to explore possible connectivity with higher order association cortices and emotional content (see papers in Part II). Patients may be restless and move during the scan. fMRI depends upon the blood oxygenation level-dependent (BOLD) effect which in turn depends upon the increase in focal cerebral blood flow that is greater than that required to match the local metabolic demand created by the neural activation response to the stimulus. This coupling mechanism is probably abnormal under pathological circumstances. Hence there is a significant failure rate at present with functional brain imaging so that a negative "scan" cannot be used as proof of the diagnosis of VS. In general, residual cortical processing in VS does not lead to those integrated processes necessary for awareness but isolated cerebral networks may remain in some cases. Early results with MCS patients suggest that, unlike VS, there is activity in the medial parietal (precuneous) and posterior cingulate cortices, areas, which may be part of the neural network subserving human awareness (see Boly et al. paper). Such findings depend upon group analysis and further refinement is necessary to detect such a network in the individual.

Although of considerable interest in general and to the individual patient when positive, functional imaging is complementary to clinical and behavioural assessment. However, with ever-faster scanners, movement artefact correction techniques, novel ligands for PET and advances in analysing the neurophysiological architecture of fMRI images in the individual patient's brain, functional imaging may in future play a more direct clinical role.

There have been significant advances in the understanding of the electrophysiological correlates of VS, MCS and coma as described (see Kobylarz & Schiff; Kotchoubey; Guerit; Schnakers et al.; and Fischer & Luauté papers). Intact thalamocortical activity is crucial for awareness as is neuro-metabolic coupling. Electrophysiological techniques are certainly easier to apply at present than functional imaging in these patients.

Finally, the therapeutic efficacy of drugs, peripheral and central electrical stimulation and, in the future, neural repair with stem cells and local instillation of growth factors are being explored (see Matsuda et al.;

Cooper et al.; and Yamamoto and Katayama papers). However, such clinical trials have been fraught with difficulty because of the international lack of consistency over diagnostic criteria and uncertainties over natural history. There will never be enough patients to qualify for a "mega" randomised controlled trial. The variability between patients means that novel trial designs will have to be developed, aided by the use of surrogate end points for specific pathological processes, if these patients are not to be denied the fruits of modern neurobiology.

REFERENCE

Royal College of Psychiatrists (2001). *Guidelines for researchers and for research ethics committees on psychiatric research involving human participants.* Council report CR82. London: Royal College of Psychiatrists.

PART II: ORGANIZATION OF PAPERS

1. Functional and structural imaging
Beuthien-Baumann et al.; Boly et al.; Owen et al.; Bekinschtein et al.

2. Electrophysiology
Kobylarz & Schiff; Kotchoubey; Guérit; Fischer & Luauté; Schnakers et al.

3. Mechanical intervention
Cooper et al.; Yamamoto & Katayama

4. Pharmaceutical intervention
Matsuda et al.

NEUROPSYCHOLOGICAL REHABILITATION
2005, 15 (3/4), 276–282

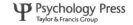

Functional imaging of vegetative state applying single photon emission tomography and positron emission tomography

Bettina Beuthien-Baumann[1], Vjera A. Holthoff[2],
and Jobst Rudolf[3]

[1]Department of Nuclear Medicine, University of Technology Dresden and
PET-Center Rossendorf, Germany
[2]Department of Psychiatry and Psychotherapy, University of Technology
Dresden, Germany
[3]Department of Neurology, Papageorgiou Hospital, Thessaloniki, Greece

Nuclear medicine techniques, such as single photon emission tomography (SPECT) and positron emission tomography (PET) have been applied in patients in a vegetative state to investigate brain function in a non-invasive manner. Parameters investigated include glucose metabolism, perfusion at rest, variations of regional perfusion after stimulation, and benzodiazepine receptor density. Compared to controls, patients in a vegetative state show a substantial reduction of glucose metabolism and perfusion. While patients post-anoxia exhibit a rather homogenous cortical reduction of glucose metabolism, patients after head trauma often show severe cortical and sub-cortical reductions at the site of primary trauma. To distinguish reduced glucose metabolism due to neuronal inactivation from neuronal loss, flumazenil-PET, an indicator of benzodiazepine receptor density, could add valuable information on the extent of brain damage. Activation studies focus on the evaluation of residual brain network, looking for processing in secondary projection fields. So far the predictive strength concerning possible recovery for the individual patient is limited, and PET and SPECT are not routine procedures in the assessment of patients in a vegetative state.

Correspondence should be addressed to Dr. Bettina Beuthien-Baumann, Klinik und Poliklinik für Nuklearmedizin, Universitätsklinikum Carl Gustav Carus, Fetscherstraße 74, 01307 Dresden, Germany. Tel: +49 351 260 2755, Fax: +49 351 260 3649. Email: b.beuthien@fz-rossendorf.de

© 2005 Psychology Press Ltd
http://www.tandf.co.uk/journals/pp/09602011.html   DOI:10.1080/09602010443000290

Single photon emission tomography (SPECT) and positron emission tomography (PET) are powerful diagnostic imaging tools which enable non-invasive assessment of regional brain function. SPECT imaging is a standard procedure in nuclear medicine departments. For brain imaging, various physiological processes, such as regional perfusion or receptor and transporter expression can be assessed in a semi-quantitative approach (Kung, Kung, & Choi, 2003). Compared to SPECT technology, PET offers a higher spatial resolution and the possibility of true quantitative assessment of physiological processes. Furthermore, positron emitters like ^{11}Carbon or ^{18}Fluorine, can be incorporated into numerous biomolecules, such as glucose analogues or amino acids which follow physiological pathways. In recent years, PET has gained wide acceptance for diagnostic applications in neurology. A vast body of literature is available on the diagnosis of epilepsy, dementia, movement disorders, brain tumour imaging, and activation studies (Cherry & Phelps, 1996; Herholz, Herscovitch, & Heiss, 2004; Herholz et al., 1999; Juhasz & Chugani, 2003; Spence, Mankoff, & Muzi, 2003; Thobois, Guillouet, & Broussolle, 2001; Van Heertum & Tikofsky, 2003).

CLINICAL RELEVANCE OF SCINTIGRAPHIC TECHNIQUES IN THE ASSESSMENT OF VS

Acute severe traumatic, toxic or anoxic brain injury inevitably results in coma, a state of loss of consciousness with the patient's eyes closed. If not resulting in death, this coma will develop into an acute vegetative state (AVS), where the patient seems awake but unaware, uncommunicative and unresponsive to his/her environment. If recovery continues, patients regain minimal responsiveness to external stimuli (the so-called "minimally conscious state") that eventually may result in full recovery of consciousness and responsiveness. Otherwise, patients may remain for a long time—even for the rest of their life span—in a persistent vegetative state (PVS). The reliable assessment of the individual patient's prognosis on the sole basis of clinical findings is difficult, and, in the early stages of the disease, often impossible. On the other hand, the probability of recovery from acute brain injury is a crucial issue in critical care medicine, as the reliable assessment of the individual prognosis of recovery from a vegetative state (VS) is mandatory for all decisions concerning initiation, prolongation or termination of extended intensive care procedures. However, clinical signs, laboratory or functional tests (e.g., electro encephalogram, evoked potentials) as well as conventional neuroimaging methods (e.g., computed tomography [CT] and magnetic resonance imaging [MRI]) only permit an indirect and incomplete estimation of the extent of structural brain damage in VS. Thus, the intention of studying patients in VS with scintigraphic techniques is to assess the true degree of functional impairment in addition to the morphological changes seen with CT or MRI. Ideally, populations tested should be homogenous with respect to the aetiology of the VS and its duration. However, most of the publications report on rather small patient groups or case reports of patients in VS of different duration and varying underlying causes. This is on the one hand due to difficulties in the examination of a patient population that often presents with vegetative irritability. On the other hand legal aspects have to be considered with the application of radioactivity to non-conscious patients that are unable to consent to this procedure.

BRAIN PERFUSION

The first scintigraphic investigation of VS patients was reported by Heiss and colleagues in 1972 (Heiss, Gerstenbrand, Prosenz, & Krenn, 1972). They performed cerebral blood flow (CBF) measurements with planar gamma camera images and ^{133}Xenon in 33 patients. Comparing the outcome of these patients with their CBF values, they found a significant correlation: Those patients who recovered had higher mean CBF values than those patients with residual deficit or patients who died. This was the first study showing the prognostic value of CBF measurements in this patient group.

Oder, Goldenberg, Podreka, and Deecke (1991) related the qualitative evaluation of perfusion SPECT with ^{99m}Tc-HMPAO of 12 patients in PVS after traumatic brain injury with their long-term outcome. A global reduction of cortical blood flow was a reliable predictor of poor long-term outcome, but the demonstration of only focal deficits did not reliably indicate a favourable outcome.

BRAIN GLUCOSE METABOLISM

The energy metabolism of the brain relies on the supply of glucose. Metabolic mapping of the brain with 18F-fluorodeoxyglucose (FDG) gives valuable information of brain function in normal conditions or in various pathological states. In VS patients, mean reductions of more than 50% of the cerebral glucose metabolism compared to normal controls were described (Beuthien-Baumann et al., 2003; De Volder et al., 1990; Levy et al., 1987; Rudolf et al., 1999a; Schiff et al., 2002; Tommasino et al., 1995). With prolonged duration of the VS, i.e., with the transition from AVS to PVS, a further reduction of glucose metabolism is observed (Rudolf et al., 1999a; Tommasino et al., 1995). Differences in the metabolic pattern can be seen according to the underlying cause. In the hypoxic brain, supratentorial glucose hypometabolism was generally homogenous (Rudolf et al., 1999a; Tommasino et al., 1995), but its accentuation in the territorial borderzones has also been described (De Volder et al., 1990). Patients with traumatic VS often show inhomogenous metabolic patterns with defects or severely reduced metabolism at the sites of primary tissue injury and reduced glucose metabolism of different degrees in the remaining cortical and sub-cortical structures. Schiff et al. (2002) investigated five patients in PVS (two patients post-hypoxia, three patients post-brain trauma) with FDG-PET. They found a wide variation of global reduction of glucose metabolism between 30–40% (hypoxic) and 45–65% (trauma) of normal controls. The post-trauma patients exhibited differing patterns of glucose metabolism, and conclusions on residual neuronal connections and individual behaviour of the patients were drawn.

Beuthien-Baumann et al. (2003) investigated 16 patients with post-traumatic PVS. They found a 25–71% reduction of grey matter glucose metabolism compared to controls. One exception was noted for the vermis cerebelli, where only an 18% reduction was found. This structure is not mentioned in other publications; this could on the one hand be due to the limited field of view of older generation PET scanners where the cerebellum was not included in the scan. On the other hand, this could be a difference between post-traumatic brain injury with relatively preserved neuronal input from the proprio-receptors and skin receptors of the periphery to the vermis cerebelli and anoxia with its more homogenous brain damage. In addition to FDG-PET, perfusion SPECT was performed. Perfusion and glucose metabolism yielded comparable patterns in both hemispheres and sub-cortical structures. One difference was noted for the cerebellum, where a relatively higher perfusion than glucose metabolism was noted. A relative preservation of the cerebellar glucose metabolism was described by Rudolf et al. (1999b). In this study of post-hypoxic patients in AVS the glucose metabolism of the cerebellum was less impaired (30% reduction compared to normal controls) than the glucose metabolism of the supra-tentorial structures (50% reduction compared to normal controls).

Although at first sight unresponsive to their surroundings, patients with locked-in syndrome (due to a lesion at the upper pontine level these patients are quadriplegic and seemingly unresponsive) are conscious and can communicate via eye contact. Levy et al. (1987) performed FDG-PET on seven patients in VS and three locked-in patients to determine the level of brain function underlying these clinical states. Locked-in patients could be discriminated from patients in VS by their near normal cerebral glucose metabolism reflecting their conscious state.

DENSITY OF CEREBRAL BENZODIAZEPINE RECEPTOR

Although FDG-PET shows the severe reduction of cerebral glucose metabolism in patients in VS, but especially post-anoxia, it does not indicate whether these changes represent functional inactivation or irreversible structural brain damage. Rudolf, Sobesky, Grond, and Heiss (2000) investigated neuronal integrity by means of PET using ^{11}C-flumazenil (FMZ), a radioligand indicating benzodiazepine receptor density. FMZ-PET was correlated to the cerebral glucose metabolism in nine patients in AVS due to hypoxia (Rudolf, Sobesky, Ghaemi, & Heiss, 2002). FMZ-PET demonstrated a considerable reduction of benzodiazepine receptor binding sites in all cortical regions, that grossly corresponded to the extent of reduction of cerebral glucose metabolism (Rudolf et al., 2000), while the cerebellum was spared from neuronal loss. In controls, cortical relative flumazenil binding was not lower than five times the average white matter activity. In AVS, nearly all values were below this threshold, without relevant overlap of the data of FMZ binding between patients and controls. During follow-up, only one patient had gained a state of minimal responsiveness, four patients had died, and four were in PVS. It was concluded, that in VS due to hypoxia the reduction of glucose metabolism represents not mere functional inactivation, but irreversible structural brain damage.

ACTIVATION STUDIES WITH ^{15}O-H$_2$O-PET

Unlike studies with FDG, flumazenil or HMPAO-SPECT, which were done to gain insight into the extent of brain damage, considerable interest has focused on the ability of the patient in VS to respond to external stimuli. These studies were based on clinical observation that some patients in VS show some response to noxious stimuli like noise or pain. As well, relatives of patients may be in doubt as to whether or not the patient may recognise their presence in some way. From a clinical point of view, responsiveness to outer stimuli excludes the diagnosis of acute or persistent VS, and corroborates the diagnosis of a minimally conscious state. A transition from VS to minimally conscious state could be interpreted as amelioration of the patient's condition, and could be predictive of further recovery. Thus, tests that document patient reactions to outer stimuli would be of utmost importance for the patients' clinical assessment and management.

De Jong, Willemsen, and Paans (1997) report on one patient whom the mother told a domestic story during perfusion PET with ^{15}O-H$_2$O. Some activation was noted in the anterior cingulate, middle temporal gyrus and right premotor cortex, which might have reflected cortical involvement in processing of emotional attributes of sound or speech, although it could not be tested whether this activation was evoked solely by the mother's voice (compared to sound alone) or would have been evoked as well by other voices. Menon et al. (1998) used, in one patient, photographs of familiar faces as a visual stimulus during perfusion PET. Activation was noted in Brodmann areas 37, 18, 19 and the cerebellum, which was cautiously interpreted as some sort of processing. This patient became responsive two months later. Owen et al. (2002) used auditory or visual stimuli in three cases. In these patients some activation in secondary cortical areas were noted in two out of three patients, the scans of the third could not be evaluated due to motion artefacts. While in a study by Laureys et al. (2002) in 15 PVS patients only activation in the primary somatosensory cortex and no activation in secondary somatosensory or association cortices was seen during stimulation of the median nerve, Kassubek et al. (2003) investigated seven patients in PVS applying pain stimulation. Activation was found not only in S1 and SII respectively posterior insular, but also in the cingulate cortex which was interpreted as residual activity of a pain-related cerebral network.

SUMMARY

Due to clinical and ethical issues, including the application of radioactivity to non-conscious patients, most of the publications report on rather small patient groups or case reports of patients in vegetative state of different duration and varying underlying causes.

While most of the studies published have concentrated on describing the degree of brain damage by measuring the reduction of glucose metabolism, the reduction of benzodiazepine density or the residual perfusion under resting conditions, recent publications have focused on the evaluation of residual brain networks by means of activation studies. Due to the so far limited predictive strength of perfusion or glucose metabolism with respect to the possible recovery for the individual patient these procedures have not yet found the way into the routine assessment of patients in the vegetative state. Activation studies could give valuable insight into residual neuronal networks. Future investigations will have to show whether benzodiazepine receptor density measurements with PET and ^{11}C-flumazenil or SPECT and ^{123}J-Iomazenil could gain importance, in particular in guiding the patient's family on what might happen to their relative.

REFERENCES

Beuthien-Baumann, B., Handrick, W., Schmidt, T., Burchert, W., Oehme, L., Kropp, J., et al. (2003). Persistent vegetative state: Evaluation of brain metabolism and brain perfusion with PET and SPECT. *Nuclear Medicine Communications, 24*, 643–649.

Cherry, S. R., & Phelps, M. E. (1996). Imaging brain function with Positron Emission Tomography. In A. W. Toga & J. C. Mazziotta (Eds.), *Brain mapping: The methods* (pp. 191–221). San Diego: Academic Press.

De Jong, B. M., Willemsen, A. T., & Paans, A. M. (1997). Regional cerebral blood flow changes related to affective speech presentation in persistent vegetative state. *Clinical Neurology and Neurosurgery, 99*(3), 213–216.

De Volder, A. G., Goffinet, A. M., Bol, A., Michel, C., de Barsy, T., & Laterre, C. (1990). Brain glucose metabolism in postanoxic syndrome: Positron emission tomographic study. *Archives of Neurology, 47*(2), 197–204.

Heiss, W.-D., Gerstenbrand, F., Prosenz, P., & Krenn, J. (1972). The prognostic value of cerebral blood flow measurement in patients with the apallic syndrome. *Journal of Neurological Sciences, 16*, 373–382.

Herholz, K., Herscovitch, P., & Heiss, W.-D. (2004). *NeuroPET: Positron emission tomography in neuroscience and clinical neurology.* Berlin: Springer.

Herholz, K., Nordberg, A., Salmon, E., Perani D., Kessler, J., Mielke, R., et al. (1999). Impairment of neocortical metabolism predicts progression in Alzheimer's Disease. *Dementia and Geriatric Cognitive Disorders, 10*, 494–504.

Juhasz, C., & Chugani, H. T. (2003). Imaging the epileptic brain with positron emission tomography. *Neuroimaging Clinics of North America, 13*, 705–716.

Kassubek, J., Juengling, F. D., Els, T., Spreer, J., Herpers, M., Krause, T., et al. (2003). Activation of a residual cortical network during painful stimulation in long-term postanoxic vegetative state: A 15O-H20 PET study. *Journal of Neurological Sciences, 212*, 85–91.

Kung, H., Kung, M., & Choi, S. (2003). Radiopharmaceuticals for Single-Photon Emission Computed Tomography brain imaging. *Seminars in Nuclear Medicine, 33*(1), 2–13.

Laureys, S., Faymonville, M. E., Peigneux, P., Damas, P., Lambermont, B., Fiore, G. D., et al. (2002). Cortical processing of noxious somatosensory stimuli in the persistent vegetative state. *NeuroImage, 17*, 732–741.

Levy, D. E., Sidtis, J. J., Rottenberg, D. A., Jarden, J. O., Strother, S. C., Dhawan, V., et al. (1987). Differences in cerebral blood flow and glucose utilization in vegetative versus locked-in patients. *Annals of Neurology, 22*(6), 673–682.

Menon, D. K., Owen, A. M., Williams, E. J., Minhas, P. S., Allen, C. M. C., Boniface, S. J., et al. (1998). Cortical processing in the persistent vegetative state. *Lancet, 352*, 200.

Oder, W., Goldenberg, G., Podreka, I., & Deecke, L. (1991). HM-PAO-SPECT in persistent vegetative state after head injury: Prognostic indicator of the likelihood of recovery? *Intensive Care Medicine, 17*, 149–153.

Owen, A. M., Menon, D. K., Johnsrude, I. S., Bor, D., Scott, S. K., Manly, T., et al. (2002). Detecting residual cognitive function in persistent vegetative state. *Neurocase, 8*, 394–403.

Rudolf, J., Ghaemi, M., Ghaemi, M., Haupt, W. F., Szelies, B., & Heiss, W.-D. (1999a). Cerebral glucose metabolism in acute and persistent vegetative state. *Journal of Neurosurgical Anesthesiology, 11*(1), 17–24.

Rudolf, J., Haupt, W. P., Szelies, B., Ghaemi, M., Beil, C., & Heiss, W.-D. (1999b). Regionaler Hirnglukosestoffwechsel im postanoxischen Coma vigile. *Aktuelle Neurologie, 26*, 81–85.

Rudolf, J., Sobesky, J., Ghaemi, M., & Heiss, W.-D. (2002). The correlation between cerebral glucose metabolism and benzodiazepine receptor density in the acute vegetative state. *European Journal of Neurology, 9*, 671–677.

Rudolf, J., Sobesky, J., Grond, M., & Heiss, W.-D. (2000). Identification by positron emission tomography of neuronal loss in acute vegetative state. *Lancet, 354*, 115–116.

Schiff, N., Ribary, U., Moreno, D. R., Beattie, B., Kronberg, E., Blasberg, R., et al. (2002). Residual cerebral activity and behavioural fragments can remain in the persistently vegetative brain. *Brain, 125*, 1210–1234.

Spence, A. M., Mankoff, D. A., & Muzi, M. (2003). Positron emission tomography imaging of brain tumors. *Neuroimaging Clinics of North America, 13*, 717–739.

Thobois, S., Guillouet, S., & Broussolle, E. (2001). Contributions of PET and SPECT to the understanding of the pathophysiology of Parkinson's disease. *Neurophysiologie Clinique/Clinical Neurophysiology, 31*, 321–340.

Tommasino, C., Grana, C., Lucignani, G., Torri, G., & Fazio, F. (1995). Regional cerebral metabolism of glucose in comatose and vegetative state patients. *Journal of Neurosurgical Anesthesiology, 7*(2), 109–116.

Van Heertum, R. L., & Tikofsky, R. S. (2003). Positron Emission Tomography and SinglePhoton Emission Computed Tomography brain imaging in the evaluation of dementia. *Seminars in Nuclear Medicine, 33*(1), 77–85.

NEUROPSYCHOLOGICAL REHABILITATION
2005, 15 (3/4), 283–289

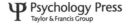

Cerebral processing of auditory and noxious stimuli in severely brain injured patients: Differences between VS and MCS

Mélanie Boly, Marie-Elisabeth Faymonville, Philippe Peigneux, Bernard Lambermont, François Damas, André Luxen, Maurice Lamy, Gustave Moonen, Pierre Maquet, and Steven Laureys

University of Liège, Belgium

We review cerebral processing of auditory and noxious stimuli in minimally conscious state (MCS) and vegetative state (VS) patients. In contrast with limited brain activation found in VS patients, MCS patients show activation similar to controls in response to auditory, emotional and noxious stimuli. Despite an apparent clinical similarity between MCS and VS patients, functional imaging data show striking differences in cortical segregation and integration between these two conditions. However, in the absence of a generally accepted neural correlate of consciousness as measured by functional neuroimaging, clinical assessment remains the gold standard for the evaluation and management of severely brain damaged patients.

Vegetative state (VS) is defined by the combination of recurring and prolonged periods of arousal and a lack of behavioural signs of awareness (ANA Committee on Ethical Affairs, 1993; Multi-Society Task Force on

Correspondence should be addressed to: Steven Laureys, M.D., Ph.D., Cyclotron Research Centre, University of Liège, Sart Tilman B35, 4000 Liège, Belgium. Tel: 00324/366.23.16, Fax: 00324/366.29.46. E-mail: steven.laureys@ulg.ac.be

This research was supported by the Fonds National de la Recherche Scientifique, (FNRS), by the Reine Elisabeth Medical Foundation, by funds of the University of Liège and the Centre Hospitalier Universitaire Sart Tilman, Liège, Belgium, and by a Tom Slick Research Award on Consciousness of the Mind Science Foundation, TX. S. Laureys and P. Maquet are Research Associate and Research Director at the FNRS.

http://www.tandf.co.uk/journals/pp/09602011.html   DOI:10.1080/09602010443000371

PVS, 1994). Minimally conscious state (MCS) patients show minimal but definite evidence of self or environment awareness but are unable to communicate (Giacino et al., 2002). Several studies underline the high frequency of misdiagnosis among VS and MCS patients (Andrews, Murphy, Munday, & Littlewood, 1996; Childs, Mercer, & Childs, 1993). Indeed, the bedside assessment of consciousness is intrinsically difficult since it can only rely on behavioural inferences. However, it is important to distinguish MCS from VS, because preliminary findings suggest there are meaningful differences in outcome (Giacino et al., 2002).

Although imaging studies cannot replace the bedside clinical assessment of these disorders of consciousness, they can help to objectively measure the cerebral activity of these patients and how it differs from normal controls. Moreover, it adds to the scientific search for the neural correlates of consciousness. Several functional imaging studies have been performed to investigate cerebral activation in response to external stimulation in VS patients (Menon et al., 1998; Owen et al., 2002; Plum, Schiff, Ribary, & Llinas, 1998; Schiff, Ribary, Plum, & Llinas, 1999; Schiff et al., 2002), yet only a few were performed in minimally conscious state patients (Bekinschtein et al., 2004; Hirsch et al., 2001). We present here recent data comparing brain activation induced by auditory and noxious stimuli in both patient populations.

AUDITORY PROCESSING

Using the $H_2^{15}O$-PET (positron emission tomography) technique, we measured changes in regional cerebral blood flow (rCBF) induced by simple auditory stimuli (clicks) in 5 MCS patients, 15 unsedated VS patients, and 15 controls (Boly et al., 2004). Controls were aged 40 ± 9 years (mean $\pm$ SD; 8 males). VS patients were aged 48 ± 17 years (12 males) and MCS patients 37 ± 12 years (3 males). They were diagnosed according to established criteria (ANA Committee on Ethical Affairs, 1993; Multi-Society Task Force on PVS, 1994, for VS and Giacino et al., 2002, for MCS), and following repetitive neurological examinations and careful anamnesis of family members and medical caregivers. Patients with uncertain diagnoses were excluded. The aetiologies of VS were: cardiorespiratory arrest ($n = 5$), diffuse axonal injury ($n = 3$), drug overdose ($n = 2$), prolonged respiratory insufficiency ($n = 2$), encephalitis with diffuse white matter injury ($n = 2$), and carbon monoxide intoxication ($n = 1$). The aetiologies of MCS were: respiratory arrest ($n = 1$), trauma ($n = 1$), encephalitis ($n = 1$), hypertensive encephalopathy ($n = 1$), and diffuse axonal injury ($n = 1$). All patients had preserved pupillary, corneal and vestibulo-ocular reflexes. Mean Glasgow Coma Scores (GCS); (Teasdale & Jennett, 1974) on admission were 4.9 $\pm$ 2.5 (range 3–13) for the VS and 5.8 $\pm$ 4.8 (range 3–14) for the MCS patients. Patients were scanned 33 $\pm$ 11 (MCS) and 36 $\pm$ 9 (VS) days after admission, while in awake periods as demonstrated by simultaneous polygraphic recordings.

During the PET data acquisition, scans were performed during rest, (left then right) auditory stimulation, and (left then right) noxious stimulation (results of the latter are described below). Each condition was repeated three times and the order of presentation was pseudorandomised. Scans obtained during left-sided stimulation were flipped. Hence, results should be interpreted as contra- and ipsilateral to the side of stimulation and not as left- or right-sided. PET data were analysed using voxel-based statistical parametrical mapping (SPM, www.fil.ion.ucl.ac.uk/spm). Data from each subject were realigned, normalised into standard stereotaxic space, and smoothed (Friston, 1997). A random-effect analysis was performed, using a two-steps procedure (Holmes & Friston, 1998). The random-effect analysis is a conservative analysis that takes into account intersubject variability, and gives results representative at the population level. A first-level analysis took into account within-subject variances related to the experimental conditions, estimated according to the general linear model at each voxel. Proportional scaling performed global flow normalisation. Primary contrasts estimated the effect of auditory stimulation versus rest in each subject. The "contrast images" obtained were then entered into a second-level analysis, separating the data into three groups (controls, MCS, VS). We then performed two conjunction analyses looking for activation (1) common to controls and VS and (2) common to controls and MCS. We also looked for the groups (MCS–VS) $\times$ condition (stimulation–rest) interaction, searching for areas less activated in VS than in MCS patients. Given our expected activation in superior temporal areas (Laureys et al., 2000), results were thresholded at small-volume-corrected $p < .05$ (20 mm diameter sphere centred on peak voxels).

A functional connectivity analysis (Friston et al., 1997; Laureys et al., 2000) was also performed, to identify areas in which activity was modulated by secondary auditory cortex (Brodmann area 42, peak activation in controls) differently in MCS versus VS patients, using a fixed-effect approach. Such a psychophysiological interaction analysis explains the activity in one cortical area in terms of an interaction between the influence of another area and a given experimental context (i.e., being a vegetative or a minimally conscious patient). A psychophysiological interaction means that the contribution (i.e., regression slope) of one area to another changes significantly with the experimental context assessed with the general linear model as employed by statistical parametric mapping (Friston, 1997). Put simply, our statistical analysis identifies brain regions that show condition-dependent differences in modulation with another (chosen) region (i.e., area 42). As we expected a large diversity of areas and no a priori areas could be suggested, p values were corrected for multiple comparisons at the cluster- or voxel-level, and results were thresholded at corrected p values <.05.

In normal subjects, stimulation increased rCBF bilaterally in areas involved in auditory processing: transverse temporal (Brodmann area 41) and superior temporal gyri (areas 42 and 22) (Figure 1a). VS patients activated bilateral area 41/42, but no significant activation was found in higher order associative area 22 (Figure 1c). The observed preservation of activation in VS patients could reflect a residual neural encoding of basic sound attributes, but with no further functional integration, as suggested in Laureys et al. (2000). In contrast, MCS patients activated similarly to controls (Figure 1b). Functional connectivity analysis showed that MCS, compared to VS, had higher interactions between auditory association area 42 and a wide cortical network known to be involved in normal auditory perception (including temporal and frontal association cortices). The activation of higher order associative cortices in MCS possibly corresponds to a more elaborate auditory processing, thought to be necessary for conscious perception (Baars, Ramsoy, & Laureys, 2003).

We recently also studied an MCS patient using complex auditory stimuli with and without emotional valence (Laureys et al., 2004). We used $H_2^{15}O$-PET imaging and SPM (fixed-effect analysis, results thresholded at uncorrected p-value <.001). Compared to meaningless noise, presentation of cries or the patient's own name produced a much more widespread activation, encompassing temporal, parietal and frontal associative areas. During the PET scanning, cognitive evoked potential recording also showed a P300 potential in response to the patient's own name and not to other names.

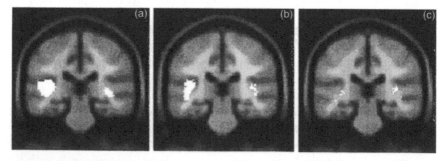

Figure 1. (a): brain areas showing an increase in regional cerebral blood flow during auditory stimulation in controls. (b) and (c): areas of increase of rCBF during auditory stimulation that are common to controls and respectively MCS patients (b) and VS patients (c). Results are projected on a coronal section of a normalised brain MRI template, 28 mm posterior to the anterior commissure line

These data suggest that MCS patients may be capable of extended cerebral processing of auditory stimuli, especially stimuli with emotional valence.

PAIN PROCESSING

Pain sensation is intrinsically a first person subjective experience and its third person evaluation is challenging in subjects that are non-communicative. Several authors have stressed the necessity of a better knowledge of brain activity in response to noxious stimuli in VS and MCS (Klein, 1997; McQuillen, 1991; Multi-Society Task Force on PVS, 1994). Noxious stimulation is also a routine clinical procedure in the bedside assessment of consciousness in brain-damaged patients. We investigated by means of $H_2^{15}O$-PET the cortical responses to noxious electrical stimulation of the median nerve at the wrist in 15 PVS patients compared to 15 controls (Laureys et al., 2002). Demographic data of controls and vegetative patients are reported above. PET data were pre-processed and analysed using SPM (random-effect analysis and functional connectivity analysis, as described above). For the random-effect analysis, three separate analyses were performed: one for the controls, one for VS patients and one interaction analysis looking at the differences of activation between VS patients and controls. Results were thresholded for the controls at whole-volume-corrected p value $<.05$, and for the patients at small-volume corrected p value $<.05$ (20 mm diameter sphere centred on peak voxels). The functional connectivity analysis looked for differences in modulation between primary somatosensory cortex and the rest of the brain in VS patients compared to controls. As we expected a large diversity of areas and no a priori areas could be suggested; results of the psychophysiological analysis were thresholded at $p < .05$ corrected for multiple comparisons.

In controls, painful stimuli activated a large set of areas known to be involved in pain processing: brainstem, thalamus, primary and secondary somatosensory cortex, insula, posterior parietal, superior temporal and anterior cingulate cortices. VS patients, despite their severe cerebral metabolic impairment, still activated brainstem, thalamus and primary somatosensory cortex. However, the functional connectivity analysis showed extended functional disconnections between primary somatosensory cortex and fronto-parietal association cortices in VS patients compared to controls. As previously described for auditory stimuli, the activation of primary somatosensory cortex in vegetative state patients was thus isolated and dissociated from higher-order associative cortices.

In sharp contrast to the VS, preliminary findings in an MCS patient show a close to normal neural activation in response to noxious stimulation. Most importantly, the MCS patient showed activation of the anterior cingulate cortex. This region is well known to be involved in pain unpleasantness or affect (Rainville et al., 1997).

CONCLUSION

Despite an apparent clinical similarity between MCS and VS, functional imaging data show striking differences in cortical segregation and integration between these two conditions. The extent of activation found in MCS patients in response to both auditory and noxious stimulation likely allows them to reach a certain level of sensory and affective perception. However, it is important to stress that these PET results were obtained at the population level and some individual VS patients may show more elaborate cerebral activation, especially when complex and meaningful stimuli are used. Cognitive evoked potential studies have indeed shown that stimulation complexity influences cerebral responsiveness in VS and MCS patients (Kotchoubey et al., 2003). Finally, in the absence of a complete understanding of the neural correlate necessary and sufficient for conscious perception it remains difficult to interpret functional imaging data in brain damaged patients as proof or disproof of their consciousness.

REFERENCES

ANA Committee on Ethical Affairs (1993). Persistent vegetative state: Report of the American Neurological Association Committee on Ethical Affairs. *Annals of Neurology, 33*, 386–390.

Andrews, K., Murphy, L., Munday, R., & Littlewood, C. (1996). Misdiagnosis of the vegetative state: Retrospective study in a rehabilitation unit. *British Medical Journal, 313*, 13–16.

Baars, B. J., Ramsoy, T. Z., & Laureys, S. (2003). Brain, conscious experience and the observing self. *Trends in Neuroscience, 26*, 671–675.

Bekinschtein, T., Leiguarda, R., Armony, J., Owen, A., Carpintiero, S., Niklison, J., et al. (2004). Emotion processing in the minimally conscious state. *Journal of Neurology, Neurosurgery, and Psychiatry, 75*, 788.

Boly, M., Faymonville, M. E., Peigneux, P., Lambermont, B., Damas, P., Del Fiore, G., et al. (2004). Auditory processing in severely brain injured patients: Differences between the minimally conscious state and the persistent vegetative state. *Archives of Neurology, 61*, 233–238.

Childs, N. L., Mercer, W. N., & Childs, H. W. (1993). Accuracy of diagnosis of persistent vegetative state. *Neurology, 43*, 1465–1467.

Friston, K. J. (1997). Analysing brain images: Principles and overview. In R. S. J. Frackowiak, K. J. Friston, C. D. Frith, R. J. Dolan, & J. C. Mazziotta (Eds.), *Human brain function* (pp. 25–41). San Diego: Academic Press.

Friston, K. J., Buechel, C., Fink, G. R., Morris, J., Rolls, E., & Dolan, R. J. (1997). Psychophysiological and modulatory interactions in neuroimaging. *Neuroimage, 6*, 218–229.

Giacino, J. T., Ashwal, S., Childs, N., Cranford, R., Jennett, B., Katz, D. I., et al. (2002). The minimally conscious state: Definition and diagnostic criteria. *Neurology, 58*, 349–353.

Hirsch, J., Kamal, A., Rodriguez-Moreno, D., Petrovich, N., Giacino, J., Plum, F., & Schiff, N. (2001). fMRI reveals intact cognitive systems in two minimally conscious patients. *Society for Neuroscience 30th Annual Meeting* (52914).

Holmes, A., & Friston, K. (1998). Generalisability, random effects and population inference. *Neuroimage, 7*, 754.

Klein, M. (1997). Perception of pain in the persistent vegetative state? *European Journal of Pain, 1*, 165–167; 167–168 discussion.

Kotchoubey, B., Lang, S., Herb, E., Maurer, P., Schmalohr, D., Bostanov, V., & Birbaumer, N. (2003). Stimulus complexity enhances auditory discrimination in patients with extremely severe brain injuries. *Neuroscience Letters, 352*, 129–132.

Laureys, S., Faymonville, M. E., Degueldre, C., Fiore, G. D., Damas, P., Lambermont, B., et al. (2000). Auditory processing in the vegetative state. *Brain, 123*, 1589–1601.

Laureys, S., Faymonville, M. E., Peigneux, P., Damas, P., Lambermont, B., Del Fiore, G., et al. (2002). Cortical processing of noxious somatosensory stimuli in the persistent vegetative state. *Neuroimage, 17*, 732–741.

Laureys, S., Perrin, F., Faymonville, M., Schnakers, C., Boly, M., Bartsch, V., et al. (2004). Cerebral processing in the minimally conscious state. *Neurology, 63*, 916–918.

McQuillen, M. P. (1991). Can people who are unconscious or in the "vegetative state" perceive pain? *Issues in Law & Medicine, 6*, 373–383.

Menon, D. K., Owen, A. M., Williams, E. J., Minhas, P. S., Allen, C. M., Boniface, S. J., & Pickard, J. D. (1998). Cortical processing in persistent vegetative state. *Lancet, 352*, 200.

Multi-Society Task Force on PVS (1994). Medical aspects of the persistent vegetative state (1). *New England Journal of Medicine, 330*, 1499–1508.

Owen, A. M., Menon, D. K., Johnsrude, I. S., Bor, D., Scott, S. K., Manly, T., et al. (2002). Detecting residual cognitive function in persistent vegetative state. *Neurocase, 8*, 394–403.

Plum, F., Schiff, N., Ribary, U., & Llinas, R. (1998). Coordinated expression in chronically unconscious persons. *Philosophical Transactions of the Royal Society of London. Series B, Biological Sciences, 353*, 1929–1933.

Rainville, P., Duncan, G. H., Price, D. D., Carrier, B., & Bushnell, M. C. (1997). Pain affect encoded in human anterior cingulate but not somatosensory cortex. *Science, 277*, 968–971.

Schiff, N., Ribary, U., Plum, F., & Llinas, R. (1999). Words without mind. *Journal of Cognitive Neuroscience, 11*, 650–656.

Schiff, N. D., Ribary, U., Moreno, D. R., Beattie, B., Kronberg, E., Blasberg, R., et al. (2002). Residual cerebral activity and behavioural fragments can remain in the persistently vegetative brain. *Brain, 125*, 1210–1234.

Teasdale, G., & Jennett, B. (1974). Assessment of coma and impaired consciousness. A practical scale. *Lancet, 2*, 81–84.

NEUROPSYCHOLOGICAL REHABILITATION
2005, 15 (3/4), 290–306

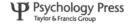

Residual auditory function in persistent vegetative state: A combined PET and fMRI study

Adrian M. Owen[1,2], Martin R. Coleman[2], David K. Menon[2],
Ingrid S. Johnsrude[1], Jennifer M. Rodd[3], Matthew H. Davis[1],
Karen Taylor[1], and John D. Pickard[2]

[1]MRC Cognition and Brain Sciences Unit, Cambridge, UK
[2]Wolfson Brain Imaging Centre and the Cambridge Coma Study Group,
Addenbrooke's Hospital, Cambridge, UK
[3]Department of Psychology, University College London, UK

In recent years, a number of studies have demonstrated an important role for functional neuroimaging in the identification of residual cognitive function in persistent vegetative state. Such studies, when successful, may be particularly useful where there is concern about the accuracy of the diagnosis and the possibility that residual cognitive function has remained undetected. Unfortunately, functional neuroimaging in persistent vegetative state is extremely complex and subject to numerous methodological, clinical and theoretical difficulties. Here, we describe the strategy used to study residual auditory and speech processing in a single patient with a clinical diagnosis of persistent vegetative state. Identical positron emission tomography studies, conducted nine months apart, revealed preserved and consistent responses in predicted regions of auditory cortex in response to intelligible speech stimuli. Moreover, a preliminary functional magnetic resonance imaging examination at the time of the second session revealed partially intact responses to semantically ambiguous stimuli, which are known to tap higher aspects of speech comprehension. In spite of the multiple logistic and procedural problems involved, these results have

Correspondence should be sent to Adrian M. Owen, MRC Cognition and Brain Sciences Unit, 15 Chaucer Road, Cambridge CB2 2EF, UK. Email: adrian.owen@mrc-cbu.cam.ac.uk

We are indebted to the Wolfson Brain Imaging Centre Team for their role in acquiring the data for the patient described in this manuscript and to Dr Roger R. Barker for his neurological assessment. We would also like to gratefully acknowledge the help of the Wellcome Trust Clinical Research Facility and the clinical and nursing staff in the University Department of Anaesthesia and in particular, Dot Chatfield, Jo Outtrim, Jurgens Nortje, and Peter Bradley.

© 2005 Psychology Press Ltd
http://www.tandf.co.uk/journals/pp/09602011.html   DOI:10.1080/09602010443000579

major clinical and theoretical implications and provide a strong basis for the systematic study of possible residual cognitive function in patients diagnosed as being in a persistent vegetative state.

INTRODUCTION

An accurate and reliable evaluation of the level and content of cognitive processing is of paramount importance for the appropriate management of patients diagnosed with persistent vegetative state (PVS). Objective behavioural assessment of residual cognitive function can be extremely difficult in these patients, as motor responses may be minimal, inconsistent, and difficult to document, or may be undetectable because no cognitive output is possible. In recent years, a number of studies have demonstrated an important role for functional neuroimaging in the identification of residual cognitive function in PVS patients. Unlike resting blood flow and glucose metabolism, which provide markers of neural capacity and potential, activation methods such as H_2 ^{15}O positron emission tomography (PET) and functional magnetic resonance imaging (fMRI) can be used to link residual neural activity to the presence of covert cognitive *function*. In short, functional neuroimaging has the potential to demonstrate distinct and specific physiological responses (changes in regional cerebral blood flow, rCBF, or changes in regional cerebral haemodynamics) to controlled external stimulation in the absence of any overt response on the part of the patient. In the first of such studies, H_2 ^{15}O PET was used to measure rCBF in a post-traumatic PVS patient during an auditorily-presented story told by his mother (de Jong, Willemsen, Paans, 1997). Compared to non-word sounds, activation was observed in the anterior cingulate and temporal cortices, possibly reflecting emotional processing of the contents, or tone, of the mother's speech. In another patient diagnosed as PVS, Menon et al. (1998) also used PET, but to study covert *visual* processing in response to familiar faces. During "experimental" scans, the patient was presented with pictures of the faces of family and close friends, while during "control" scans scrambled versions of the same images were presented which contained no meaningful visual information whatsoever. Previous imaging studies in healthy volunteers have shown such tasks to produce robust activity in the right fusiform gyrus, the so-called human "face area" (e.g. Haxby et al., 1991, 1994). The same visual association region was activated in the PVS patient when the familiar face stimuli were compared to the meaningless visual images (Menon et al., 1998; Owen et al., 2002). In other cohort studies, both noxious somatosensory stimuli (Laureys, Majerus, & Moonen, 2002) and auditory stimuli (Boly et al., 2004; Owen et al., 2002) have also been shown to systematically activate appropriate cortical regions in patients meeting the clinical criteria for PVS.

In this study we combined $H_2{}^{15}O$ PET with fMRI to study covert auditory processing in a patient with a probable clinical diagnosis of PVS. The decision to use auditory (language) stimuli was made, in part, on the basis of partially preserved brainstem auditory evoked responses (BAER). In an initial PET study, a hierarchical auditory processing test of graded complexity was employed (Davis & Johnsrude, 2003; Scott, Blank, Rosen, & Wise, 2000). This task allows neural responses to the processing of the linguistic content of spoken sentences (words and meanings) to be examined, relative to their more general acoustic properties. Preserved speech-related cortical responses were observed and on this basis a decision was made to reassess the patient following an interval of approximately nine months, during which time there was no significant change in his clinical condition. First, an identical PET study was carried out to ascertain whether the preserved cortical responses observed during the first session were still evident. Second, an fMRI study was conducted, using the phenomenon of semantic ambiguity to examine activity in regions of the brain that are involved in the semantic aspects of speech comprehension, in particular the processes of activating, selecting and integrating contextually appropriate word meanings (Rodd, Davis, & Johnsrude, in press). When words have more than one meaning, contextual information must be used to identify the appropriate meaning. For example, for the sentence "The boy was frightened by the loud bark", the listener must work out that the ambiguous word "bark" refers to the sound made by a dog and not the outer covering of a tree. This requires additional processing by those brain regions involved in activating and selecting contextually appropriate word meanings (Rodd et al., in press).

MATERIALS AND METHODS

Case history

The patient was a 30-year-old male with a diagnosis of basilar thrombosis and a posterior circulation infarction. In early June 2003, he collapsed with a severe headache and quickly became unresponsive. By the following day, he was drowsy, with a left partial Horner's syndrome, horizontal nystagmus, right hemiparesis and bilateral upgoing plantars. An MRI scan revealed an infarction of the left pons, cerebellum and posterior thalamus, which was still clearly evident at the time of the first PET scan four months post-ictus (Figure 1). Consciousness fluctuated for the next few days until the patient became unconscious with absent dolls eyes movement. At that stage, one week post-ictus, angiography revealed severe basilar stenosis. Two recombinant tissue plasminogen activator infusions produced some improvement,

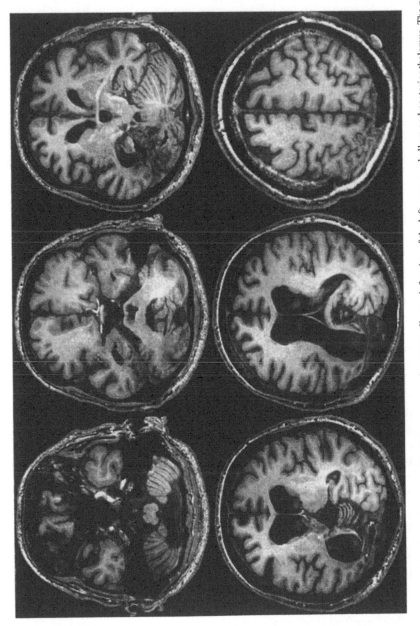

Figure 1. Structural MRI taken in October 2003 (4 months post-ictus) revealing an infarction of the left pons, cerebellum and posterior thalamus. The patient's left hemisphere appears left of figure.

293

although, following a brief spell of partial recovery after the anaesthesia had worn off, he deteriorated into a deep state of unconsciousness. Three weeks post-ictus the patient left the intensive care unit and to date he has not recovered. During the acute care period a BAER and a passive mismatch negativity (MMN) odd-ball paradigm were conducted. The BAER revealed preserved responses bilaterally from the pons and midbrain, although the onset of the midbrain component and consequently peak III–V interpeak interval was increased bilaterally. An MMN superior temporal N1 response was also observed, however, an N2 discriminating response was absent. Following sequential multidisciplinary assessment a diagnosis of PVS was made.

In October 2003, four months post-ictus, a decision was made to investigate the possibility of residual cognitive functions using PET and a novel language intelligibility task. Nine months later an identical PET activation study was performed, both to assess the reproducibility of the technique and to establish whether there had been any significant deterioration in cortical activity. On the same day, an event-related fMRI study was performed using the phenomenon of semantic ambiguity to examine activity in regions of the brain that are involved in the semantic aspects of speech comprehension. Informed written assent for participation was obtained for the patient from the next-of-kin after the nature of the study and possible consequences had been fully explained. The study was approved by the Cambridgeshire Local Research and Ethics Committee.

Stimuli and testing conditions

Auditory intelligibility (PET studies).   In the two PET studies, the patient underwent a spoken language comprehension task. This involved the use of 189 declarative English sentences, on a range of topics, comprising 5–17 words (1.7–4.3 s in duration) taken from the test sentences used in a previous study (Davis & Johnsrude, 2003). A form of distortion (speech in noise) was generated by adding a continuous pink-noise background to these sentences at three signal-to-noise ratios (-1, -4, or -6 dB), using Praat software (www.praat.org). This form of distortion disrupts both the spectral and temporal properties of speech, while preserving the duration, amplitude and overall spectral composition of the original. In a previous study using the same stimuli (Davis & Johnsrude, 2003), participants' word report scores (calculated as the proportion of words per sentence that were reported correctly) and the rated intelligibility of stimuli were reliably correlated ($r = .99$, $p < .001$). Within each condition there were three trials. Thus, there were three "high intelligibility" trials, three "medium intelligibility" trials and three "low intelligibility" trials (totalling nine stimulus presentations in the experimental phase). Within conditions, the three trials varied *in content only*; the signal-to-noise ratio remained the same but the sentences differed.

Each trial comprised 21 declarative "speech in noise" sentences, with a 1 s gap between each sentence. The total time taken to play each trial was approximately 100 s. The study also contained a control condition (also undertaken three times) during which no stimuli were presented. In total therefore, 12 scans were performed (3×3 experimental conditions; 1×3 control condition).

Each PET scan lasted 90 s and the stimuli were initiated 5 s before scanning began. The scans were separated by 8 min and the order in which the conditions were administered was pseudorandomly arranged.

Semantic ambiguity (fMRI study). There were two experimental conditions (high-ambiguity sentences and low-ambiguity sentences) and a low-level noise baseline condition. There were 59 items in each of these three conditions. The high-ambiguity sentences all contained at least two ambiguous words (e.g., there were *dates* and *pears* in the fruit bowl). The ambiguous words were either homonyms (two meanings that have the same spelling and pronunciation; e.g., 'bark'), or homophones (two meanings that have the same pronunciation but different spelling; e.g., "knight"/"night"). Each high-ambiguity sentence was matched to a low-ambiguity sentence that had the same number of words and the same syntactic structure but contained words with minimal ambiguity (e.g., there was beer and cider on the kitchen shelf). The two sets of sentences were matched for the number of syllables, physical duration, rated naturalness, rated imageability, and the log-transformed mean frequency of the content words in the CELEX database (Baayen, Piepenbrock, & Gulikers, 1995). The imageability and naturalness scores came from pretests in which groups of healthy participants listened to the sentences and rated how imageable or natural they were on a 9-point Likert scale (Rodd et al., in press).

A set of 59 sentences that had not been used as experimental stimuli, but were matched for number of syllables, number of words and physical duration to the experimental sentences, were converted to signal-correlated noise (Schroeder, 1968) using Praat software. These stimuli had the same spectral profile and amplitude envelope as the original speech, but since all spectral detail was replaced with noise they were entirely unintelligible and they were used as a low-level baseline condition.

A sparse imaging technique was used (Hall et al., 1999), to minimise interference from scanner noise. The patient was played a single sentence (or noise-equivalent) in the 7.4 s silent period before a single 1.6 s scan. The timing of stimulus onset and offset was jittered relative to scan onset by temporally aligning the midpoint of the stimulus item (0.6 to 2.2 s after sentence onset) with a point that was 5 s before the mid-point of the subsequent scan.

There were 59 trials of each sentence type and an additional 21 silent trials for the purpose of monitoring data quality. The experiment was divided into three sessions of 66 sentences. Sentences were pseudorandomised to ensure that the three experimental conditions and rest scans were evenly distributed among the three sessions, and that each condition occurred equally often after each of the other conditions. The sentences were presented diotically using a high-fidelity auditory stimulus-delivery system incorporating flat-response electrostatic headphones inserted into sound-attenuating ear defenders (Palmer, Bullock, & Chambers, 1998). To further attenuate scanner noise, the patient wore insert earplugs. DMDX software running on a Windows 98 PC (Forster & Forster, 2003) was used to present the stimulus items.

Image acquisition and data analysis

PET scans were obtained with the General Electrics Advance system, which produces 35 image slices at an intrinsic resolution of approximately $4.0 \times 5.0 \times 4.5$ mm. The patient underwent two separate PET investigations, comprising 12 scans each. Using the bolus $H_2{}^{15}O$ methodology, rCBF was measured during the 12 separate scans. For each scan, the patient received a 20 s intravenous bolus of $H_2{}^{15}O$ through a forearm cannula at a concentration of 300 Mbq ml^{-1} and a flow rate of 10 ml min^{-1}. With this method, each scan provides a static image of rCBF integrated over a period of 90 s from when the tracer first enters the cerebral circulation. The 12 PET scans were realigned using the first scan as a reference, normalised for global CBF value and averaged within each session for each activation state (experimental task and control task). The images were then smoothed using an isotropic Gaussian kernel at 16 mm. Finally, a simple ANCOVA (analysis of covariance) model was fitted to the data at each voxel, as implemented by the method of Statistical Parametric Mapping (SPM99, Wellcome Department of Imaging Neuroscience, London, UK), with a condition effect for each of the conditions, using global CBF as a confounding covariate. A 3D MRI volume ($256 \times 256 \times 128$ pixels, 3 mm thick) was acquired and resliced so as to be coregistered with the PET data. The significance of a given rCBF difference was assessed by application of an intensity threshold to the SPM images (Worsley, Evans, Marrett, & Neelin, 1992; Worsley et al., 1996). This threshold, based on 3D Gaussian random field theory, predicts the likelihood of obtaining a false positive in an extended 3D field.

The fMRI imaging data was acquired using a Bruker Medspec (Ettlingen, Germany) 3-Tesla MR system with a head gradient set. A total of 198 echoplanar image volumes were acquired over three 12-min sessions. Each volume consisted of 21×4 mm thick slices with an interslice gap of 1 mm; FOV: 25×25 cm; matrix size, 128×128, TE = 27 ms; acquisition time 1.6 s; actual TR = 9 s. Acquisition was transverse-oblique, angled away from the eyes, and covered all of the brain.

The data were pre-processed and analysed using Statistical Parametric Mapping software (SPM99, Wellcome Department of Imaging Neuroscience, London, UK). Pre-processing steps included within-subject realignment, and spatial smoothing using a Gaussian kernel of 12 mm. Analysis was conducted using a single General Linear Model in which each scan within each session (after excluding two initial dummy volumes) was coded for whether it followed the presentation of signal correlated noise, a low-ambiguity or a high-ambiguity sentence. Each of the three scanning runs was modelled separately within the design matrix. Additional columns encoded subject movement (as calculated from the realignment stage of preprocessing) as well as a constant term for each of the three scanning runs.

Determination of a priori defined regions of interest. Each study was designed to test anatomically specific hypotheses as both of the tasks used are known to produce well-documented, specific, robust and reproducible activation patterns in normal volunteers (Davis & Johnsrude, 2003; Rodd et al., in press). The graded complexity speech task used in the PET studies has been shown previously to produce activity, related to the intelligibility of the presented stimuli, in the left anterior and superior temporal lobe (Davis & Johnsrude, 2003; Scott et al., 2000). Importantly, this task also includes a "silence" baseline condition, making a more general comparison of speech (collapsed across different levels of background noise) versus silence possible. Many previous studies in healthy volunteers have shown that such comparisons produce bilateral activity in an extensive region of the superior temporal gyrus, incorporating Heschel's gyrus and the planum temporale (Davis & Johnsrude, 2003; Mummery, Ashburner, Scott, & Wise, 1999; Scott et al., 2000). The semantic ambiguity task has been used previously in healthy volunteers to investigate the network of brain regions that is involved in computing the meaning of speech (Rodd et al., in press). Relative to low-ambiguity sentences, high-ambiguity stimuli produce increases in signal intensity in the left posterior inferior temporal cortex and inferior frontal gyri bilaterally. Again, this task also incorporated two baseline conditions involving either silence or signal correlated noise, making the more general comparison of speech perception (irrespective of ambiguity) versus acoustically-controlled non-speech stimuli as well as silence possible. Previous studies in healthy volunteers have shown that such comparisons produce bilateral (although commonly stronger in the dominant hemisphere), activity in the superior and middle temporal gyri (Davis & Johnsrude, 2003; Mummery et al., 1999; Rodd et al., in press; Scott et al., 2000).

In spite of this background, single subject studies using PET or fMRI are rare and, compared to the commonly used group designs, are very under-powered. Accordingly, for the comparisons described above, a directed search was conducted within the regions identified by the studies in healthy volunteers and the threshold for reporting a peak was set at $p < .001$, uncorrected for multiple comparisons. For the rest of the brain an exploratory search involving all peaks within the grey matter (volume 600 cm^3) was conducted and the threshold for reporting a peak was set at $p < .05$, corrected for multiple comparisons.

RESULTS

Auditory intelligibility (PET studies)

During the first PET study, 4 months post-ictus, the comparison of speech (collapsed across the three levels of intelligibility) with the silence baseline condition revealed significant foci of activation over the left and right superior temporal planes (see Figure 2, top left) suggesting that basic auditory processes were probably functional.

With this in mind, a second comparison was made comparing low intelligibility sentences with high intelligibility sentences in order to isolate any residual activity related specifically to the comprehension of spoken language. This comparison revealed two peaks in the superior and middle temporal gyri of the left hemisphere (see Figure 2, bottom left). Although neither of these peaks approaches whole-brain conventional levels of corrected significance, they are well within the region that has been shown to be activated in healthy volunteers during this same task (Davis & Johnsrude, 2003). The results of additional comparisons, between the high and medium intelligibility conditions, for example, were entirely consistent with, but did not add to, these results, yielding peaks of activation that were weaker, but at similar co-ordinates.

During the second PET study, 13 months post-ictus, the comparison of speech (collapsed across the three levels of intelligibility) with the silence baseline condition revealed several foci of activation over the superior and middle temporal gyri of the left and right hemispheres (see Figure 2, top right), suggesting again that basic auditory processes were probably functional.

The second comparison, comparing low intelligibility sentences with high intelligibility sentences revealed two peaks in the brain in the superior and middle temporal gyrus of the left hemisphere (see Figure 2, bottom right). Although not significant, these peaks are well within the region found to be activated in healthy volunteers during this same task (Davis & Johnsrude, 2003). Similarly, the activation foci are extremely close to those regions that were activated by the same comparison in the patient, nine months earlier (see Figure 2, bottom left).

In the semantic ambiguity fMRI study, the contrast between all the speech conditions (irrespective of ambiguity) plus the signal correlated noise versus silence baseline yielded a pattern of activation very similar to the speech versus silence contrast of the initial PET investigation, although all of these

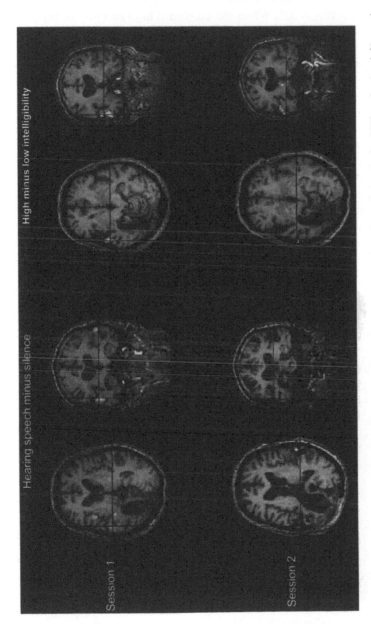

Figure 2. Activation data from the two PET sessions, nine months apart. (1) Hearing speech minus silence during the first PET session (top left) reveals activity bilaterally in the superior temporal gyrus. (2) Hearing speech minus silence during the second PET session (bottom left) reveals very similar activity bilaterally in the superior temporal gyrus. (3) High intelligibility speech minus low intelligibility speech during the first PET session (top right) reveals activity predominantly in the left superior temporal gyrus. (4) High intelligibility speech minus low intelligibility speech during the second PET session (bottom right) reveals very similar activity predominantly in the left superior temporal gyrus. The patient's left hemisphere appears left of figure.

299

changes were statistically significant. Thus, large areas of activity were observed bilaterally in the middle and superior temporal gyri all of which survived correction at $p < .05$. When the combined high and low ambiguity sentences were compared to signal correlated noise, significant changes in signal intensity were again observed, bilaterally, in the middle and superior temporal gyri (see Figure 3, upper panel), a pattern which is very similar to that observed in healthy volunteers (see Figure 3 lower panel; see also Rodd et al., in press). This activity, although distributed over a larger area of the temporal cortex, incorporates that region that was activated in the comparison between high and low intelligibility sentences in both of the previous PET studies in this same patient (see Figure 2). In addition to the temporal lobe foci, an area of significantly increased activity was also seen in the left inferior frontal gyrus (see Figure 3).

For the high-ambiguity sentences compared to low-ambiguity sentences no statistically significant increases in signal intensity were observed anywhere in the brain when a conservative whole brain correction method was employed. A directed search within the predicted left posterior inferior temporal cortices and the inferior frontal gyrus, bilaterally, was then conducted

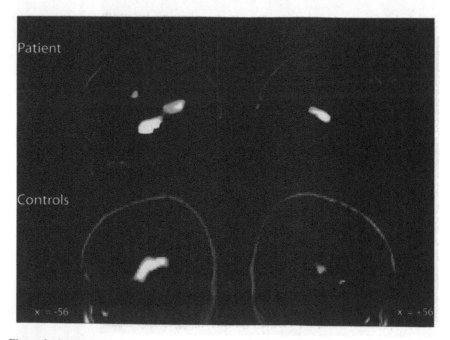

Figure 3. fMRI data from the hearing speech (ambiguous plus unambiguous sentences) minus signal correlated noise contrast. In both the patient (top) and a group of healthy volunteers (bottom; from Rodd et al., in press) a very similar pattern of signal intensity changes is observed in the superior temporal lobe, bilaterally.

using a regions of interest (ROI) generated from an independent data set obtained previously in healthy volunteers (Rodd et al., in press). Because the data from the patient were not spatially normalised, it was necessary to use anatomical landmarks identified by one member of the research team (DKM) who was blind to the hypothesis, to identify the appropriate regions for analysis in the patient. The ROI analysis revealed responses in the patient that were well within the normal range in the left posterior inferior temporal region, but there was no evidence for the predicted changes in the inferior frontal gyrus in either hemisphere (Figure 4).

DISCUSSION

In this exploratory study, we investigated how longitudinal functional neuro-imaging might be used to investigate residual auditory processing in a single

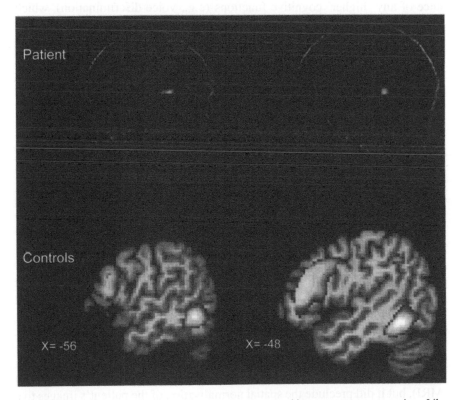

Figure 4. fMRI data for the ambiguous sentences versus unambiguous sentences comparison. Like controls (bottom; from Rodd et al., in press), the patient exhibited significant signal intensity changes in the left posterior inferior temporal cortex, but (unlike controls), not in the inferior frontal gyrus.

patient meeting the clinical criteria for PVS. Two established auditory paradigms, involving speech intelligibility and semantic ambiguity, respectively, were employed during two (repeated) PET activation studies and one fMRI investigation. The results clearly illustrate that functional neuroimaging has the potential to demonstrate distinct and specific physiological responses to controlled external stimulation in the absence of any overt response on the part of the patient. They also clearly demonstrate, however, that the technique poses a number of unique methodological, ethical and procedural problems. For example, like most patients diagnosed as PVS, motor responses were minimal in the patient studied here and by definition could not be elicited directly (e.g., wilfully) by external stimulation. In addition, even if we had assumed *a priori* that some level of residual cognitive processing did exist, there was no reliable mechanism for ensuring that the presented stimuli were actually *perceived* by the patient. Many PVS patients suffer serious damage to auditory and/or visual input systems, which may impede performance of any 'higher' cognitive functions (e.g., voice discrimination), which place demands on these "lower" sensory systems (e.g., hearing). In both of the paradigms selected here (speech intelligibility and semantic ambiguity), the various levels of processing assessed were designed to have broadly similar basic acoustic and sensory properties; thus, any differences observed *between* those levels could not be attributed to a basic lack of perception on the part of the patient. Like patients with any form of serious brain damage, PVS may also be accompanied by a significant reduction in attention span (assuming some level of cognitive processing remains), which may further complicate the assessment of higher cognitive functions. Again, in the current study, the paradigms were chosen such that different levels of each task made similar demands on attention. For example, in healthy volunteers, the ambiguity in the sentences used in the fMRI study goes largely unnoticed (Rodd et al., in press). The additional semantic processes that are required for the comprehension of ambiguous sentences are invoked relatively "automatically", without healthy participants reporting that they were aware of the increased difficulty of comprehension. Thus, semantic ambiguity appears to recruit additional comprehension processes that may be dependent on the inferior temporal and frontal regions without these processes being deliberately and consciously invoked.

Finally, data processing of functional neuroimaging data may also present challenging problems in patients with PVS. In the current study, for example, the presence of focal pathology did not complicate co-registration of functional data (PET and fMRI) to anatomical data (e.g., acquired using structural MRI), but it did preclude the spatial normalisation of the patient's images to a healthy reference brain. Under these circumstances statistical assessment of activation patterns is anatomically imprecise and activation foci could not be localised in terms of standard stereotaxic coordinates.

Notwithstanding these methodological and theoretical caveats, the current study yielded compelling evidence for high level residual auditory processing in the PVS patient. Thus, at four months post-ictus, a comparison of speech sounds with silence yielded activity bilaterally in a region of the superior temporal gyrus very similar to that which has been activated using similar comparisons in healthy volunteers. More importantly, a comparison of high intelligibility sentences with low intelligibility sentences designed to isolate any residual activity related specifically to the comprehension of spoken language revealed two foci in the patient in the superior and middle temporal gyri of the dominant (left) hemisphere. While it was not possible to relate these foci to control data within standard stereotaxic space (because spatial normalisation of the damaged brain was not possible) a qualitative comparison with data from healthy volunteers revealed remarkable similarity between the two (Davis & Johnsrude, 2003). More importantly perhaps, the pattern of activation observed during the first PET study was both qualitatively and quantitatively similar to that observed nine months later when an identical procedure was carried out. Although anatomical and global blood flow factors preclude direct statistical comparisons between the two sessions, examination of Figure 2 reveals a startling similarity between the activation patterns observed in temporal-lobe auditory areas in both cases. In short, notwithstanding qualitative differences that are well within the range that would be expected given normal inter-subject variability, the pattern of activation observed in the patient during the two PET sessions was similar to that observed in healthy awake control volunteers while performing identical tasks.

This finding has a number of important theoretical and clinical implications. First and foremost, it suggests that whatever level of residual cognitive activity existed in the patient, it was persistent across time and remains, at least until 13 months post-ictus. Second, the results suggest that some level of speech comprehension is preserved in this patient; the different activation patterns observed could not simply be due to the perception of sounds in general as the basic acoustic properties of the stimuli were well matched across conditions. However, whether the responses observed reflected speech comprehension per se (i.e., understanding the contents of spoken language), or a more basic response to the acoustic properties of intelligible speech that distinguish it from less intelligible speech could not be determined on the basis of this data alone.

The fMRI study in the same patient both confirmed and extended the PET investigations. Thus, a comparison of speech with signal correlated noise revealed bilateral changes in signal intensity in the middle and superior temporal gyri that, unlike the PET data, survived statistical correction for multiple comparisons (Figure 3). This finding suggests that in future, fMRI may provide a statistically more robust approach to the assessment of PVS patients using functional neuroimaging. The findings also add to the corpus of data in this patient suggesting that some level of speech comprehension was intact despite the clinical diagnosis. The comparison of ambiguous versus unambiguous sentences in this patient partially confirmed this suggestion still further and, in addition, suggests that some of the semantic aspects of speech comprehension are partially preserved. Thus, signal intensity changes within the normal range were observed in the posterior inferior temporal lobe when ambiguous sentences were compared with unambiguous sentences, although (unlike healthy volunteers), consistent activation was not observed in the inferior frontal gyrus. These results suggest that some of the processes involved in activating and selecting contextually appropriate word meaning may be intact in the patient, despite his clinical diagnosis of PVS.

The question therefore arises as to whether the presence of some "normal" activation in this patient indicates some level of "awareness" similar to that which (presumably) exists in healthy volunteers when performing similar tasks. One possibility, which must be considered, is that the diagnosis of PVS was unwarranted in this case and the patient was in fact at a stage of recovery which, while eluding conventional diagnosis, nevertheless yielded patterns of activation that were similar to those seen in healthy control volunteers. If that were the case, then the possibility of "minimal awareness" as an accompaniment to, and partial explanation for, the neural changes observed cannot be ruled out. Notwithstanding this possibility, definitive judgements regarding "awareness" or "consciousness" in this and similar patients are difficult based on the data presented here, although a number of clear conclusions can be drawn. For example, it is clear that the patient was perceiving something more complex than pure sound (as indexed by the significantly increased activity in response to speech relative to signal correlated noise), confirming that some component of the *perception* of speech was relatively preserved. Second, the fact that a significant response was observed to speech of increasing intelligibility suggests that these perceptual processes are recruited more strongly for speech that can be more readily understood. These results could be interpreted as suggesting that *comprehension* may also have been relatively preserved. One piece of evidence that supports this final conclusion was our observation of a significant response to ambiguous sentences, showing that some *semantic* aspect of sentences can alter neural activity; in other words, not only did the patient's brain recognise speech as speech, but it was also being processed at a level sufficient to detect when words with multiple meanings were presented. Whether this semantic activity can also be elicited in other situations in which sentences are not consciously perceived (e.g., during sleep) remains a critical issue for future investigations with normal volunteers.

In summary, there is a clear need to improve our characterisation of the clinical syndrome of PVS, not only to redefine diagnosis, but also to stratify patients in terms of the depth and breadth of residual cognitive functioning. This has major implications, not only for prognosis, but also for possible responses to novel therapies that may emerge in the future. The use of functional neuroimaging in this context will clearly continue to present logistic and procedural problems. However, the detection and elucidation of residual cognitive function in this group of patients has such major clinical and scientific implications that such an effort is clearly justified.

REFERENCES

Baayen, R. H., Piepenbrock, R., & Gulikers, L. (1995). *The CELEX Lexical Database* [CD-ROM]. Linguistic Data Consortium, University of Pennsylvania, Philadelphia, PA.

Boly, M., Faymonville, M. E., Peigneux, P., Lambermont, B., Damas, P., Del Fiore, G., Degueldre, C., Franck, G., Luxen, A., Lamy, M., Moonen. G., Maquet, P., & Laureys, S. (2004). Auditory processing in severely brain injured patients: Differences between the minimally conscious state and the persistent vegetative state. *Archives of Neurology, 61*, 233–238.

Davis, M. H., & Johnsrude, I. S. (2003). Hierarchical processing in spoken language comprehension. *Journal of Neuroscience, 23*(8), 3423–3431.

de Jong, B., Willemsen, A. T., & Paans, A. M. (1997). Regional cerebral blood flow changes related to affective speech presentation in persistent vegetative state. *Clinical Neurology and Neurosurgery, 99*, 213–216.

Forster, K. I., & Forster, J. C. (2003). A Windows display program with millisecond accuracy. *Behavior Research Methods Instruments & Computers, 35*, 116–124.

Hall, D. A., Haggard, M. P, Akeroyd, M. A., Palmer, A. R., Summerfield, A. Q., Elliott, M. R., Gurney, E. M., & Bowtell, R. W. (1999). "Sparse" temporal sampling in auditory fMRI. *Human Brain Mapping, 7*, 213–223.

Haxby, J. V., Grady, C. L., Horwitz, B., Ungerleider, L. G., Mishkin, M., Carson, R. E., Herscovitch, P., Schapiro, M. B., & Rapoport, S. I. (1991). Dissociation of object and spatial visual processing pathways in human extrastriate cortex. *Proceedings of the National Academy of Science USA, 88*, 1621–1625.

Haxby, J. V., Horwitz, B., Ungerlieder, L. G., Maisog, J. M., Pietrini, P., & Grady, C. L. (1994). The functional organization of human extrastriate cortex: A PET-rCBF study of selective attention to faces and locations. *Journal of Neuroscience, 14*, 6336–6353.

Laureys, S., Majerus, S., & Moonen, G. (2002). Assessing consciousness in critically ill patients. In J. L. Vincent (Ed.), *Yearbook of intensive care and emergency medicine* (pp. 715–727). Heidelberg: Springer-Verlag.

Menon, D. K., Owen, A. M., Williams, E. J., Kendall, I. V., Downey, S. P. M. J., Minhas, P. S., Allen, C. M. C., Boniface, S., Antoun, N., & Pickard, J. D. (1998). Cortical processing in the persistent vegetative state revealed by functional imaging. *Lancet, 352*, 200.

Mummery, C. J., Ashburner, J., Scott, S. K., & Wise, R. J. S. (1999). Functional neuroimaging of speech perception in six normal and two aphasic subjects. *Journal of the Acoustical Society of America, 106*, 449–456.

Owen, A. M, Menon, D. K., Johnsrude I. S., Bor, D., Scott, S. K., Manly, T., Williams, E. J., Mummery, C., & Pickard, J. D. (2002). Detecting residual cognitive function in persistent vegetative state. *Neurocase, 8*, 394–403.

Palmer, A. R., Bullock, D. C., & Chambers, J. D. (1998). A high output, high-quality sound system for use in auditory fMRI. *NeuroImage, 7*, S359.

Rodd, J. M., Davis, M. H., & Johnsrude, I. S. (in press). The neural mechanisms of speech comprehension: fMRI studies of semantic ambiguity. *Cerebral Cortex* [Epub ahead of print, Jan 5].

Schroeder, M. R. (1968). Reference signal for signal quality studies. *Journal of the Acoustic Society of America, 44*, 1735–1736.

Scott, S. K., Blank, C., Rosen, S., & Wise, R. J. S. (2000). Identification of a pathway for intelligible speech in the left temporal lobe. *Brain, 123*, 2400–2406.

Worsley K. J., Evans A. C., Marrett, S., & Neelin, P. (1992). Determining the number of statistically significant areas of activation in subtracted activation studies from PET. *Journal of Cerebral Blood Flow and Metabolism, 12*, 900–918.

Worsley, K. J, Marrett, S., Neelin, P., Vandal, A. C., Friston, K. J., & Evans, A. C. (1996). A unified statistical approach for determining significant signals in images of cerebral activation. *Human Brain Mapping, 4*, 58–73.

NEUROPSYCHOLOGICAL REHABILITATION
2005, 15 (3/4), 307–322

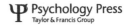

Assessing level of consciousness and cognitive changes from vegetative state to full recovery

Tristan Bekinschtein, Cecilia Tiberti, Jorge Niklison, Mercedes Tamashiro, Melania Ron, Silvina Carpintiero, Mirta Villarreal, Cecilia Forcato, Ramon Leiguarda, and Facundo Manes

Institute for Neurological Research (FLENI), Buenos Aires, Argentina

Although investigations addressing cognitive recovery from the vegetative state have been reported, to date there have been no detailed studies of these patients combining both neuropsychology and functional imaging to monitor and record the recovery of consciousness. This paper describes the recovery of a specific vegetative state (VS) case. The patient (OG) remained in the vegetative state for approximately two months, increasing her level of awareness to a minimally conscious state, where she continued for approximately 70 days. In the course of the ensuing 18 months, she was able to reach an acceptable level of cognitive functioning, with partial levels of independence. Throughout this two year period, she received continuous cognitive evaluation, for which several different tools were applied including coma and low functioning scales, full cognitive batteries, and structural and functional magnetic resonance imaging (MRI). We present here preliminary data on fMRI using a word presentation paradigm before and after recovery; we also discuss the difficulty of how to determine level of consciousness using the tools currently available, and the subsequent improvement in different cognitive domains. We confirm that accurate diagnosis and proper cognitive assessment are critical for the rehabilitation of patients with disorders of consciousness.

Correspondence should be sent to Facundo Manes, Cognitive Neurology Section, Neurology Department, Institute for Neurological Research (FLENI), Montañeses 2325 (C1428AQK), Buenos Aires, Argentina. Tel: (54) 11 5777 3200 ext 2802, Fax: (54) 11 5777 3209. Email: fmanes@fleni.org.ar

http://www.tandf.co.uk/journals/pp/09602011.html   DOI:10.1080/09602010443000443

INTRODUCTION

Disorders of consciousness can be categorised in terms of degree of patient awareness into different levels: (1) coma (very low arousal level and no awareness); (2) vegetative state (VS; higher level of arousal without awareness of self or environment); and (3) minimally conscious state (MCS; full arousal level and inconsistent but reproducible evidence of awareness) (Multi-Society Task Force on PVS, 1994; Giacino et al., 2002). However, these conditions can also be considered as a single awareness level continuum, ranging from coma to high minimally conscious state. Accurate diagnosis is crucial in low awareness patients, because of the potential effect on patient prognosis, as well as the way in which the families and/or caregivers perceive the condition.

New imaging techniques such as positron emission tomography (PET) and functional magnetic resonance imaging (fMRI) have been used to assess brain function in VS and MCS patients (see Laureys, Owen, & Schiff, 2004 for a recent review). Menon et al. published results from a patient in VS showing fusiform gyrus activity, indistinguishable from what was observed in control groups after presentation of facial stimuli (Menon et al., 1998). Recently, Laureys and coworkers reported increased activity in the auditory temporal area and related structures after click stimulation in VS patients, with decreased functional connectivity (Laureys et al., 2000). Higher brain activity was also found in MCS patients as compared to VS (Boly et al., 2004). Our group has recently reported a case of MCS that showed decreased temporal auditory cortex activity after speech stimuli presentation and increased amygdala activity while hearing a voice with emotional valence (Bekinschtein et al., 2004). To our knowledge, there are no reports of functional imaging during both VS and after recovery using complex stimuli.

The cognitive assessment plays a key role in the management of these patients with disorders of consciousness, due to the fact that even minimal improvement or change in behaviour may influence treatment and prognosis. However, simple cognitive tests traditionally used in clinical practice are insufficient to capture the subtle changes that may occur under different states of consciousness. The Rancho Los Amigos Scale or the Glasgow Coma Scale (GCS; Teasdale, Knill-Jones, & van der Sande, 1978) offer limited sensitivity compared to changes that can be detected using other more extended scales, such as the Coma Rating Scale (CRS; Giacino, Kalmar, & Whyte, 2004; Giacino, Kezmarsky, DeLuca, & Cicerone, 1991) or the Wessex Head Injury Matrix (WHIM; Shiel et al., 2000). These extended scales cover different cognitive and physiological responses, allowing improvement in different cognitive domains to be easily detected when patients are followed for weeks or even months (Wilson, Harpur, Watson, & Morrow, 2002).

To date, few detailed investigations addressing cognitive recovery from the vegetative state have been described. Barbara Wilson et al. have published one case in which a patient, having remained in VS/MCS for six months, underwent several cognitive assessments after recovery (Wilson, Gracey, & Bainbridge, 2001). This patient showed a slow pattern of cognitive improvement, only partly dependent on physical recuperation. Unfortunately, the data presented by Wilson's group lacked behavioural assessment while in VS and MCS and functional imaging after recovery. Other authors have used only limited cognitive assessments, and cognitive recovery was tested to a minimum degree (Passler & Riggs, 2001).

The objective of this study was, therefore, to redress this imbalance in the literature and to monitor and record the recovery of consciousness in a brain-injured patient (OG); initially diagnosed as vegetative, from very low functioning to high cognitive ability levels, combining a breadth of neuropsychological assessments with structural and functional imaging.

CASE REPORT

OG was 20 years old when she sustained a motor vehicle accident. She was transferred almost immediately, unconscious, to the nearest regional hospital. Six hours later she was admitted to FLENI Intensive Care Unit with a Glasgow Coma Scale (GCS) score of 3. On arrival the patient presented decerebration, bilateral decorticate posturing and unreactive right, and hyporeactive left pupils. On day 2, a computed tomography (CT) scan showed subarachnoideal haemorrhages and small concussions in the right frontal and left temporoparietal regions. She subsequently developed hydrocephalus and required ventriculoperitoneal shunt decompression. A follow-up CT scan on day 6 showed partial haemorrhagic lesions on the left side of the pons, as well as in the upper left cerebellum and right frontal subcortical regions. Hypodense lesions were also observed in the region surrounding the left catheter. A third CT scan on day 23 revealed a decrease in lesion size, with persistent limited bifrontal tissue hypodensities in the cortical and subcortical regions. These findings were confirmed through structural MRI on day 30. During the first month, both a tracheotomy and a gastrostomy were performed. The patient also presented central fever, tachycardia, hypertension and pneumonia during the acute phase of her condition. Only after the patient was clinically stable was she admitted to the FLENI Rehabilitation Centre (day 50) where she immediately began physical and occupational therapy, together with a complete multisensory stimulation programme. Methylphenidate and dopaminergic agonists were subsequently introduced aiming to improve arousal and other attentional mechanisms (Matsuda et al., 2003; Richer & Tell, 2003). For the first four months, patient level of consciousness was assessed using coma or low functioning assessment scales, and for the ensuing year and a half, Addenbrooke's Cognitive

Examination was used for patient cognitive status follow up. Also, two full cognitive batteries were administered during this second period and two fMRI studies were undertaken, the first during the VS phase, and the second after partial recovery.

Methods

Patient consciousness level was assessed following the Multi-Society Task Force on PVS Guidelines (1994) and the recent clinical definition of MCS (Giacino et al., 2002). Also, as behavioural assessment tools, the JFK Coma Recovery Scale (CRS; Giacino et al., 1991) was applied weekly, or every two weeks, and the Wessex Head Injury Matrix (WHIM; Shiel et al., 2000) was administered monthly. In addition, the Functional Independence Measure (FIM; Granger, Deutsch, & Linn, 1998) and Disability Rating Scale (DRS; Rappaport, Herrero-Backe, Rappaport, & Winterfield, 1989), were used both to monitor degree of disability and as measures of clinical outcome. All assessments were carried out by the same examiners, both for each scale and for the entire duration of the study.

Initial cognitive status of the patient was monitored using Bedside Language Assessment (BLA), a screening test battery developed at our centre specifically for low functioning patients; comprising spontaneous language tests, yes/no responses to specific questions, repetition tests, writing tests and reading tests. The maximum score for the BLA is 25/25 and patients with severe cognitive deficits, but capable of communication, usually reach this score. Once a ceiling effect for the BLA is observed, it is replaced with Addenbrooke's Cognitive Examination (ACE), which then became the cognitive tool that was need to follow OG's cognitive recovery. This test has six components evaluating separate cognitive domains: (1) orientation, (2) attention, (3) memory, (4) verbal fluency, (5) language, and (6) visual-spatial abilities (Mathuranath et al., 2000). Also, a complete cognitive evaluation was conducted on two separate occasions. The battery included the following tests: Raven's Progressive Matrices, the Rivermead Behavioural Memory Test (Wilson, Cockburn, Baddeley, & Hiorns, 1989), the Rey List, Logical Memory Test, Rey-Osterreith Complex Figure Test, the Wechsler Adult Intelligence Scale (WAIS III)—Digits Span, Vocabulary, Letter Number, and the Reitan Trail Making Test.

A Frontal Assessment Battery (FAB; Dubois, Slachevsky, Litvan, & Pillon, 2000) was used as a screening battery for frontal function three times during this study. FAB performance gives a composite global score, which evaluates the severity of the dysexecutive syndrome, and may suggest a descriptive pattern of executive dysfunction in a given patient. It consists of six subtests exploring conceptualisation, mental flexibility, motor programming, sensitivity to interference, inhibitory control and environmental autonomy, and takes approximately 10 minutes to administer.

An fMRI study was performed during VS and after recovery, including a 5 minute passive auditory task, consisting of 30-second blocks of silence, white noise and simple words as stimuli. The BOLD images were acquired using a T2-weighted gradient echo sequence (TR 3 s, 8 mm slice thickness), on a General Electric Signa CVI 1.5T system. Five slices covering the temporal lobe region were acquired both during stimulation periods and at rest. The data were analysed with SPM2 (developed by members and collaborators of the Wellcome Department of Imaging Neuroscience, London, UK). EPI images underwent slice-timing, realign and smooth processing, without normalisation because of the major differences occurring in brain tissue in the VS and after TBI. Activation maps were co-localised following co-registration with the corresponding anatomical T1-IR volume. A corrected significance threshold of $p < .05$ and an uncorrected p value of $< .001$ were used for comparative analysis.

Treatment

From day 50 until day 113 after trauma OG followed an integrative multisensory programme at the rehabilitation institute. The multidisciplinary team included an occupational therapist (OP), a physical therapist (PT), and a speech language pathologist (SPL). This approach is based on the application of combined visual, acoustic, tactile, taste and smell stimulation. Acoustic stimulation included reading familiar literature to the patient, playing her favourite music or bells, or exposing her to familiar voices; visual stimulation included showing her bright colourful objects or familiar items or pictures; olfactory stimulation involved exposure to familiar smells both pleasant and unpleasant; tactile stimulation included feeling objects of different texture and/or temperature, and buco-facial massage; kinaesthetic and proprioceptive stimulation included both vestibular and proprioceptive stimuli. General goals for this stage were to increase arousal and alertness, enhance recognition of the environment, and improve posture and body movement capacity. During this first rehabilitation period she underwent two two-hour sessions a day.

On day 114, a cognitive rehabilitation programme was started, where different goals were established depending on the degree of recovery already achieved. Initially, the focus was on sustained attention and orientation (daily individual 30 minute sessions). Higher cognitive functions including memory, executive functions, and abstract reasoning were addressed at a later stage. As an outpatient, she received both individual and group therapy, in an attempt to solve problems in daily living (such as memory deficits or social skills issues). As part of group therapy, she also began, and continues to attend, weekly group sessions on understanding brain injury (since May 2003). Under a holistic approach, OG began cognitive-behavioural therapy sessions (from February 2004), in order to address "emotional reactions". Cognitive (thoughts associated with emotions), behavioural (increasing activity) and emotional techniques (identification and expression of emotions) were all used to improve her ability to identify, express and recognise emotional reactions and states. Currently, she continues to work on these deficits.

Results

From VS to MCS. The patient arrived at the FLENI ICU presenting a GCS score of 3 (day 1). On the following day she received sedation lasting five days. Once discontinued (day 6), the GCS score fluctuated between 3 and 7 throughout the day. For the next 44 days the GCS score ranged between 4 and 9. When the patient was finally discharged to the rehabilitation clinic on day 50, she presented a score of 8, localising painful stimuli, eye opening responses to pain, but still lacking verbal response capacity or any sign of awareness.

The CRS and WHIM results are summarised in Figure 1. The CRS captured a few changes in OG's level of consciousness. Between days 66 and 108, total CRS values ranged between 17/25 and 19/25, with inconsistent responses to simple commands, corresponding therefore to a minimally

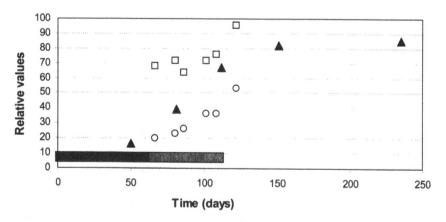

Figure 1. CRS, DRS and WHIM performance over time. CRS and DRS data are from days 66 to 122 post-trauma, WHIM data are from days 51 to 235. The values are converted to 0–100 scale for each assessment tool. Triangles are used to show WHIM data, open circles for DRS data and open squares for CRS data. The estimated periods in which the patient was diagnosed as VS or MCS are shown in the horizontal bar (dark grey for VS and light grey, for MCS)

conscious state. Also, she was able to track nearby moving objects, and erratically move one hand to touch the other. Arousal level, as measured by the CRS, fluctuated between the ability to maintain her eyes open for 15–30 minutes (days 66 to 86), to being able to do so only for a few minutes on days 101 and 108, and finally on day 122, she was able to maintain a certain degree of sustained attention. The patient recovered verbal reflexes on day 66, presenting spontaneous vocalisation on days 80 and 86, later expressing isolated words, sometimes abusive (swearing) on days 101 and 108 (CRS 19/25), and finally yes/no responses on day 122, but still lacking spontaneous speech.

On day 122 considerable improvement in awareness level was observed, the patient scored 24/25 on tests for movement reproduction prompted by simple commands, as well as for object recognition; more importantly, she began to show clear signs of communication, e.g., saying no to the therapist (MT) whenever she was asked to show how to move her lower limbs. At this stage the ceiling effect clearly revealed the limitations of CRS when evaluating this patient in high MCS, fortunately the improvement was readily captured by other tools.

The Wessex Head Injury Matrix was first administered on arrival of the patient at the rehabilitation centre (day 51), two weeks prior to the first CRS assessment. At the time, with a score of 10/62, OG could not follow simple commands but sustained visual pursuit was observed, a sign of transition from VS to MCS (Giacino & Trott, 2004). One month later (day 81), the patient was able to inconsistently follow simple commands, and she was therefore diagnosed as being in MCS (with a WHIM score of 24/62). On day 112, having reached scores of 41/62, the patient began to show sporadic signs of communication, as observed whenever she was forced to choose an object, or vocalising to protest forcibly against a blood extraction, even being able to name one of the nurses. The first Bedside Language Assessment taken on day 105 showed a very low score of 8/25, with 5 points for repetition, 2 points for spontaneous language, and 1 point for an yes/no question. By that time she was showing highly complex behaviour for an MCS patient, probably in high MCS or emerging from this state. This was also reflected in the patient's CRS score of 24/25 on day 122, and her WHIM score of 41/62 on day 112, both indicating some degree of communication.

Disability rating measures. As a measure of disability degree, the Disability Rating Scale was administered and assessed on the same days as the CRS; both results are shown in Figure 1. From days 66 to 122, OG presented spontaneous eye opening. During the first two assessments (on days 66 and 80) she manifested no communication ability and finally, on day 86, she began to show signs of verbal response, but remained incomprehensible. As expected, scale application revealed motor withdrawal in response to noxious stimuli (greater than a simple reflex) on day 66, noxious localisation a few days later and command-following capacity on the last day (122). Cognitive independent self-care skills remained absent until day 108, and on day 122 were classified as minimal. OG continued to be totally dependent on others until day 108. Yet, by day 122, she had become moderately independent (she was back at home by then). Total agreement between the DRS and the CRS scale was observed; the main difference being absence of ceiling effect for the DRS (see Figure 1).

The Functional Independence Measure (FIM) proved to be the best assessment instrument to make an appropriate follow up, and accurately reflected OG's rate of recovery during the period from September 2002 to June 2004 (Figure 2). The first 130 days showed scores in the lower third of the scale, middle values were registered between days 131 and 230, reflecting an improvement in almost all items except social adjustment; and from day 231 to 683, the FIM was only able to detect minor improvements in self-care, sphincter control and cognition.

Recovery from MCS. In January 2003 the second Bedside Language Assessment (BLA), on day 162, confirmed the presence of significant recovery with a very high score of 24/25, so Addenbrooke's Cognitive Examination (ACE) was immediately performed, with a score of 50/100 (see Table 1). This corresponded to clear deficits in all cognitive domains. Despite profound deficits in memory, attention, motor skills and other cognitive functions, she could consistently communicate with staff, relatives, and friends. Three months later, on day 235, the last WHIM scale was performed

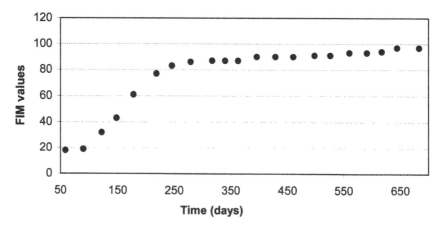

Figure 2. FIM performance over time from days 59 to 683 post-trauma. Circles are used to show FIM data, top FIM score is 126

TABLE 1
OG's Addenbrooke's Cognitive Examinations from January 2003 to July 2004

	January 2003	May 2003	June 2003	January 2004	July 2004
Day	162	270	302	492	690
ACE	50	74	81	87	95
MMSE	17	27	28	29	30
Orientation	7	10	10	10	10
Attention	3	7	8	8	8
Memory	15	25	25	28	35
Fluency	6	5	8	8	9
Language	18	24	27	28	28
Praxis abilities	1	3	3	5	5

Total ACE and MMSE values and sub-values for each cognitive domain are shown. Highest possible scores for ACE domains are: 100 for total score; 10 for orientation; 8 for attention; 35 for memory; 14 for fluency; 28 for language; and 5 for praxis abilities

with a score of 52/62. All unassigned points corresponded to motor tasks that the patient was unable to execute. However, she had scored top points in all other domains, demonstrating that the WHIM was no longer useful for cognitive recovery follow up monitoring. The second ACE was administered 4 months (day 270) after the first, with improvement in all domains, but most especially in language and memory skills, jumping from 15/35 to 25/35, and 18/30 to 24/30, respectively (total score of 74/100). One month later (day 302) as her cognitive recovery continued, she scored 81/100 in the ACE (MMSE of 28).

Cognitive recovery.   Patient cognitive recovery dynamics are described in Table 1 and the detailed cognitive analysis in Table 2. A sustained improvement in her cognitive abilities has been observed between days 162 to 690, as shown from the five ACEs performed during this period. Between the first (50/100) and the second ACE (74/100), clear progress in all cognitive domains could be seen. The third ACE (day 302) showed some improvements in language, attention and fluency, compared to the second assessment. Seven months later, the fourth ACE (day 527) only showed slight progress in memory, language and praxis abilities.

A lack of sensitivity for the ACE was observed at this time and it became necessary to assess in detail the different cognitive domains. Therefore, two full cognitive evaluations were conducted on days 307–314 and 520–527 (June 2003 and January 2004), the results can be seen in Table 2.

Full cognitive assessment suggested that OG was impaired in delayed recall in the Logical Memory Test, but not in immediate recall or recognition (see Table 2). Both the immediate and delayed recall improved during the second assessment marking significant progress in OG's anterograde

TABLE 2
OG's results for first (June 2003) and second (January 2004) full cognitive assessments,
and WAIS-III and FAB for June 2003, January 2004 and July 2004

Test		June 2003	January 2004	July 2004
Wechsler Adult Intelligence Scale III				
Forward digits		8	8	8
Backward digits		2	4	6
Digit Span (Aged scale score)		5	7	8
FAB (Frontal Assessment Battery)		*14/18*	*18/18*	*17/18*
Ravens Coloured Progressive		25/36	28/36	
Matrices (Raw Score)				
Wechsler Memory Scale—Revised				
Logical Memory (Prose Recall)				
Immediate Recall	Mean (SD) 27.4 (9.6)	20	27	
Delayed Recall	Mean (SD) 19.8 (6.7)	13	26	
Recognition		18/20	19/20	
Rey Auditory—Verbal Learning Test				
Recall	Mean (SD) 52.3 (8.0)	36	35	
Delayed Recall	Mean (SD) 1.1 (2.7)	6	3	
Recognition	Mean (SD) 13.5 (1.6)	1	9	
Rey-Osterreith Complex Figure				
Copy	Mean (SD) 33.9 (1.5)	could not complete	34	
Delayed Recall	Mean (SD) 21.8 (6.5)		10.5	
Recognition			correct	
Rivermead Behavioural Memory Test				
Screening Score		8 (Poor memory)	9 (Poor memory)	
Standardised Profile Score		17 (Poor memory)	19 (Poor memory)	
Trail Making Test				
Part A	Mean (SD) 27.4 (9.6)	250 sec	177sec	
Part B	Mean (SD) 58.7 (15.9)	discontinued at 300 s	308 sec	
Wisconsin Card Sorting Test		cancelled		
Categories				6/6
Total errors				1

long-term memory capacity. Very limited learning capacity was evidenced on either cognitive evaluations (no learning curve) as seen with the Rey List. However, significant recognition improvement was observed in the second assessment. This enhanced cue recall capacity suggests some degree of recovery for memory storage ability. Finally, the Rivermead Behavioural Memory Test, built up to detect impairment of everyday memory functioning and to monitor changes following treatment for memory difficulties, showed poor memory results on both evaluations.

Visuospatial and praxis abilities were assessed with the Rey-Osterreith Complex Figure. Unfortunately, OG was unable to draw for the first evaluation due to right hand motor impairment. However, after intense physical therapy, she managed to copy the figure within normal limits. Deficit in verbal and visual memory were present. Scores for delayed recall of Rey figure were only half of normal values. Also, as for other test results, she was able to recognise the figure correctly.

Coloured Raven Matrices were used to assess intelligence. However, the patient was too slow to complete a full Raven test and unable to give a correct response for the analogical reasoning items. She did show a better performance during the second assessment, but still within impairment range.

Executive and frontal functions were assessed using the Frontal Assessment Battery, the WAIS-III, Trail Making Test A and B and WCST (Table 2). The Immediate Memory Span revealed small but consistent working memory improvement. Trail Making Test performance observed during patient recovery was indicative of some degree of set shifting and working memory capacity. Further complementary information was obtained with the Wisconsin Card Sorting Test (WCST). Unable to perform the test in the first evaluation, the patient surprisingly completed six of six categories during the second assessment, thus presenting strong evidence of partial executive function recovery after seven months of therapy.

Brain activation after word presentation. Both fMRI results are shown in Figure 3.The first was completed while the patient was in VS (September 2002), and the second after recovery (May 2003). Word vs. silence comparison showed a small area of left temporal activation in the transverse temporal gyrus and superior temporal gyrus during the vegetative state. However, much stronger bilateral temporal activation was observed after recovery (speech and auditory areas) with some degree of frontal activity as well. This second scan activation pattern was similar to the one of normal subjects (Bekinschtein & Manes, unpublished data). Transverse temporal gyrus and superior temporal gyrus focal activity was slightly higher after recovery than while in VS. However, activation variability was much higher in VS (see Figure 4). Extended spread of activation to other areas from superior

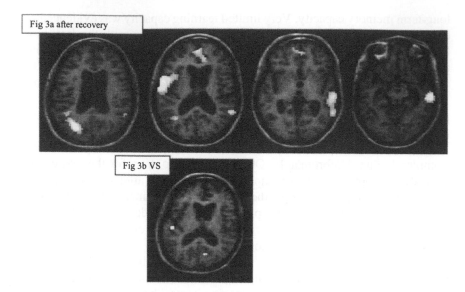

Figure 3. Brain activation after word presentation (words vs. silence contrast). Fig. 3a OG's brain activity after recovery (May 2003) showing large bilateral activation in the temporal cortex, bilateral parietal activation stronger on the left and bilateral medial prefrontal cortex activation (corrected $p < .05$); Fig. 3b brain activity while in vegetative state (September 2002) showing left transverse and superior temporal gyri activation and striate cortex activation near the precuneus (uncorrected $p < .001$). Global maximum for this contrast is in both, VS and recovered states, in the left superior temporal gyrus (being more posterior in VS). The activation maps are superimposed on 3D-T1 images according to each scan

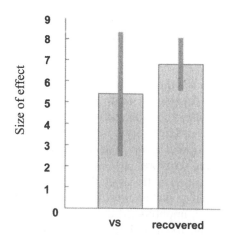

Figure 4. Left superior temporal gyrus activity after words vs. silence contrast. The bars show the mean values and standard error of the higher activity voxel for each state of consciousness

temporal gyrus to middle temporal gyrus, temporoparietal and frontal regions, also suggested integrated brain processing after recovery.

DISCUSSION

This work adds to growing evidence that full cognitive recovery from the vegetative or minimally conscious state is possible, and demonstrates the need for the development of new tests, better able to capture both degree and rate of recovery in this type of patient. This study also showed several findings: (1) the WHIM Scale was able to capture several different awareness levels, ranging from VS to MCS to partial recovery; (2) the CRS allowed mapping of both MCS and high MCS; (3) the BLA and ACE overlapped with WHIM, when used to unmask differences during the cognitive recovery curve, and (4) the ACE proved to be a good brief cognitive assessment tool for recovery monitoring once a degree of communication is attained.

In comparison to previous studies on patients transitioning from very low functioning states to high cognitive capabilities, two strengths arising from this investigation merit consideration. First, whereas previous authors (Wilson et al., 2001) had no information regarding assessment tools like the WHIM or CRS, in this case both were included from VS to recovery and different cognitive and functional scales were also examined. Second, this work included MRI data during VS and after recovery.

Although it is important to understand the limitations of the neuropsychological tools employed, assessment of cognitive function is critical, and may influence decisions about level of care or treatment provided.

Once the patient had reached a relatively high score in the ACE (81/100), full cognitive assessment was performed. Strikingly, the comparatively small differences observed between the third and fourth ACE tests contrasts with the enhanced cognitive abilities found during full cognitive evaluation, where the tests clearly captured the degree of cognitive improvement gained between these two points in time.

Seven months later, a second assessment showed improvement in all cognitive domains, particularly memory and language. The patient has recently achieved a normal score in the ACE (95/100). Despite the fact she is still experiencing social skills deficits, this result demonstrates an almost complete recovery.

As it has been clearly established in clinical practice, significant spontaneous recovery frequently occurs during the subacute period (Wilson et al., 2002; Giacino & Trott, 2004). Furthermore, two other favourable factors were also presented in this case; that is to say, the patient's young age, and the fact that she received immediate medical assistance after the accident. Although fluctuations were observed during the acute and subacute period, in the end there was a clear trend towards higher levels of consciousness (from GCS 3–5 to GCS 7–9 in 50 days). On day 51 the patient received methylphenidate, and this was replaced one week later by levodopa, coinciding with transition from VS to MCS, as documented using the Wessex Head Injury Matrix (days 50 to 81). Unlike the WHIM, the CRS had to be interrupted on two separate occasions because the patient lacked the arousal level necessary to complete the test. A few weeks later (day 66), the first full CRS was completed; also, because it was administered more often than the WHIM, the CRS evaluations were able to show improvement in different aspects of the MCS, and even register the fluctuations observed during this period. The DRS performed during recovery showed similar results to the CRS but without registering fluctuations, probably because the DRS measures more general features of recovery. Although DRS (not CRS) could have been used to follow the recovery for a longer period, FIM was the tool finally selected to measure the patient's functional recovery.

Day 112, the point at which she was able to call a nurse by name, was considered the beginning of exiting the minimally conscious state. Some might argue that the day of the first BLA (day 105) could be taken as the end of the MCS, but on day 108 the patient was not able to communicate spontaneously (CRS score was 19/25). This would, therefore, appear to represent more a fluctuation in awareness level, rather than a clear-cut end to the MCS. From day 112 until now, patient cognitive status has continued to show uninterrupted improvement. The fMRI study revealed particular physiological features in this patient. It was able to capture increased cortical activity during a passive word listening task, showing small but consistent focal processing in VS, as compared to the large bilateral cortical processing observed after recovery. The first assessment showed limited cortical activation, probably residual, automatic and unconscious. This result was expected due to the very limited behavioural responses demonstrated by the patient in September 2002. This activation pattern coincides with recent findings concerning differences in brain activity observed between VS patients, MCS patients and control subjects (Boly et al., 2004). Also, the increased variability (Figure 4) in the focal temporal activity (STG-TTG/ Brodmann area 22) revealed qualitative differences in the cortical processing during these two states of consciousness. It is important to note that OG's recovered brain activity was very similar to that seen in controls, suggesting good functional and physiological recovery 10 months after the accident, and 5 months after abandoning the MCS. Several studies have highlighted the need for careful, repeated and reliable assessment of patients with impaired levels of consciousness (McMillan & Herbert, 2004; Lombardi et al., 2002; Lippert-Gruner, Wedekind, & Klug, 2003). Once again, we confirm the need for appropriate cognitive supervision after leaving MCS, since this could shed light on recovery mechanisms activated during consciousness disorders. Although the patient's cognitive abilities were meticulously assessed, the clear deficit in social skills persisting to date was not captured either by ACE tests, nor even a full cognitive assessment. Cognition abilities with theory of mind tasks, decision-making tasks, social performance tests and an expanded cognitive assessment, to further characterize post-traumatic vegetative patients after recovery remain under evaluation at this time. This study suggest that the cognitive recovery in patients with disorders of consciousness is a continual process rather than a step-by-step phenomenon and confirms that a good recovery assessment should include objective measures of behavioural, cognitive and functional domains, and neurophysiological data to support the diagnosis.

REFERENCES

Bekinschtein, T., Leiguarda, R., Armony, J., Owen, A., Carpintiero, S., Niklison, J., et al. (2004). Emotion processing in the minimally conscious state. *Journal of Neurology, Neurosurgery, and Psychiatry, 75*(5), 788.

Boly, M., Faymonville, M. E., Peigneux, P., Lambermont, B., Damas, P., Del Fiore, G., et al. (2004). Auditory processing in severely brain injured patients: Differences between the minimally conscious state and the persistent vegetative state. *Archives of Neurology, 61*(2), 233–238.

Dubois, B., Slachevsky, A., Litvan, I., & Pillon, B. (2000). The FAB: A Frontal Assessment Battery at bedside. *Neurology, 55*(11), 1621–1626.

Giacino, J. T., Ashwal, S., Childs, N., Cranford, R., Jennett, B., Katz, D. I., et al. (2002). The minimally conscious state: Definition and diagnostic criteria. *Neurology, 58*(3), 349–353.

Giacino, J. T., Kalmar, K., & Whyte, J. (2004). The JFK Coma Recovery Scale—Revised: Measurement characteristics and diagnostic utility. *Archives of Physical Medicine Rehabilitation, 85*(12), 2020–2029.

Giacino, J. T., Kezmarsky, M. A., DeLuca, J., & Cicerone, K. D. (1991). Monitoring rate of recovery to predict outcome in minimally responsive patients. *Archives of Physical Medicine Rehabilitation, 72*(11), 897–901.

Giacino, J. T., & Trott, C. T. (2004). Rehabilitative management of patients with disorders of consciousness: Grand rounds. *Journal of Head Trauma Rehabilitation, 19*(3), 254–265.

Granger, C. V., Deutsch, A., & Linn, R. T. (1998). Rasch analysis of the Functional Independence Measure (FIM) Mastery Test. *Archives of Physical Medical Rehabilitation, 79*(1), 52–57.

Laureys, S., Faymonville, M. E., Degueldre, C., Fiore, G. D., Damas, P., Lambermont, B., et al. (2000). Auditory processing in the vegetative state. *Brain, 123*(8), 1589–1601.

Laureys, S., Owen, A. M., & Schiff, N. D. (2004). Brain function in coma, vegetative state, and related disorders. *Lancet Neurology, 3*(9), 537–546.

Lippert-Gruner, M., Wedekind, C., & Klug, N. (2003). Outcome of prolonged coma following severe traumatic brain injury. *Brain Injury, 17*(1), 49–54.

Lombardi, F., Taricco, M., De Tanti, A., Telaro, E., & Liberati, A. (2002). Sensory stimulation of brain-injured individuals in coma or vegetative state: Results of a Cochrane systematic review. *Clinical Rehabilitation, 16*(5), 464–472.

Mathuranath, P. S., Nestor, P. J., Berrios, G. E., Rakowicz, W., & Hodges, J. R. (2000). A brief cognitive test battery to differentiate Alzheimer's disease and frontotemporal dementia. *Neurology, 55*(11), 1613–1620.

Matsuda, W., Matsumura, A., Komatsu, Y., Yanaka, K., & Nose, T. (2003). Awakenings from persistent vegetative state: Report of three cases with Parkinsonism and brain stem lesions on MRI. *Journal of Neurology, Neurosurgery and Psychiatry, 74*(11), 1571–1573.

McMillan, T. M., & Herbert, C. M. (2004). Further recovery in a potential treatment withdrawal case 10 years after brain injury. *Brain Injury 18*(9), 935–940.

Menon, D. K., Owen, A. M., Williams, E. J., Minhas, P. S., Allen, C. M., Boniface, S. J., & Pickard, J. D. (1998). Cortical processing in persistent vegetative state. Wolfson Brain Imaging Centre Team. *Lancet, 352*(9123), 200.

Multi-Society Task Force on PVS (1994). Medical aspects of the persistent vegetative state, 1. *New England Journal of Medicine, 330*, 1499–1508.

Passler, M. A., & Riggs, R. V. (2001). Positive outcomes in traumatic brain injury-vegetative state: Patients treated with bromocriptine. *Archives of Physical Medical Rehabilitation, 82*(3), 311–315.

Rappaport, M., Herrero-Backe, C., Rappaport, M. L., & Winterfield, K. M. (1989). Head injury outcome up to ten years later. *Archives of Physical Medical Rehabilitation, 70*(13), 885–892.

Richer, E., & Tell, L. (2003). Indications, efficacy and tolerance of drug therapy in view of improving recovery of consciousness following a traumatic brain injury. *Ann Readapt Med Phys, 46*(4), 177–183.

Shiel, A., Horn, S. A., Wilson, B. A., Watson, M. J., Campbell, M. J., & McLellan, D. L. (2000). The Wessex Head Injury Matrix (WHIM) main scale: A preliminary report on a scale to assess and monitor patient recovery after severe head injury. *Clinical Rehabilitation, 14*(4), 408–421.

Teasdale, G., Knill-Jones, R., & van der Sande, J. (1978). Observer variability in assessing impaired consciousness and coma. *Journal of Neurology, Neurosurgery and Psychiatry, 41*(7), 603–610.

Wilson, B., Cockburn, J., Baddeley, A., & Hiorns, R. (1989). The development and validation of a test battery for detecting and monitoring everyday memory problems. *Journal of Clinical, Experimental and Neuropsychology, 11*(6), 855–870.

Wilson, B. A., Gracey, F., & Bainbridge, K. (2001). Cognitive recovery from "persistent vegetative state": Psychological and personal perspectives. *Brain Injury, 15*(12), 1083–1092.

Wilson, F. C., Harpur, J., Watson, T., & Morrow, J. I. (2002). Vegetative state and minimally responsive patients—regional survey, long-term case outcomes and service recommendations. *NeuroRehabilitation, 17*(3), 231–236.

NEUROPSYCHOLOGICAL REHABILITATION
2005, 15 (3/4), 323–332

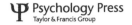

Neurophysiological correlates of persistent vegetative and minimally conscious states

Erik J. Kobylarz and Nicholas D. Schiff

Weill Medical College of Cornell University, New York, USA

The evaluation of patients after severe brain injury is a complex process for the clinician, even with the information provided by a detailed neurological examination. The clinical examination often does not provide sufficient information to fully evaluate these patients due to several factors. Limited and inconsistent motor responses may obscure expression of greater cognitive capacities. More importantly, evaluation of the functional integrity of the cerebral cortical, thalamic and basal ganglia system is poorly indicated by the clinical examination in many patients. Neurophysiological studies provide a complementary set of objective data for evaluating brain-injured patients, as well as predicting and following the course of their recovery. This additional information can be of great importance since vegetative patients may be difficult to distinguish clinically from those in the minimally conscious state. This is important because the latter category of patients may have a significantly better prognosis for recovery in the initial phase of injury. Electrodiagnostic and imaging studies can help the practitioner to determine the degree of preserved and recovering neurological function. In this review we will assess the various neurophysiological studies currently at our disposal to evaluate and follow the clinical course of patients who have suffered severe brain injuries.

In this review we discuss neurophysiological studies of patients in the vegetative state (VS) and preliminary studies of patients meeting diagnostic criteria for the recently defined minimally conscious state (MCS; Giacino et al., 2002). Neurophysiological correlates have been more comprehensively evaluated for VS than for MCS, at least in part due to the relatively recent definition of the latter state. Therefore, this review will be primarily focused on the neurophysiological studies of patients in the persistent

Correspondence should be sent to Erik J. Kobylarz, Department of Neurology and Neuroscience, Weill Medical College of Cornell University, 1300 York Avenue, New York, NY, USA 10021. Tel: (212) 746 6575, Fax: (212) 746-8050. Email: ejk2001@med.cornell.edu

© 2005 Psychology Press Ltd
http://www.tandf.co.uk/journals/pp/09602011.html   DOI:10.1080/09602010443000605

vegetative state with the expectation that as corresponding studies of MCS patients become available, they will provide further insight into the pathophysiology of this condition. It is likely that the complementary information derived from different neurophysiological studies, such as electroencephalography (EEG) and evoked potentials (EPs), will enhance the determination of the neurological status, clinical course and outcome prediction of patients following severe brain injuries. Here, however, we will focus on the use of neurophysiological methods to improve the understanding of underlying pathophysiology of the severely injured brain.

NOSOLOGY

Patients in VS following a severe brain injury show a very limited recovery of cyclical arousal. VS patients remain unresponsive and their cyclical arousal pattern is limited to an eyes open "wakeful" appearance alternating with an eyes closed "sleep-like" state (Jennett & Plum, 1972). Otherwise, VS is identical to coma in that patients demonstrate no evidence of awareness of self or their environment. A VS that lasts more than one month is arbitrarily defined as a persistent vegetative state (PVS). It is estimated that the chance of further recovery after VS lasting longer than three months after an anoxic injury or one year after a traumatic brain injury is less than 1 in 1000, and is thus considered permanent (Jennett, 2002). The permanent vegetative state is often the clinical sequelae of diffuse anoxic cerebral injury or severe head trauma (Multi-Society Task Force on PVS, 1994).

The minimally conscious state (MCS) has been recently defined as a state of severely altered consciousness with demonstration of minimal, but definite behavioural evidence of awareness of self or the environment. It differs from PVS by the presence of inconsistent, but clearly discernible, behavioural evidence of consciousness (Giacino et al., 2002). MCS patients may exhibit intermittent behavioural fragments, such as simple verbalisation or context-appropriate gestures, or sustained visual fixation. It is essential to distinguish this condition from PVS due to the potential for a more favourable outcome in the initial stages of the illness (Giacino & Kalmar, 1997). When patients exhibit consistent, reliable functional communication (regaining more than the ability to follow simple commands), they are considered to have emerged from MCS. Due to the wide range of behavioural patterns of patients within MCS, there exists a need for further refinement of this diagnostic category and association with quantitative neurophysiological criteria.

EEG IN THE VEGETATIVE STATE

A variety of awake electroencephalography (EEG) patterns have been reported in patients in VS. These include focal or diffuse continuous slowing in the theta (4–7.5 Hz) and/or delta (1–3.5 Hz) frequency ranges, intermittent delta rhythms, and attenuation of the EEG signal, which can be of a very severe degree such that the EEG is essentially isoelectric (Hansotia, 1985; Li, Wei, & Guo, 1993). In addition, epileptiform activity can occur, such as focal sharp waves, whether or not the patient has documented electrographic seizures. Alpha-theta coma and spindle coma EEG patterns are also reported in PVS. The EEG can provide prognostic information for severely brain-injured patients. Kane and colleagues found a highly significant correlation between the initial EEG grade (i.e., degree of abnormality) and clinical outcome (Glasgow Outcome Score) in comatose patients 6 and 12 months after brain injury (Kane, Moss, Curry, & Butler, 1998).

The normal diurnal and nocturnal EEG pattern fluctuations, as well as the reactivity of the EEG to stimuli can be affected by severe brain injury. In a study of 12 PVS patients, Isono and colleagues found that the diurnal EEG patterns typically did not vary significantly during the course of the day and that no changes were noted when PVS patients were subjected to noxious sensory stimuli (Hansotia, 1985; Isono et al., 2002). Behavioural arousal in VS indicates preservation of brainstem systems. The cyclic variability and reactivity of the EEG, however, are associated with the interaction of brainstem arousal systems and other cerebral systems supporting attention and other cognitive processes and, thus more directly reflects the integrity of corticothalamic systems. The upper brainstem-mesencephalic component of the reticular activating system and thalamus, where overwhelming injuries may lead to permanent VS (see Schiff et al., 2002), play a key role in these interactions. Many of the EEG changes, which normally occur during the different stages of sleep, are absent in PVS patients, such as rapid eye movements (REM), sleep spindles and vertex waves. In some PVS patients sleep EEGs show diffuse low voltage slow waves immediately following sleep onset. The slow waves can remain unchanged during the sleep period or gradually increase in amplitude with time. In other PVS patients there are no discernible fluctuations in the EEG during sleep compared with that during wakefulness (Isono et al., 2002). The diminution or absence of EEG fluctuation during the sleep–wake cycle, particularly when there is a coexisting evoked potential abnormality (see below), can serve as an indicator of the severity of brainstem dysfunction and VS patient's prognosis for recovery (Cheliout-Heraut, Rubinsztajn, Ioos, & Estournet, 2001).

Besides evaluating the EEG in the time domain, power spectrum and coherence analysis of the EEG has been used to evaluate various brain pathophysiological conditions. Power spectra analysis quantitates the relative amplitudes of the various frequencies that comprise the EEG signal. Changes in the EEG power spectrum after severe brain injury may have prognostic value. Kane et al. (1998) found highly significant correlations between six month and one year post-injury Glasgow Outcome Scores and left frontal-central beta and left central-temporal alpha and beta activity power in comatose patients. Coherence is a measure of cross-correlation in the frequency domain. Coherence analysis of the EEG has been used to study patients with a variety of pathological conditions (Leocani & Comi, 1999). It is proposed that coherence provides an index of the integrity of inter-regional networks and communication between cortical areas, as well as with subcortical structures (e.g., thalamus and basal ganglia) that mediate this connectivity (Davey, Victor, & Schiff, 2000; Nunez, Wingeier, & Silberstein, 2001). Therefore, EEG coherence may serve as a better prognostic indicator for recovery after brain injury than power spectral analysis (Thatcher et al., 1991). Kane and colleagues (1998) found a significant reduction of the mean interhemispheric coherence of the EEG for all regions in comatose patients compared to normal healthy control subjects. However, they found no correlation between the degree of interhemispheric coherence and outcome scales at six months and one year post-injury. This is in contrast to the study by Thatcher and colleagues (1991) that identified coherence and phase measurements as the best predictors of functional outcome one year following closed head injury. Davey et al. (2000) performed power spectra and coherence analysis of the EEG in a PVS patient who had suffered severe damage predominantly to the right subcortical grey matter structures after a series of intraparenchymal haemorrhages from an arteriovenous malformation. EEG power spectra computed for each bilateral hemispheric region (frontal, central and parieto-temporal) showed only slight differences between the two hemispheres; there was relatively greater power of the lower frequencies and diminished power of the higher frequencies throughout the more damaged right cerebral hemisphere. In contrast, a marked reduction of coherence over the entire damaged right hemisphere was demonstrated, which was most evident frontally where the brain injury was most severe. This study provides a correlate of the impact of subcortical grey matter structures on the EEG as well as insight into the thalamic contribution to organised cerebral activity.

EEG IN THE MINIMALLY CONSCIOUS STATE

A few reports of EEG findings in MCS patients are available. Observed EEG abnormalities depend on the location and type of cerebral lesions and include diffuse or focal slowing, often in the theta and delta frequency range, disorganisation (e.g., absence, diminution and/or decreased reactivity of the posterior dominant rhythm, and diminished or absent sleep spindles) (Boly et al., 2004). Bilateral, but predominantly ipsilesional polymorphic theta activity represented the most prominent abnormality in awake EEGs from two MCS patients we studied. This abnormal slow activity was most apparent in the electrodes nearest to the respective lesions. There was also disorganisation of the background, predominantly in the more severely injured hemisphere, with an attenuated and slow posterior dominant ("alpha") rhythm. Asleep EEG from our MCS patients showed continuous polymorphic slowing, which was more apparent near the cerebral lesions. The sleep spindles were also attenuated, less frequent and less well formed in the more severely affected hemisphere, particularly if the lesions involved the parasaggital regions (Kobylarz, Kamal, & Schiff, 2003).

We performed similar power spectra and coherence analyses of the EEG from an MCS patient to that utilised by Davey and colleagues (2000). For our MCS patients the EEG power spectra revealed generally few significant differences between corresponding hemispheric regions in the asleep and awake states (see Figure 1). Notably, there was slightly decreased EEG power for nearly all frequencies in the right frontal region during wakefulness. In the central-temporal regions there was slightly decreased EEG power on the right during wakefulness for several frequency ranges, most prominently from approximately 20–30 Hz and 40–50 Hz. These differences in

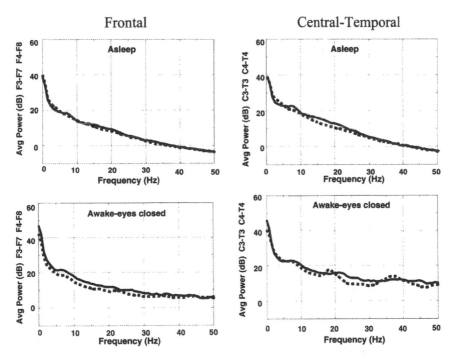

Figure 1. Regional asleep (above) and awake (below) EEG power spectra compared between the left (solid line) and right (dashed line) hemispheres from an MCS patient with post-traumatic right frontal lobe encephalomalacia and a right thalamic infarct. Frontal region, electrodes F3/F7 (left) and F4/F8 (right); central region, electrodes C3/T3 (left) and C4/T4 (right) (from Kobylarz, Kamal, & Schiff, 2003)

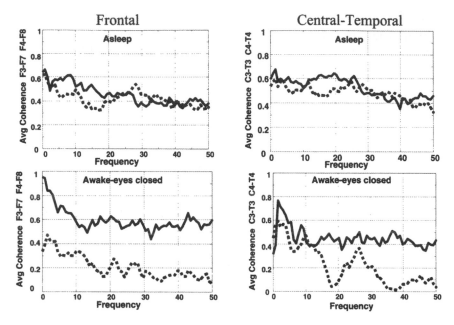

Figure 2. Regional asleep (above) and awake (below) EEG coherence compared between the left (solid line) and right (dashed line) hemispheres from an MCS patient with post-traumatic right frontal lobe encephalomalacia and a right thalamic infarct. Frontal region, electrodes F3/F7 (left) and F4/F8 (right); central region, electrodes C3/T3 (left) and C4/T4 (right) (from Kobylarz, Kamal, & Schiff, 2003)

regional power correlated with the underlying structural brain injury. There was also notably reduced coherence over the right hemisphere in this MCS patient (see Figure 2). The reduction was more marked across the entire right hemisphere for this patient in the awake state, but was also present to a lesser degree in the right frontal and central-temporal regions during sleep (Kobylarz et al., 2003).

EPs IN THE VEGETATIVE STATE

Evoked potentials (EPs) are affected to varying degrees in VS patients. Although brainstem auditory evoked potentials (BAEPs) can be normal in VS patients (Hansotia, 1985), the BAEP waveforms can also be attenuated, delayed or absent, depending on the location and degree of brainstem injury (Li et al., 1993). Isono et al. (2002) reported such abnormalities in waveforms III and V, corresponding to the superior olivary complex (pons) and lateral lemiscal-inferior colliculus (pons-midbrain) auditory responses for PVS patients.

Similarly, somatosensory evoked potentials (SEPs) have been found to be abnormal in PVS patients with delay and attenuation, or even absence of the

N20 cortical response to median nerve stimulation (Hansotia, 1985; Isono et al., 2002; Li et al., 1993). Rothstein and colleagues studied the prognostic value of EEGs and median nerve SEPs in patients with hypoxic-ischaemic coma lasting six or more hours (Rothstein, Thomas, & Sumi, 1991). They found that bilateral absence of median SEP cortical responses and/or a malignant EEG abnormality (e.g., low amplitude non-reactive delta slowing, burst suppression, alpha coma or isoelectric) predicted an unfavourable outcome or death without awakening in greater than 80% and 40% of patients with these neurophysiological abnormalities, respectively. However, comatose patients with normal or delayed central conduction time (CCT, time difference between cervical and cortical SEP responses) and benign (normal, theta slowing or frontal rhythmic delta) or uncertain (diffuse non-reactive or reactive delta slowing, epileptiform discharges) EEG patterns had an uncertain prognosis that included recovery of consciousness, entry into PVS or death without awakening. The spinal components of somatosensory evoked potential responses are remarkably resilient in amplitude and latency in comparison to the cortical responses, despite systemic changes that may occur due to metabolic derangements, anaesthesia and even brain death (Hansotia, 1985). Therefore, the cortical responses and, specifically the CCT are better indices of cerebral injury, recovery and prognosis after severe brain injury (Hume, Cant, & Shaw, 1979). For the patients who awakened after PVS, cortical SEP and EEG findings did not distinguish between patients who recovered completely from those who had varying degrees of motor or cognitive impairment.

Magnetoencephalography (MEG) is a unique functional imaging technique, which provides spatiotemporal identification of the sources of brain activation. Schiff and colleagues applied MEG to study auditory and somatosensory evoked responses in PVS patients (Schiff et al., 2002). They found that the auditory and somatosensory MEG responses were delayed, attenuated and incomplete, or absent for various frequency bands compared to those for normal subjects. These results correlated with the local abnormalities of the corresponding positron emission tomography (PET) imaging studies. The use of PET studies to evaluate brain-injured patients are described further below.

IMAGING STUDIES OF THE VEGETATIVE STATE

Imaging techniques can also provide useful information to study the neurophysiology of patients with severe brain injuries. Brain metabolism can be quantified by fluorodeoxyglucose-positron emission tomography (FDG-PET) imaging. Cerebral metabolic rates measured by FDG-PET correlate with neuronal firing rates in cerebral structures (Eidelberg et al., 1997). FDG-PET imaging has shown that glucose utilisation is significantly reduced in PVS patients globally (Levy et al., 1987; Rudolf et al., 1999) and regionally (Tomassino et al., 1995) in comparison with age-matched controls. Levy and colleagues (1987) hypothesised that the decrease in glucose metabolism is evidence of a loss of cognitive function in PVS.

Studies employing ^{15}O-radiolabelled PET (^{15}O- PET) allow for measurements of brain activation in response to transient stimuli to be compared with baseline resting conditions. Laureys et al. (2002b) studied ^{15}O- PET cerebral activation patterns in response to noxious somatosensory stimuli in 15 PVS patients. PVS patients showed brain activations in the contralateral thalamus and primary somatosensory cortex, but not secondary somatosensory insular or anterior cingulate cortices activated in normal subjects presented with the same stimuli (Laureys et al., 2002b). In addition, Laureys and colleagues reported ^{15}O- PET abnormalities in the bilateral frontal and parieto-temporal association cortices in PVS patients using a similar strategy employing auditory click stimuli (Laureys et al., 2002a). The absence of activation of the sensory association regions and their functional connections with the higher level cortices is significant, since these are felt to be necessary for conscious perception.

IMAGING STUDIES OF THE MINIMALLY CONSCIOUS STATE

As with PVS, MCS patients often have PET imaging abnormalities related to their brain injury, although some characteristics of their studies appear more like those of normal subjects. Quantitative (FDG-PET) measurements of regional cerebral metabolic rates averaged 40–50% of normal values over the entire brain for both of our MCS patients (Kobylarz et al., 2003). However, Boly and colleagues (2004) determined similar ^{15}O-radiolabelled PET responses to auditory stimuli for patients in MCS compared to healthy control subjects. When subjected to auditory (click) stimulation, there was activation of the bilateral superior temporal gyri (Brodmann areas 41, 42, and 22). In contrast, for PVS patients activation was limited to bilateral Brodmann areas 41 and 42 (Laureys et al., 2000). The ^{15}O-radiolabelled PET responses to auditory stimuli with emotional valence (i.e., infant cries and patient's own name) in an MCS patient showed more widespread activation than that for meaningless noise (Laureys et al., 2004). The activation patterns were comparable to those from normal control subjects. Bekinschtein et al. (2004) recently reported evidence of emotion processing in an MCS patient who suffered a severe traumatic brain injury using functional magnetic resonance imaging (fMRI). When they played a recording of the patient's mother's voice, fMRI demonstrated activation of the amygdala and the insula, subcortical structures related to emotion, which later spread to the inferior frontal gyrus. In their study, stronger functional connectivity between the secondary auditory cortex and temporal and prefrontal cortices, and thus for higher order integrative processes necessary for conscious auditory perception in MCS patients compared with those in PVS.

DISCUSSION

Severely brain-injured patients pose a unique set of diagnostic and management challenges to the clinician, both in the initial evaluation as well as during the subsequent course of recovery. The more traditional information provided by the neurological examination can be limited, given the physically debilitated state of these patients. Neurophysiological studies provide an additional set of useful, reliable indices to assess and follow patients with severe brain injury. In addition to using conventional parameters provided by the EEG and evoked potentials, quantitative analyses of these signals, such as in the frequency domain with power spectra and coherence, can also provide useful information. In conjunction with analyses of electrophysiological studies, more recently developed imaging techniques, such as PET and fMRI will provide additional information regarding preservation and recovery of brain activity and intracerebral networks both at rest and in response to stimulation. All of these neurophysiological techniques will enhance our understanding of the pathophysiology of the entire spectrum of severe brain injuries as well as mechanisms supporting or limiting further recovery.

REFERENCES

Bekinschtein, T., Niklison, J., Sigman, L., Manes, F., Leiguarda, R., Armony, J., et al. (2004). Emotion processing in the minimally conscious state. *Journal of Neurology, Neurosurgery and Psychiatry, 75*, 788.

Boly, M., Faymonville, M., Damas, P., Lambermont, B., Del Fiore, G., Degueldre, C., et al. (2004). Auditory processing in severely brain injured patients: Differences between the minimally conscious state and the vegetative state. *Archives of Neurology, 61*, 233–238.

Cheliout-Heraut, F., Rubinsztajn, R., Ioos, C., & Estournet, B. (2001). Prognostic value of evoked potentials and sleep recordings in the prolonged comatose state of children. Preliminary data. *Neurophysiology Clinics, 31*(5), 283–292.

Davey, M. P., Victor, J. D., & Schiff, N. D. (2000). Power spectra and coherence in the EEG of a vegetative patient with severe asymmetric brain damage. *Clinical Neurophysiology, 111*(11), 1949–1954.

Eidelberg, D., Moeller, J. R., Kazumata, K., Antonini, A., Sterio, D., Dhawan, V., et al. (1997). Metabolic correlates of pallidal neuronal activity in Parkinson's disease. *Brain 120*(8), 1315–1324.

Giacino, J. T., Ashwal, S., Childs, N., Cranford, R., Jennett, B., Katz, D. I., et al. (2002). The minimally conscious state: Definition and diagnostic criteria. *Neurology, 58*(3), 349–353.

Giacino, J. T., & Kalmar, K. (1997). The vegetative and minimally conscious states: A comparison of clinical features and functional outcome. *Journal of Head Trauma Rehabilitation, 12*(4), 36–51.

Hansotia, P. L. (1985). Persistent vegetative state. Review and report of electrodiagnostic studies in eight cases. *Archives of Neurology, 42*(11), 1048–1052.

Hume, A. L., Cant, B. R., & Shaw, N. A. (1979). Central somatosensory conduction time in comatose patients. *Annals of Neurology, 5*, 379–384.

Isono, M., Wakabayashi, Y., Fujiki, M. M., Kamida, T., & Kobayashi, H. (2002). Sleep cycle in patients in a state of permanent unconsciousness. *Brain Injury, 16*(8), 705–712.

Jennett, B. (2002). *The vegetative state: Medical facts, ethical and legal dilemmas.* New York: Cambridge University Press.

Jennett, B., & Plum, F. (1972). Persistent vegetative state after brain damage: A syndrome in search of a name. *Lancet, 1*(7753), 734–737.

Kane, N. M., Moss, T. H., Curry, S. H., & Butler, S. R. (1998). Quantitative electroencephalographic evaluation of non-fatal and fatal traumatic coma. *Electroencephalography and Clinical Neurophysiology, 106*(3), 244–250.

Kobylarz, E. J., Kamal, A., & Schiff, N. D. (2003). *Power spectrum and coherence analysis of the EEG from two minimally conscious patients with severe asymmetric brain damage.* [Abstract]. Association for the Scientific Study of Consciousness Annual Meeting.

Laureys, S., Antoine, S., Boly, M., Elincx, S., Faymonville, M. E., Berre, J., et al. (2002a) Brain function in the vegetative state. *Acta Neurologicala Belgica, 102*(4), 177–185.

Laureys, S., Faymonville, M. E., Degueldre, C., Fiore, G. D., Damas, P., Lambermont, B., et al. (2000). Auditory processing in the vegetative state. *Brain, 123*(8), 1589–1601.

Laureys, S., Faymonville, M. E., Peigneux, P., Damas, P., Lambermont, B., Del Fiore, G., et al. (2002b). Cortical processing of noxious somatosensory stimuli in the persistent vegetative state. *Neuroimage, 17*(2), 732–741.

Laureys, S., Perrin, F., Faymonville, M. E., Schnakers, C., Boly, M., Bartsch, V., et al. (2004). Cerebral processing in the minimally conscious state. *Neurology, 63*(5), 916–918.

Leocani, L., & Comi, G. (1999). EEG coherence in pathological conditions. *Journal of Clinical Neurophysiology, 16*(6), 548–555.

Levy, D. E., Sidtis, J. J., Rottenberg, D. A., Jarden, J. O., Strother, S. C., Dhawan, V., et al. (1987). Differences in cerebral blood flow and glucose utilization in vegetative versus locked-in patients. *Annals of Neurology, 22*(6), 673–682.

Li, S., Wei, J., & Guo, D. (1993). Persistent vegetative state: Clinical and electrophysiologic observations of 5 cases. *Chinese Medical Science Journal, 8*(2), 101–106.

Multi-Society Task Force on PVS (1994). Medical aspects of the persistent vegetative state (1). *New England Journal of Medicine, 330*(21), 1499–1508.

Nunez, P. L., Wingeier, B. M., & Silberstein, R. B. (2001). Spatial-temporal structures of human alpha rhythms: Theory, microcurrent sources, multiscale measurements, and global binding of local networks. *Human Brain Mapping, 13*(3), 125–164.

Rothstein, T. L., Thomas, E. M., & Sumi, S. M. (1991). Predicting outcome in hypoxic-ischemic coma: A prospective clinical and electrophysiologic study. *Electroencephalography and Clinical Neurophysiology, 79*(2), 101–107.

Rudolf, J., Ghaemi, M., Ghaemi, M., Haupt, W. F., Szelies, B., & Heiss, W. D. (1999). Cerebral glucose metabolism in acute and persistent vegetative state. *Journal of Neurosurgical Anesthesiology, 11*(1), 17–24.

Schiff, N., Ribary, U., Moreno, D., Beattie, B., Kronberg, E., Blasberg, R., et al. (2002). Residual cerebral activity and behavioral fragments in the persistent vegetative state. *Brain, 125*, 1210–1234.

Thatcher, R. W., Cantor, D. S., McAlaster, R., Geisler, F., & Krause, P. (1991). Comprehensive predictions of outcome in closed head-injured patients. The development of prognostic equations. *Annals of the New York Academy of Science, 620*, 82–101.

Tomassino, C., Grana, C., Lucignani, G., Torri, G., & Ferrucio, F. (1995). Regional metabolism of comatose and vegetative state patients. *Journal of Neurosurgical Anesthesiology, 7*(2), 109–116.

NEUROPSYCHOLOGICAL REHABILITATION
2005, 15 (3/4), 333–356

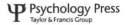

Apallic syndrome is not apallic: Is vegetative state vegetative?

Boris Kotchoubey

*Institute of Medical Psychology and Behavioural Neurobiology,
Eberhardt-Karls-University of Tübingen, Germany*

Initial conceptualisation about the nature of vegetative state (VS) assumed at least temporary loss of the entire cortical functioning. Since a broad range of stimulus-related cortical activations was demonstrated in VS patients, this simplified idea is not tenable any longer, but no alternative concept emerges instead. Two recent hypotheses, empirically testable and well grounded, could fill this vacuum: (1) In VS, isolated cortical areas may work, but their integration into a distributed network is lacking. (2) In VS, complex stimulus processing is limited to primary sensory and motor areas; the co-ordination between them and the secondary and tertiary areas is lacking. To test these hypotheses, we estimated the frequency of occurrence of late event-related potential components P3 and N400, presumably indicating activity of complex distributed networks including high-level sensory and associative areas. Both components occurred in VS with above-chance frequencies, but less frequently than in two control groups. Besides these frequent normal brain activations, some VS patients exhibit highly significant but abnormal activations, whose functional meaning remains unclear. A methodological analysis leads to the conclusion that any neurophysiological assessment of VS patients is biased toward under-, rather than over-estimation, of their remaining information processing abilities.

Correspondence should be addressed to Boris Kotchoubey, Institute of Medical Psychology and Behavioral Neurobiology, Eberhardt-Karls-University of Tübingen, Gartenstr. 29, 72074 Tübingen, Germany. Tel: 49 7071 2974221, Fax: 49 7071 295956.
Email: boris.kotchoubey@uni-tuebingen.de
The author thanks Simone Lang, Vladimir Bostanov, Niels Birbaumer, Petra Maurer, Manfred Schneck, Dieter Schmalohr, and Ellen Stec.
The study was supported by the German Research Society (Deutsche Forschungsgemeinschaft) in the SFB 550.

INTRODUCTION

When Jennett and Plum (1972) described this most severe neurological state, they gave their article the subtitle, "A syndrome in search of a name". They knew that a name is not just a sign. *Nomen est omen*. In each name there is always a hidden theory, an explanation of a phenomenon. And this is danger-ous, because we often give names before we can test this explanation, and when it proves to be wrong, the name is wrong too.

The condition was first discovered by Ernst Kretschmer (1940) who baptized it as the "apallic syndrome", meaning "without cortex" (Greek *pallium*—cortex). In other words, Kretschmer assumed that all functions of the cerebral cortex are lacking; he spoke about panagnosia and panapraxia. Thirty-two years later, Jennett and Plum (1972) already supposed that Kretschmer's assumption might be incorrect. The term they proposed, "vege-tative state", does not mention any neurophysiological function, either corti-cal or subcortical. Instead, the point is the patient's mental life. This life, according to Jennett and Plum (more exactly, according to their term), is like the life of a plant. This implies that all most important life functions (breathing, circulation, metabolism) and even sleep–wakefulness are present, but there is no experience, and even the elementary sensations of colour, light, pain, etc., are lacking. Patients can respond to stimuli, but these reactions are purely automatic and unrelated to any mental experience of those stimuli.

Now, another 32 years have passed since Jennett and Plum (1972), the period equal to that separating their article from that of Kretschmer. Because the term "vegetative" does not speak about brain functions, but rather, about mental states (or the lack thereof), data from brain physiology cannot directly test the implicated model. Nevertheless, these data can throw a light on the nature of the phenomenon.

GENERAL MORPHOPHYSIOLOGICAL DATA

In addition to classical (e.g., Arceni, Nereantiu, & Carp, 1981; Blumberg, Jones, & North, 1989; Dougherty, Rawlinson, Levy, & Plum, 1981; Dalle Ore et al., 1987) and more recent morphological studies (e.g., Jennett, Adams, Murray, & Graham, 2001; Kinney & Samuels, 1994; Walter, 2000), magnetic resonance (MR) tomography has been used (Kampfl et al., 1998a, 1998b) to analyse morphological patterns in persistent vegetative state (PVS). The two most typical lesions concern the thalamus and the cortical white matter (diffuse axonal injury). Large multifocal or diffuse lesions of cortical grey matter (e.g., laminar necrosis) have also been found, particularly in patients with anoxia. In traumatic head injury patients cortical structures can be spared. Additionally, there are numerous other, less frequent localisations of lesions also leading to PVS, such as damage to middle brain involving the black substance and other dopaminergic nuclei (e.g., Matsuda et al., 2003).

Another set of data is devoted to brain metabolism. On average, the metabolic activity in both cortical and subcortical regions in PVS patients is reduced by more than one-half compared with that in healthy awake individuals (Laureys et al., 1999, 2002b; Levy et al., 1987; Rudolf, 2000; Rudolf, Ghaemi, Haupt, Szelies, & Heiss, 1999; Tommasino et al., 1995). This level approximately corresponds to the brain activity in slow wave sleep. In the cortex, the metabolic rate in PVS can even be lower than in coma.

Can this be taken as a proof of the "vegetativeness" of the brain state? Probably not, because the large difference in means is counter-effected by the considerable variance among both PVS patients and healthy subjects. Even in a standard control group of young students one can find an individual with a metabolic rate as low as in PVS (Agardh, Rosén, & Ryding, 1983; Laureys et al., 2002a). Likewise, an overlap was found between PVS patients and other neurological patients who definitely possessed conscious awareness (DeVolder et al., 1990).

Both morphological and metabolism data are compatible with the idea that the consciousness in *most* patients diagnosed as PVS is *severely disturbed*. However, this statement is not identical to, *all* PVS patients are *completely unconscious*. Jennett (2002) underscores the fact that the term PVS does not mean any "severe disorder" of consciousness, but rather, the total absence of any conscious experience including elementary sensation and primitive feelings of pleasure versus displeasure. From his point of view there is no such thing as a "partial vegetative state". But a proof of the complete and certain loss of consciousness is very difficult and requires a much better knowledge about the neuromorphological foundations of consciousness than we presently possess.

The data about general changes in brain metabolism may be misleading because they do not take into account the differences between local activity in different cortical regions. The frequent presence among PVS patients of axonal injury combined with relatively intact cortical grey matter may indicate that local cortical circuits can remain functionally active, but separated from each other so that larger networks are out of work. Accordingly, Plum and colleagues (Plum, Schiff, Ribary, & Llinas, 1998; Schiff, Ribary, Plum, & Llinas, 1999; Schiff et al., 2000) reported patients with isolated regions of high cortical activity on a background of decreased activity in most cortical regions. These active areas varied from patient to patient, which is in line with the idea that there is no "PVS-specific" localisation of brain damage.

The meaning of such isolated activity is difficult to understand. There is no similar condition in healthy subjects which would allow a putative interpretation of its functional significance in relation to mental activity or the lack thereof. From a logical point of view, therefore, it is important to avoid a circular inference: Neuromorphological and physiological abnormalities found in PVS patients are the cause for the lack of mental activity and subjective experience, because we know that these patients possess neither mental activity nor subjective experience. And we know that they do not have mental activity and subjective experience because they exhibit neuromorphological and physiological deficits necessarily leading to this loss.

To avoid this circularity, a judgement of the presence or absence of conscious experience in a PVS patient or group of patients can only be based on those data about the neurophysiological organisation of this experience which are obtained in independent studies—*not* in PVS studies. An example of such an independent data set is the data on brain mechanisms of pain perception. Convergent evidence has been obtained in recent imaging studies indicating the brain areas most consistently related to processing of pain: the primary and secondary somatosensory cortex, the middle and posterior insula, the parietal operculum, the anterior cingulate gyrus, and possibly supplementary motor area (e.g., Alkire, White, Hsieh, & Haier, 2004; Casey, 2000; Garcia-Larrea, Frot, & Valeriani, 2003; Niddam et al., 2003; Peyron, Laurent, & Garcia-Larrea, 2000; Peyron et al., 2002); other authors add the orbitofrontal and prefrontal cortex (Coghill, McHaffie, & Yen, 2003; Lotze, Flor, Grodd, Larbig, & Birbaumer, 2001), or some brainstem structures such as nucleus accumbens or pontine nuclei (Bingel et al., 2003; Zhang et al., 2003). Regardless of the remaining controversies between the studies, it can be stated that the list of brain regions most probably representing pain do not coincide with the list of the regions most frequently damaged in PVS. The only exception is the thalamus, appearing in both lists. If this structure is critical, one should expect preserved pain sensation in the subpopulation of PVS patients with purely cortical damage (Klein, 1997). However, the only study investigating brain responses to pain stimuli in PVS found significant changes of glucose metabolism in the thalamus as well as the primary somatosensory cortex in every patient, although no response was obtained from the insula and anterior cinguli (Laureys et al., 2002b). Of course, the complexity of the relationship between pain experience and brain activity does not allow a simple conclusion on the intact pain sensation on an intact morphological or physiological basis. However, it is difficult to regard these data as evidence for the widespread belief that PVS patients cannot have any subjective experience of pain.

FUNCTIONAL TASKS

More interesting, as compared with the rest condition or simple stimulation, are brain responses of PVS patients to cognitive tasks. Such tasks usually entail two conditions: an experimental condition (EC) with more complex stimuli and a control condition (CC) with simpler stimuli. Varying the complexity of stimulus feature(s), which distinguish between EC and CC, we can, in principle, build a battery of hierarchically organised test situations checking different levels of brain information processing (Kotchoubey, Lang, Bostanov, & Birbaumer, 2002).

As a rule, studies employed meaningful stimuli (e.g., familiar faces or human speech) as the EC, and comparable meaningless stimuli (e.g., irregular visual patterns or sounds) as the CC. Most studies have been done using the technique of positron emission tomography (PET) as an index of differential brain activation in EC and CC. Several groups reported PVS patients whose patterns of regional blood flow varied consistently as a function of stimulation in the visual (Menon et al., 1998; Owen et al., 2002) as well as the auditory modalities (de Jong, Willemsen, & Paans, 1997; Laureys et al., 2000a; Owen et al., 2002). These data suggest that at least in some PVS patients, high-level information processing operations (i.e., the processing of stimulus meaning) can take place. Unfotunately, most studies used single cases or small patient samples. Thus it remains unclear as to how far they were typical PVS patients; alternatively, one might think of rare exceptional cases or even diagnostic errors.

However, these data gave a rise to two important hypotheses concerning the possible mechanisms of PVS. Laureys et al. (2000a) developed a method of assessment of correlations between metabolic responses in different functionally related brain regions and showed that even though five VS patients had adequate activation of the auditory association cortex during acoustical stimulation, the correlation between the activity in this region and in the hippocampus was negative, instead of a positive correlation characterising healthy controls. These authors also described a patient who recovered from an acute VS and whose correlations between the activity of different brain regions were restored in parallel with clinical recovery (Laureys et al., 2000b). These results indicate that an important feature of PVS may be disconnection between different regions rather than the lack of activity in some particular regions.

Another hypothesis was based on the finding of a larger (17 patients) study, that meaningful acoustic stimulation elicited in PVS a stimulus-specific activation in the primary auditory cortex only, but not in the secondary auditory cortex. In minimally conscious state, in contrast, the secondary areas and the associative cortex did respond to the stimulation, like in the healthy control group (Boly et al., 2004).

Interestingly, this hypothesis reminds one of the old "apallic" concept claiming that in PVS only subcortical structures are able to adequately respond to stimuli, while the cortex is (morphologically, or at least functionally) dead. Likewise, the new hypothesis also postulates a neuroanatomical borderline of brain activity in PVS, but this borderline is now being drawn between the primary and secondary sensory cortical areas—rather than between the cortex and subcortical nuclei.

This hypothesis could be tested using event-related brain potentials (ERPs).

ERPs IN PATIENTS WITH SEVERE DISORDERS OF CONSCIOUSNESS

EEG waves time-locked to particular events, e.g., sensory stimuli, are referred to as evoked potentials. Their short latency components reflect propagation of sensory signals from receptors via ascending pathways to the cortex. Later components, in contrast, are of cortical origin. Of special importance are components that appear between 100 and 1000 ms post-stimulus, which are referred to as event-related potentials (ERPs). They constitute a unique non-invasive technique to obtain information about how the cortex processes signals and prepares actions (Coles, Gratton, & Fabiani, 1990; Picton & Hillyard, 1988). Both neuropsychological tests and relatively slow brain imaging techniques like PET deliver the result of a chain of many processing operations. In contrast, ERP waves are supposed to manifest single members of this processing chain. The ERP method permits one to follow stimulus processing in real time at all levels of complexity. Furthermore, ERPs can be recorded immediately at a patient's bedside, even at home; patients do not need to be transported to a laboratory. This allows examination of a larger group of patients as compared with technically more complex PET examinations.

Some ERP components such as the auditory N1 and P2, the mismatch negativity (Näätänen, 2000), or visual P1 and N1, are largely generated by the primary sensory cortical areas. In the present context other ERP components, called P3 and N400, are more important, since they require co-ordinated activity of several cortical regions.

P3 is a large positive wave with a latency of about 300–500 ms, elicited in response to all kinds of target stimuli. Although the entire complexity of the brain mechanisms participating in the generation of P3 remains unclear, a widespread network including the temporal and parietal cortex, the hippocampus, and possibly the cingular cortex, should play a large role in this process (Anderer, Pasqual-Marqui, Semlitsch, & Saletu, 1998; Halgren, Baudena, Clarke, & Heit, 1995; Knight & Scabini, 1998; Molnar, 1994; Polich & Squire, 1993; Puce & Bladin, 1991; Scheffers, Johnson, & Ruchkin, 1991; Tarkka & Stokic, 1998; Yamagushi & Knight, 1991). Rare unexpected stimuli can also yield another variety of P3, called P3a (270–350 ms latency), which is mainly of frontal origin (Knight, 1996; Spencer, Dien, & Donchin, 1999, 2001). The P3a is regarded as reflecting just noticing the stimulus difference, or automatic "surprise", whereas the parieto-central "P3 properly" (or P3b) indicates that stimulus relevance (or "targetness") is processed (Polich, 1991; Polich & Comerchero, 2003; Pritchard, 1981; Verleger, Jaskowsky, & Wauschkuhn, 1994).

The simplest paradigm to obtain a P3 is the "oddball paradigm" in which two stimuli or two stimulus classes are presented with unequal frequencies. In our examination of PVS patients we used two oddball experiments. In the first one two chords were randomly presented with the probabilities of .85 and .15. In the second experiment the chords were replaced with vowels/o/and/i/. The methodology of these experiments is described elsewhere (Kotchoubey et al., 2001; Neumann & Kotchoubey, 2004). (To save space, in the present text I have omitted the methodological details of stimulus presentation and data analysis whenever they have already been described in previous publications.)

P3 and P3-like ERP waves are discussed as a possible outcome predictor in acute coma (Fischer et al., 1999; Gott, Rabinovicz, & DiGiorgio, 1991; Guerit et al., 1999; Kane, Curry, Butler, & Cummings, 1993; Kane, Butler, & Simpson, 2000; Signorino et al., 1997). They consistently occur in patients with locked-in syndrome (Onofrj, Melchionda, Thomas, & Fulgente, 1996; Onofrj et al., 1997), even in a patient who was totally locked-in including the complete gaze paralysis for many years (Kotchoubey, Lang, Bostanov, & Birbaumer, 2003a). These waves were also described in akinetic mutism (Kotchoubey, Schneck, Lang, & Birbaumer, 2003b). Previous studies reporting a P3 in patients who were possibly (Rappaport, McCandless, Pond, & Krafft, 1991) or surely in PVS (Witzke & Schönle, 1996), concur with the PET data described above. However, in contrast to the rigorous PET studies, clinical ERP studies suffer from the subjectivity of visual evaluation for the presence versus absence of the sought brain activity (e.g., P3).

The N400 is a usual brain response to verbal and other *meaningful* stimuli. Its main attribute is the inverse relationship between its amplitude and the strength of the semantic context in which these stimuli are embedded (Van Petten, 1995). Accordingly, the N400 is a unique measure for context violation (Kutas, 1997) whose presence indicates that at least some of the brain mechanisms responsible for the analysis of word meaning (semantics) are intact. In our PVS examinations the semantic mismatch was produced in two experiments. In the Sentence experiment 50 short sentences with semantically correct and highly expected end words were presented as a CC (e.g., I drink coffee with milk and sugar), and 50 sentences with semantically meaningless end words (e.g., I drink coffee with milk and shoes) served as the EC (Kutas & Hillyard, 1980). In the Word Pair experiment 50 semantically closely related word pairs (e.g., moon–sun) and 50 unrelated word pairs (e.g., man–sun) were used (Bentin, Kutas, & Hillyard, 1993). All stimuli, spoken by a female voice, were presented through earphones, with the onset-to-onset intervals within word pairs or sentences being 600–1000 ms. The intervals between pairs were 1.2 s, and those between sentences 2 s. In both experiments semantically unrelated words are known to elicit a negative ERP component with a latency of about 400 ms, therefrom the name N400. Studies using intracranial electrodes (McCarthy, Nobre, Bentin, & Spencer, 1995), magnetoencephalography (Halgren et al., 2002; Mäkelä et al., 2001), and functional magnetic resonance imaging (fMRI) (Kuperberg et al., 2003; Rossel, Price, & Nobre, 2003) converge on the fact that the N400 critically depends on the activity of the anterior medial temporal lobe, inferior frontal regions and temporo-parietal junctions, with some authors adding the lateral frontal cortex (Halgren et al., 2002), the left posterior fusiform area, as well as motor and pre-motor regions (Kiehl, Laurens, & Liddle, 2002).

PATIENTS AND RECORDING

We examined 50 PVS patients, aged 18–76 years (mean 42), 15 females, from five hospitals for neurological rehabilitation in southwest Germany. The inclusion criteria were (1) age > 14 years, (2) normal auditory brainstem evoked potentials at least on one side, and (3) no pharmacological sedation. The duration since accident varied between 5 weeks and 57 months (mean 6.2 months). The PVS was caused by head injury (19 patients), anoxia (15), subarachnoidal haemorrhage (11), and intraventricular haemorrhage (3 patients). It should be noted that the patients may not be a representative sample from the PVS population. PVS patients are usually admitted to hospital when either the diagnosis or therapy or prognosis is unclear. Thus one may suppose that many severe patients, e.g., with permanent VS who remain at home were not included in our sample.

The PVS group was compared with two control groups. Control group 1 contained 12 patients with very severe diffuse brain damage (aged 15–61, three females) who were consistently able to communicate. Control group 2 included 20 age-matched healthy subjects (10 females) without any history of neurological disease. The study was approved by the Ethical Committee of the University of Tübingen, Medical Faculty. Subjects were examined with informed consent of their own (control groups) or their legal representatives (the PVS group).

The EEG was recorded at patients' bedside from nine recording sites (international 10–20 system), referred to two mastoid electrodes which were linked via a 15 kΩ shunt. The EEG was digitised at 250 Hz and band-filtered between 0.3 and 70 Hz (with an additional notch filter at 50 Hz). The vertical and horizontal electro-oculogram was recorded in a bipolar manner and used for off-line artefact correction. ERPs were averaged separately for each condition (i.e., rare and frequent stimuli in oddballs; and semantically related and unrelated stimuli in semantic experiments). Trials still containing artefacts after artefact correction were dismissed. An experiment was valid if each condition contained at least 35 artefact-free trials.

In contrast to previous ERP studies in which the presence of a component was evaluated per visual inspection, we applied, to each subject and each experiment, a strict statistical evaluation technique developed in our group (Bostanov, 2004; Bostanov & Kotchoubey, 2004) and based on continuous wavelet transformation of ERP waveforms. Three possible ERP outcomes were distinguished: (1) no response: the lack of significant differences between EC and CC; (2) normal response: a significant difference expected according the extant data, i.e., P3 in oddball experiments and the N400 in semantic mismatch experiments; (3) abnormal response: a significant difference between the conditions, which, however, was not expected on the basis of previous data. Mostly, this was an ERP component of the opposite polarity, e.g., a slow negative deflection to rare oddball stimuli instead of the expected positive wave. The significance level was set at .05. As regards normal responses, statistical tests were one-tailed because only one particular polarity was expected. For abnormal responses, because "everything significant" was counted, two-tailed tests were applied. Finally, for middle-latency ERP components N1 and P2, which did not distinguish between conditions, the significance of their difference from zero was evaluated. Figure 1 illustrates the types of responses recorded in our sample.

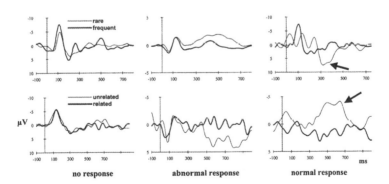

Figure 1. Examples of ERP responses in PVS patients. Top row: oddball with musical tones (chords). Bottom row: word pair experiment. For simplicity, only data recorded at Cz are presented. Negativity is plotted upwards. Normal responses (P3 and N400) are pointed by arrows. Both normal and abnormal responses were statistically significant, but the former were similar in their polarity and morphology to the responses recorded in healthy subjects, whereas the latter were not. ERP components delayed for 100–200 ms compared to control subjects were still regarded as normal because it is known that even a mild brain injury can lead to such latency delays. In the left column, note clear middle-latency ERP responses to both stimulus conditions, but no difference between conditions; such instances were regarded as no-responses

OCCURRENCE OF COMPLEX INFORMATION
PROCESSING IN PVS

Either the N1 or P2 wave, or both, was clearly seen in 45 of 50 PVS patients. They attained significance in 37 patients, indicating that the primary cortical processing was preserved (see also Figure 1, top row). In oddball with tonal stimuli (chords), a significant P3 was found in 13 out of 47 valid experiments. If we suppose, for simplicity, that 5% of all findings can be significant by chance (in fact, the exact figure is always lower than 5%), the P3 wave occurrence was clearly above chance: $\chi^2(1) = 7.80, p < .01$. The same holds true for P3 to vowels, 12 out of 45 valid experiments; $\chi^2(1) = 6.68, p < .01$, the N400 in the word pair experiment, 10 of 44; $\chi^2(1) = 5.79$, $p < .05$, and the N400 to sentences, 9 of 39; $\chi^2(1) = 5.19, p < .05$.

In addition to these normal responses, several patients (6 to 10) exhibited abnormal responses in the form of polarity inversion. These inverted responses occurred with an above-chance frequency in oddball with chords, 10 out of 47; $\chi^2(1) = 4.70$, $p < .05$, and approached significance in oddball with vowels, 9 out of 47: $\chi^2(1) = 3.11$, $p < .10$. In the semantic experiments this frequency did not differ from chance.

Despite the above-chance frequencies of normal ERP responses in PVS patients, these frequencies were lower than in control groups. Abnormal responses, in contrast, were less frequent in control group 1 and disappeared in control group 2 (healthy subjects). These differences, presented in Figure 2, were significant in all experiments, chords: $\chi^2(4) = 22.8, p < .0001$; vowels: $\chi^2(4) = 31.99, p < .0001$; sentences: $\chi^2(4) = 18.49, p < .001$; word pairs: $\chi^2(4) = 13.79, p < .01$. Moreover, even the small control group 1, which consisted of patients with very severe brain damage, was superior in terms of P3 frequency as compared with the PVS group: $\chi^2(1) = 4.17$, and $\chi^2(1) = 5.01$, for chords and vowels, respectively; both $ps < .05$.

Within the PVS group, several factors were explored for their possible effects on ERP responses. The occurrence of the ERP components did not vary as a function of age, gender, and the time elapsed since the accident. The causal factor, in contrast, was significant, because patients with anoxic brain damage were consistently less responsive in the semantic experiments than patients with vascular lesions, $\chi^2(2) = 8.22$, and $\chi^2(2) = 7.55$, for word pairs and sentences, respectively; both $ps < .05$. The same tendency showed itself in the oddball experiments too, but it did not reach significance (Figure 3, top).

These chi-square data are not exact because, when we take all aetiological groups and the three kinds of responses separately, some groups become very small. However, if we combine normal and abnormal responses, anoxic patients remain significantly less responsive in the word pair experiment than both vascular, $\chi^2(1) = 7.22$, $p < .01$, and traumatic, $\chi^2(1) = 3.12$,

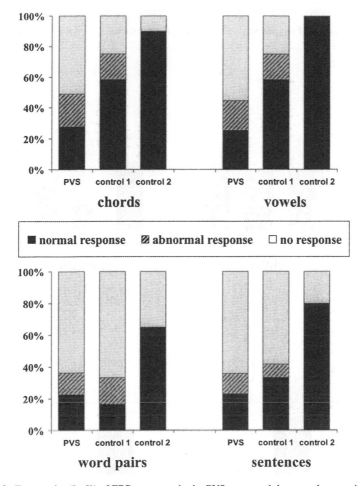

Figure 2. Frequencies (in %) of ERP responses in the PVS group and the control groups in oddball experiments (top) and semantic experiments (bottom)

$p < .07$, brain lesions. Alternatively, we can use Fisher's exact test for 2×2 tables (Agresti, 1992), which, again, results in highly significant differences between vascular and anoxic patients as in terms of the N400 ($p = .0005$), all responses in the semantic experiments ($p = .006$), and between trauma and anoxia patients in terms of the N400 ($p = .01$). Moreover, the oddball P3 also tends to occur more frequently in vascular than anoxic patients ($p = .10$).

Morphological classification of the patients was very difficult due to a very high variability of the localisations of damage. On the basis of CT and MR tomography data, the sample was roughly classified according to the size of the lesion (moderate versus large), the left- versus right-side prevalence,

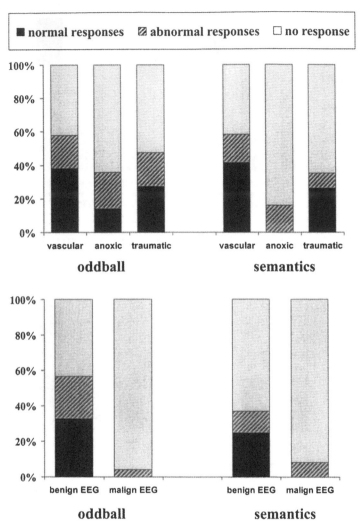

Figure 3. Frequencies (in %) of ERP responses in PVS patients as a function of aetiology (top) and the pattern of the background EEG. "Benign EEG" implies the presence of distinct rhythmic activity in the theta or low-alpha band. "Malign EEG" entails patients with flat EEG as well as large-amplitude slow (1–2.5 Hz) delta-waves. The data of the two oddball experiments and two semantic experiments are collapsed together

and the patients with cortical versus subcortical (basal ganglia, thalamus, pons, and the middle brain) lesions. The frequency of occurrence of the P3 component in the oddball experiment with vowels varied as a function of the size of the lesion: $\chi^2(2) = 7.52, p < .05$. Patients whose lesions were substantially larger on the right than the left side ($N = 13$) exhibited at least one

N400 significantly more often than the patients with the opposite pattern of lateralisation ($N = 15$): $\chi^2(1) = 4.00$, $p < .05$; see Figure 4. Normal ERP responses in the word pair experiment were also significantly more frequent in patients with purely subcortical lesions than in patients with cortical lesions: $\chi^2(1) = 6.82$, $p < .01$.

The type of the rest EEG was the most powerful factor related to the occurrence of the ERP components (Figure 3, bottom). Almost all significant ERP responses were obtained in a subgroup of PVS patients with a "benign" EEG patterns, that is, with prevailing theta (4–7 Hz) or slow alpha (8–9 Hz) activity which did not respond or weakly responded to light. No one significant normal response and only three significant abnormal responses (one slow negativity in an oddball paradigm and two slow positive shifts in the sentence paradigm) were found among 12 patients having a "malign" EEG pattern, that is, cither a flat EEG or dominant and widespread delta activity (1–2.5 Hz). According to Fisher's exact significance test, all the differences were significant with $p \leq .009$. One patient with malign EEG demonstrated an apparent P3 wave in the oddball with chords, but the significance of this wave did not attain our criterion ($p = .12$). A comparison between the type of EEG and the aetiology revealed slightly more patients with brain anoxia among "malign" EEG (47%) versus "benign" EEG (26%), but this difference was not significant.

Since the ERP effects occasionally observed in PVS patients with the malign EEG do not statistically deviate from chance, this subgroup can be regarded as virtually ERP-nonresponsive. If we relate the obtained response frequencies to the remaining subgroup of 38 benign EEG patients rather than to the whole group of 50 patients, this results in 34% (tonal stimuli) or 32% (vowels) of patients having a P3 (both $ps < .01$), and 26% (word pairs) or 24% (sentences) of patients having an N400 (both $ps < .02$). In addition, abnormal responses in oddball experiments were obtained in 24% patients ($p < .01$), and in semantic experiments in 12% patients (not significantly different from chance).

The final question is, whether taking normal and abnormal responses into account reveals something new as compared with normal responses only. In other words, is it not simpler to ignore the abnormal responses and to regard them just as non-responses, as we always did for simplicity in our previous studies? On the one hand, significant abnormal responses were not very frequent in semantic experiments. Probably this was the reason why only normal responses significantly correlated with the morphology of the lesion, and abnormal responses did not. On the other hand, in the oddball experiments one-fourth of patients with the benign EEG exhibited abnormal responses. Yet more important, subdividing PVS patients into those with and without normal ERP responses did not result in a significant association between the four experiments. That is, having a P3 in an oddball experiment

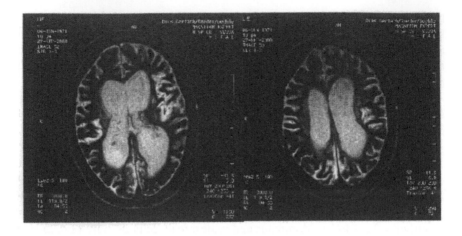

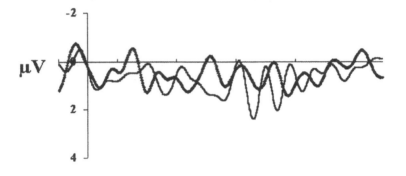

(a)

Figure 4 (above and opposite). Examples of two PVS patients with prevailing left-hemispheric (a) and right-hemispheric (b) lesions following subarachnoidal haemorrhages. Below: the patients' ERPs in response to semantically related (bold line) and unrelated (meaningless; thin line) end words in the sentence experiment. Negativity is up. Arrow indicates the N400 to semantically unrelated words

does not increase the probability of having a P3 in the other experiment; having a P3 in either experiment does not increase the probability of having an N400, etc. The situation changes when both normal and abnormal responses are taken into consideration. The responsiveness in oddball with chords significantly predicts the responsiveness in oddball with vowels: $\chi^2(2) = 7.71$, $p < .05$. Patients having significant responses in the oddball experiments also tend to respond in the word pair experiment: $\chi^2(2) = 5.25$, $p < .08$. Finally, the responsiveness in the word pair experiment predicts that in the sentence experiment: $\chi^2(2) = 22.76$, $p < .001$.

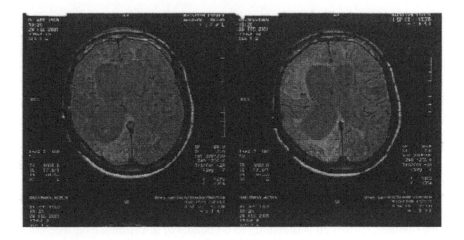

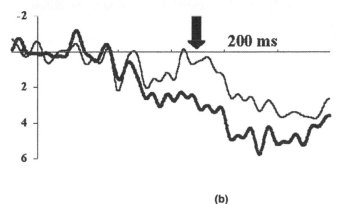

(b)

Figure 4. Continued

WHY DO WE UNDERESTIMATE OUR PATIENTS' COGNITIVE CAPACITIES

Due to the nature of statistical assessment, in each particular patient there is a remaining probability to obtain a (false) positive result by chance. Another factor contained in almost all methods of analysis of EEG as well as PET and fMRI is voluntary selection of relevant time windows or regions of interest. This preselection can further increase the probability of obtaining a false positive result. The technique employed here minimised the effect of this factor (see Bostanov, 2004, for technical details).

Much longer is the list of factors having the opposite effect. First, a healthy individual sometimes does not manifest all normal brain responses typical for group data. As shown in Figure 2, semantic ERP components are lacking in a considerable number of healthy subjects with normal semantic comprehension. Thus a lack of a late ERP component does not necessarily imply the lack of the corresponding function.

Second, fluctuations in arousal/alertness may be particularly strong in neurological patients with severe brain injuries. A critical ERP test may occasionally be performed during a period of low activation, yielding a negative result. Some time earlier or later the same patient might manifest a clear ERP component.

Third, apart of arousal fluctuations, there can be a continuous response decrement due to habituation or a decrease of attention during an experiment which lasted, as a rule, about 5 min each. In particular, a considerable drop of alertness during these 5-min sessions may be expected in patients with frontal lobe damage. Clearly, it is one thing to be unable to discriminate between two stimuli, and another thing to be unable to maintain attention to the difference between these stimuli during 5 min.

Fourth, the conventional statistics are characterised by considerable asymmetry between the Type I and Type II errors. The α-level of .05 may be related to a ß-level as high as .50, which means that about one-half of the positive results may be missed. Usually this asymmetry between H0 and H1 is justified by the necessity to be cautious in accepting new results. This argument sounds well in the basic science, but in the clinical testing this bias is questionable. Here the null hypothesis asserts that a given patient cannot perform some cognitive operation, while the alternative hypothesis asserts that he or she can. Why should we a priori believe in the former more than the latter?

These problems are more or less common for all neurophysiological techniques which are (or can be) used for the assessment of the remaining information processing in the brain of severely damaged patients. Apart of this, there are particular problems arising with different techniques. The fMRI, for instance, is related to a high stress due to loud noise, which can considerably interfere with a patient's cognitive performance. On the other hand, the ERP technique employed in this study is based on the averaging procedure necessary to improve the signal/noise ratio. This averaging implies that patients not only display an expected brain activation, but also that this activation is phase-locked to stimulus onset. Severe brain pathology can increase the variability of response timing (latency jitter), thus an ERP component can be lacking in the average waveform even if it appeared on many single trials.

All this means that our data across the whole sample are biased towards false negatives, that is, any technique of cognitive neuroscience suffers from the tendency to underestimate the abilities of the examined patients. It would be cautious, therefore, to regard the data reported above as the lower limit of the patients' real processing capacities.

DISCUSSION

The most recent and well-substantiated hypotheses concerning the neurophysiological bases of the persistent vegetative state relate this condition to (1) the lack of activity of secondary sensory and associative areas despite the remaining activity of the primary sensory areas; and (2) the lack of activity of large distributed cortical networks despite intact local cortical activity (Boly et al., 2004; Laureys et al., 1999, 2000b; Schiff et al., 1999, 2000).

The present results indicate, first, that components of event-related brain potentials (ERP) which manifest the activity of complex cortical networks in the temporal, parietal, and probably frontal lobes, occur in PVS patients with above-chance probabilities. This finding concurs with some reliable single-case observations of stimulus-related variation in regional cerebral blood flow in PVS (e.g., Owen et al., 2002). The novelty of our finding is that such cortical activation is frequent—at least, in some subgroups of PVS patients.

The results indicate, second, that although the frequencies of those late ERP components in PVS are higher than expected, they are still lower than even in a group of comparable severely brain-damaged, but conscious and communicating, patients, not to mention the group of healthy subjects. This suggests that those ERP components can be used as one of the measures of high-level cortical activity in patients with severe brain damage.

The results demonstrate, third, the existence of two subgroups of PVS patients in which the occurrence of the ERP components P3 and N400 is significantly lower than in other patients with the same diagnosis—in fact, this occurrence does not differ from the chance level. These are, (1) patients with the malign EEG pattern which included flat EEG or diffuse delta activity and (2) patients with anoxic brain damage. As regards the former factor, the lack or deep suppression of the oscillatory activity above 3 Hz may indicate a collapse of basic thalamo-cortical loops whose functioning appears to be necessary for cognitive processing operations (Schiff & Plum, 2000). This finding is in line with the ideas of the critical role of the thalamo-cortical oscillations underlying elementary consciousness (Llinas, Ribary, Contreras, & Pedroarena, 1998; Schiff & Plum, 2000; Steriade, 2000; Tononi & Edelman, 2000).

As regards the latter factor, patients with anoxic brain damage are frequently considered as the most severe subgroup of all PVS patients in terms of the extent of their damage, the decrement of brain metabolism, and prognosis (e.g., Adams, Graham, & Jennett, 2000; Falk, 1990; Heindl & Laub, 1996; Rudolf et al., 1999; Sazbon et al., 1990); but see, in contrast, a recent report of Shah, Al-Adawi, Dorvlo, and Burke (2004). In our study patients with anoxia displayed fewer significant responses, and, particularly, much fewer normal responses than patients with other (i.e., vascular or traumatic) aetiologies. A possible explanation, suggested by Adams et al. (2000), is that anoxia (rather than a mechanical injury and, perhaps, a stroke) results in irreversible neuronal loss. Therefore, one may speculate that in some patients with other aetiologies, in which more cell bodies remained intact, partial regeneration of axons with time (most of our patients were chronic) have led to partial restoration of thalamo-cortical connections, but not so in patients with brain anoxia.

To sum up, we can putatively suggest the existence of two subtypes of VS, one with relatively intact, and the other with completely broken down, thalamo-cortical links. It is possible that cortical functions are really absent in the latter group, as hypothesised by Kretschmer (1940), but they are consistently present in the former. It is also possible that the former subtype is caused by brain anoxia more frequently than by head injury or stroke.

Finally, our data show that in addition to normal (or close-to-normal) patterns of stimulus-related brain activation, PVS patients frequently display completely different patterns which may never appear in normal controls, at least in a waking state. A frequent abnormal pattern observed in this study was slow negative waves in response to rare stimuli in the oddball paradigms, instead of the expected P3. Apparently similar ERPs to rare stimuli have been reported in sleep stage 2 (Loewy et al., 2000; Salisbury & Squires, 1992; Winter, Kok, Kenemans, & Elton, 1995) and anaesthesia (Yppärilä et al., 2002). Several authors (Atienza, Cantero, & Escera, 2001; Loewy et al., 2000; Sallinen, Kaartinen, & Lyytinen, 1997) noted similarities between these waveforms and K-complexes, which are classical cortical responses to stimuli in sleep stage 2 and can well distinguish between frequent and rare stimuli (Perrin, Bastuji, Mauguiére, & García-Larrea, 2000). At present, a hypothesis about common mechanisms between abnormal oddball responses in PVS and K-complexes in sleep remain a speculation. But although we do not know how to interpret such abnormal response patterns, they should not be simply ignored as "no responses". The correlations between the four experimental paradigms employed in this study demonstrate that the data are more consistent (thus leading to a better individual assessment) when both normal and abnormal response patterns are taken into account.

CONCLUSION

A great achievement of the philosophy of science in the 20th century was the acceptance of the idea that a good scientific theory must be testable (Lakatos, 1976; Popper, 1963). In other words, the theory must make clear which empirical findings, if observed, would contradict it and lead to its refusal. The apallic hypothesis, claiming that the entire cerebral cortex in PVS is "switched off", was a good scientific hypothesis because its empirical predictions were clear-cut: no cortical activity specifically related to complex stimuli should be observed. This made it possible to test this hypothesis and to falsify it: large parts of the cortex in PVS remain active. The vegetative hypothesis, which does not speak about brain functions, but rather, about mental processes (subjective experience), cannot be falsified in its present form, because those subjective events are first-person events and, hence, they can never be proved nor disproved by any third person observation. But a scientific idea which cannot be disproved by any objective data is meaningless (Platt, 1964).

In the present study, ERP signs of stimulus processing involving broadly distributed cortical structures in temporal, parietal and frontal lobes were found in a substantial fraction of PVS patients. These findings broaden our knowledge about these patients' capacities, but they do not necessarily indicate that the patients possess elements of subjective experience, since even those complex information processing operations can run outside conscious awareness (e.g., Perrin, Bastuji, & Garcia-Larrea, 2002; Portas et al., 2000).

However, if we finally admit that mental processes and conscious experience should anyway be related to brain function (and I do not know any neurologist who negates this), we should one day develop testable neurophysiological criteria (may be preliminary) of which level of brain activity would be incompatible with the definition of vegetative state. The vegetative hypothesis should be made testable and refutable, and it should be refuted whenever its own criteria are reached.

REFERENCES

Adams, J. H., Graham, D. I., & Jennett, B. (2000). The neuropathology of the vegetative state after an acute brain insult. *Brain, 123*(7), 1327–1338.

Agardh, C. D., Rosén, I., & Ryding, E. (1983). Persistent vegetative state with high cerebral blood flow following profound hypoglycemia. *Annals of Neurology, 14*, 482–486.

Agresti, A. (1992). A survey of exact inference for contingency tables. *Statistical Science, 7*, 131–177.

Alkire, M. T., White, N. S., Hsieh, R., & Haier, R. (2004). Dissociable brain activation responses to 5-Hz electrical pain stimulation: A high-field functional magnetic resonance imaging study. *Anesthesiology, 100*(4), 939–946.

Anderer, P., Pasqual-Marqui, R. D., Semlitsch, H. V., & Saletu, B. (1998). Electrical sources of P300 event-related brain potentials revealed by low resolution electromagnetic tomography. 1. Effects of normal aging. *Neuropsychobiology, 37*(1), 20–27.

Arceni, S., Nereantiu, F., & Carp, N. (1981). Persistent vegetative state after multiple trauma: A clinicopathologic study. *Acta Neurochirurgica, 59*, 45–53.

Atienza, M., Cantero, J. L., & Escera, C. (2001). Auditory information processing during human sleep as revealed by event-related brain potentials. *Clinical Neurophysiology, 112*, 2031–2045.

Bentin, S., Kutas, M., & Hillyard, S. A. (1993). Electrophysiological evidence for task effects on semantic priming in auditory word processing. *Psychophysiology, 30*, 161–169.

Bingel, U., Quante, M., Knab, R., Bromm, B., Weiller, C., & Buchel, C. (2003). Single trial fMRI reveals significant contralateral bias in responses to laser pain within thalamus and somatosensory cortices. *Neuroimage, 18*(3), 740–748.

Blumberg, P. C., Jones, N. R., & North, J. B. (1989). Diffuse axonal injury in head trauma. *Journal of Neurology, Neurosurgery, and Psychiatry, 52,* 838–841.

Boly, M., Faymonville, M. E., Peigneux, P., Lambermont, B., Damas, P., Del Fiore, G., et al. (2004). Auditory processing in severely brain injured patients: Differences between the minimally conscious state and the persistent vegetative state. *Archives of Neurology, 61*(2), 233–238.

Bostanov, V. (2004). BCI competition 2003—Data sets Ib and IIB: Feature extraction from event-related brain potentials with the Continuous Wavelet Transform and the *t*-value scalogram. *IEEE Transactions of Biomedical Engineering, 51*(6), 1057–1061.

Bostanov, V., & Kotchoubey, B. (2004). Recognition of affective prosody: Continuous wavelet measures of event-related brain potentials to emotional exclamations. *Psychophysiology, 41,* 259–268.

Casey, K. L. (2000). Concepts of pain mechanisms: The contribution of functional imaging of the human brain. *Progress in Brain Research, 129,* 277–287.

Coghill, R. C., McHaffie, J. G., & Yen, Y. F. (2003). Neural correlates of interindividual differences in the subjective experience of pain. *Proceedings of the National Academy of Sciences of the USA, 100,* 8538–8542.

Coles, M. G. H., Gratton, G., & Fabiani, M. (1990). Event-related potentials. In J. T. Caccioppo, L. G. Tassinari, & R. E. Petty (Eds.), *Tutorials in psychophysiology: Physical, social, and inferential elements* (pp. 413–455). Cambridge, England: Cambridge University Press.

Dalle Ore, G., Gerstenbrand, F., Lücking, G. H., Peters, G., & Peters, U. H. (Eds.). (1987). *The apallic syndrome.* Berlin: Springer.

de Jong, B. M., Willemsen, A. T. M., & Paans, A. M. J. (1997). Regional cerebral blood flow changes related to affective speech presentation in persistent vegetative state. *Clinical Neurology and Neurosurgery, 99,* 213–216.

Dougherty, J. H., Rawlinson, D. G., Levy, D. E., & Plum, F. (1981). Hypoxic-ischemic brain injury and the vegetative state: Clinical and neuropathologic correlation. *Neurology, 31,* 991–997.

DeVolder, A. G., Goffinet, A. M., Bol, A., Michel, C., de Barsy, T., & Laterre, C. (1990). Brain glucose metabolism in post-anoxic syndrome: Positron emission tomography study. *Archives of Neurology, 47,* 197–204.

Falk, R. H. (1990). Physical and intellectual recovery following prolonged hypoxic coma. *Postgraduate Medical Journal, 66,* 384–386.

Fischer, C., Morlet, D., Bouchet, P., Luaute, J., Jourdan, C., & Salord, F. (1999). Mismatch negativity and late auditory evoked potentials in comatose patients. *Clinical Neurophysiology, 110*(9), 1601–1610.

Garcia-Larrea, L., Frot, M., & Valeriani, M. (2003). Brain generators of laser-evoked potentials: From dipoles to functional significance. *Neurophysiologie Clinique, 33*(4), 279–292.

Gott, P. S., Rabinovicz, A. L., & DiGiorgio, C. M. (1991). P300 auditory event-related potentials in nontraumatic coma: Association with Glasgow Coma Score and awakening. *Archives of Neurology, 48*(12), 1267–1270.

Guerit, J. M., Verougstraete, D., Tourtchaninoff, M., Debatisse, D., & Witdoeckt, C. (1999). ERPs obtained with the auditory oddball paradigm in coma and altered states of consciousness: Clinical relationships, prognostic value and origin of components. *Clinical Neurophysiology, 110,* 1260–1269.

Halgren, E., Baudena, P., Clarke, J. M., & Heit, G. (1995). Intracerebral potentials to rare target and distractor auditory and visual stimuli. II. Medial, lateral, and posterior temporal lobe. *Electroencephalography and clinical Neurophysiology, 94*(4), 229–250.

Halgren, E., Dhond, R. P., Christensen, N., Van Petten, C., Marinkovic, K., Lewine, J. D., & Dale, A. M. (2002). N400-like magnetoencephalography responses modulated by semantic context, word frequency, and lexical class in sentences. *Neuroimage*, *17*(3), 1106–1116.

Heindl, U. T., & Laub, M. C. (1996). Outcome of persistent vegetative state following hypoxic or traumatic brain injury in children and adolescents. *Neuropediatrics*, *27*, 94–100.

Jennett, B. (2002). *The vegetative state*. Cambridge, UK: University Press.

Jennett, B., Adams, J. H., Murray, L. S., & Graham, D. I. (2001). Neuropathology in vegetative and severely disabled patients after head injury. *Neurology*, *56*(4), 486–490.

Jennett, B., & Plum, F. (1972). Persistent vegetative state after brain damage: A syndrome in search of a name. *Lancet*, *1*, 734–737.

Kampfl, A., Franz, G., Aichner, F., Pflauser, B., Haring, H.-P., Felber, S., et al. (1998a). The persistent vegetative state after closed head injury: Clinical and magnetic resonance imaging findings in 42 patients. *Journal of Neurosurgery*, *88*, 809–816.

Kampfl, A., Schmutzhard, E., Franz, G., Pflauser, B., Haring, H.-P., Ulmer, H., et al. (1998b). Prediction of recovery from post-traumatic vegetative state with cerebral magnetic-resonance imaging. *Lancet*, *351*, 1763–1767.

Kane, N. M., Curry, S. H., Butler, S. R., & Cummings, B. H. (1993). Electrophysiological indicator of awakening from coma. *Lancet*, *341*, 688.

Kane, N. M., Butler, S. R., & Simpson, T. (2000). Coma outcome prediction using event-related potentials: P3 and mismatch negativity. *Audiology and Neuro-Otology*, *5*, 186–191.

Kiehl, K. A., Laurens, K. R., & Liddle, P. F. (2002). Reading anomalous sentences: An event-related fMRI study of semantic processing. *Neuroimage*, *17*, 842–850.

Kinney, H. C., & Samuels, M. A. (1994). Neuropathology of the persistent vegetative state: A review. *Journal of Neuropathology and Experimental Neurology*, *53*(6), 548–558.

Klein, M. (1997). Perception of pain in the persistent vegetative state? *European Journal of Pain*, *1*, 165–168.

Knight, R. T. (1996). Contribution of human hippocampal region to novelty detection. *Nature*, *383*, 256–259.

Knight, R. T., & Scabini, D. (1998). Anatomic bases of event-related potentials and their relationship to novelty detection in humans. *Journal of Clinical Neurophysiology*, *15*(1), 3–13.

Kotchoubey, B., Lang, S., Baales, R., Herb, E., Maurer, P., Mezger, G., et al. (2001). Brain potentials in human patients with severe diffuse brain damage. *Neuroscience Letters*, *301*, 37–40.

Kotchoubey, B., Lang, S., Bostanov, V., & Birbaumer, N. (2002). Is there a mind? Psychophysiology of unconscious patients. *News in Physiological Sciences*, *17*, 38–42.

Kotchoubey, B., Lang, S., Bostanov, V., & Birbaumer, N. (2003a). Cortical processing in Guillain-Barre syndrome after years of total immobility. *Journal of Neurology*, *250*, 1121–1123.

Kotchoubey, B., Schneck, M., Lang, S., & Birbaumer, N. (2003b). Event-related brain potentials in a patient with akinetic mutism. *Neurophysiologie Clinique*, *33*, 23–30.

Kretschmer, E. (1940). Das apallische Syndrom. *Zeitschrift für gesamte Neurologie und Psychiatrie*, *169*, 576–579.

Kuperberg, G. R., Holcomb, P. J., Sitnikova, T., Greve, D., Dale, A. M., & Caplan, D. (2003). Distinct patterns of neural modulation during the processing of conceptual and syntactic anomalies. *Journal of Cognitive Neuroscience*, *15*(2), 272–293.

Kutas, M. (1997). Views on how the electrical activity that the brain generates reflects the functions of different language structures. *Psychophysiology*, *34*, 383–398.

Kutas, M., & Hillyard, S. A. (1980). Reading senseless sentences: Brain potentials reflect semantic incongruity. *Science*, *207*, 203–205.

Lakatos, I. (1976). *Proofs and refutations*. Cambridge, UK: University Press.

Laureys, S., Goldman, S., Phillips, C., Van Bogaert, P., Aerts, J., Luxen, A., et al. (1999). Impaired effective cortical connectivity in vegetative state: Preliminary investigation using PET. *Neuroimage, 9*, 377–382.

Laureys, S., Faymonville, M. E., Degueldre, C., DelFiore, G., Damas, P., Lambermont, B., et al. (2000a). Auditory processing in vegetative state. *Brain, 123*(8), 1589–1601.

Laureys, S., Faymonville, M. E., Luxen, A., Lamy, M., Franck, G., & Maquet, P. (2000b). Restoration of thalamocortical connectivity after recovery from persistent vegetative state. *Lancet, 355*(9217), 1790–1791.

Laureys, S., Antoine, S., Boly, M., Elincx, S., Faymonville, M. E., Berre, J., et al. (2002a). Brain function in the vegetative state. *Acta Neurologica Belgica, 102*, 177–185.

Laureys, S., Faymonville, M. E., Peigneux, P., Damas, P., Lambermont, B., Del Fiore, G., et al. (2002b). Cortical processing of noxious somatosensory stimuli in the persistent vegetative state. *Neuroimage, 17*(2), 732–741.

Levy, D. E., Sidtis, J. J., Rottenberg, D. A., Jarden, J. O., Strother, S. C., Dhawan, V., et al. (1987). Differences in cerebral blood flow and glucose utilization in vegetative versus locked-in patients. *Annals of Neurology, 22*, 673–682.

Llinas, R., Ribary, U., Contreras, D., & Pedroarena, C. (1998). The neuronal basis for consciousness. *Philosophical Transactions of the Royal Society of London. B: Biological Sciences, 353*, 1841–1849.

Loewy, D. H., Campbell, K. B., de Lugt, D. R., Elton, M., & Kok, A. (2000). The mismatch negativity during natural sleep: Intensity deviants. *Clinical Neurophysiology, 111*, 863–872.

Lotze, M., Flor, H., Grodd, W., Larbig, W., & Birbaumer, N. (2001). Phantom movements and pain. An fMRI study in upper limb amputees. *Brain, 124*, 2268–2277.

Mäkelä, A. M., Mäkinen, V., Nikkilä, M., Ilmoniemi, R. J., & Tiitinen, H. (2001). Magneto-encephalographic (MEG) localization of the auditory N400m: Effects of stimulus duration. *Neuroreport, 12*(2), 249–253.

Matsuda, W., Matsumura, A., Komatsu, Y., Yanaka, K., & Nose, T. (2003). Awakenings from persistent vegetative state: Report of three cases with Parkinsonism and brain stem lesions on MRI. *Journal of Neurology, Neurosurgery and Psychiatry, 74*(11), 1571–1573.

McCarthy, G., Nobre, A. C., Bentin, S., & Spencer, D. D. (1995). Language-related field potentials in the anterior-medial temporal lobe: I. Intracranial distribution and neural generators. *Journal of Neuroscience, 15*, 1080–1089.

Menon, D. K., Owen, A. M., Williams, E. J., Minhas, P. S., Allen, C. M., & Boniface, S. J. (1998). Cortical processing in persistent vegetative state. *Lancet, 352*, 200.

Molnar, M. (1994). On the origin of the P3 event-related potential component. *International Journal of Psychophysiology, 17*, 129–144.

Mutschler, V., Chaumeil, S. G., Marcoux, L., Wioland, N., Tempe, J. D., & Kurtz, D. (1996). Etude du P300 auditif chez des sujets en coma post-anoxique. Donnees preliminaires. *Neurophysiologie Clinique, 26*, 158–163.

Näätänen, R. (2000). Mismatch negativity (MMN): Perspectives for application. *International Journal of Psychophysiology, 37*(1), 3–10.

Neumann, N., & Kotchoubey, B. (2004). Assessment of cognitive functions in severely paralysed and severely brain damaged patients: Neuropsychological and electrophysiological methods. *Brain Research Protocols, 14*, 25–36.

Niddam, D. M., Yeh, T. C., Wu, Y. T., Lee, P. L., Arendt-Nielsen, L., Chen, A. C., et al. (2003). Event-related functional MRI study on central representation of acute muscle pain induced by electrical stimulation. *Neuroimage, 17*(3), 1437–1450.

Onofrj, M., Melchionda, D., Thomas, A., & Fulgente, T. (1996). Reappearance of event-related P3 potential in locked-in syndrome. *Cognitive Brain Research, 4*, 95–97.

Onofrj, M., Thomas, A., Paci, C., Scesi, M., & Tombari, R. (1997). Event related potentials recorded in patients with locked-in syndrome. *Journal of Neurology, Neurosurgery and Psychiatry, 63*, 759–764.

Owen, A. M., Menon, D. K., Johnsrude, I. S., Bor, D., Scott, S. K., Manly, T., et al. (2002). Detecting residual cognitive function in persistent vegetative state. *Neurocase, 8*(5), 394–403.

Perrin, F., Bastuji, H., Mauguiére, F., & García-Larrea, L. (2000). Functional dissociation of the early and late portions of human K-complexes. *Neuroreport, 11*(8), 1637–1640.

Perrin, F., Bastuji, H., & Garcia-Larrea, L. (2002). Detection of verbal discordances during sleep. *Neuroreport, 13*(10), 1345–1349.

Peyron, R., Laurent, B., & Garcia-Larrea, L. (2000). Functional imaging of brain responses to pain. A review and meta-analysis. *Neurophysiologie Clinique, 30*(5), 263–288.

Peyron, R., Frot, M., Schneider, F., Garcia-Larrea, L., Mertens, P., Barral, F. G., Sindou, M., et al. (2002). Role of opercularinsular cortices in human pain processing. *Neuroimage, 17*(3), 1336–1346.

Picton, T. W., & Hillyard, S. A. (1988). Endogenous event-related potentials. In T. W. Picton (Ed.), *Human event-related potentials* (Vol. 3, pp. 361–426). Amsterdam: Elsevier.

Platt, J. R. (1964). Strong inference. *Science, 146*(3642), 347–353.

Plum, F., Schiff, N., Ribary, U., & Llinas, R. (1998). Coordinated expression in chronically unconscious persons. *Philosophical Transactions of the Royal Society, London, 353*, 1929–1933.

Polich, J. (1991). P300 in clinical applications: Meaning, method, and measurement. *American Journal of EEG Technology, 31*, 201–231.

Polich, J., & Comerchero, M. D. (2003). P3a from visual stimuli: Typicality, task, and topography. *Brain Topography, 15*, 141–152.

Polich, J., & Squire, L. R. (1993). P300 from amnestic patients with bilateral hippocampal lesions. *Electroencephalography and Clinical Neurophysiology, 86*, 408–417.

Popper, K. R. (1963). *Conjectures and Refutations.* London: Routledge and Kegan Paul.

Portas, C. M., Krakow, K., Allen, P., Josephs, O., Armony, J. L., & Frith, C. D. (2000). Auditory processing across the sleep-wake cycle: Simultaneous EEG and fMRI monitoring in humans. *Neuron, 28*, 991–999.

Pritchard, W. S. (1981). Psychophysiology of P300. *Psychological Bulletin, 89*, 506–540.

Puce, A., & Bladin, P. F. (1991). Scalp and limbic P3 event-related potentials in the assessment of patients with temporal lobe epilepsy. *Epilepsia, 32*(5), 629–634.

Rappaport, M., McCandless, K. L., Pond, W., & Krafft, M. C. (1991). Passive P300 response in traumatic brain injury patients. *Journal of Neuropsychiatry and Clinical Neurosciences, 3*(2), 180–185.

Rossel, S. L., Price, C. J., & Nobre, A. C. (2003). The anatomy and time course of semantic priming investigated by fMRI and ERPs. *Neuropsychologia, 41*(5), 550–564.

Rudolf, J. (2000). Beitrag der Positronen – Emissionstomographie zur diagnostischen Zuordnung und prognostischen Einschätzung postanoxischer Hirnschäden. *Fortschritte der Neurologie und Psychiatrie, 68*(8), 344–351.

Rudolf, J., Ghaemi, M., Haupt, W. F., Szelies, B., & Heiss, W. D. (1999). Cerebral glucose metabolism in acute and persistent vegetative state. *Journal of Neurosurgical Anesthesiology, 11*, 17–24.

Salisbury, D., & Squires, N. K. (1992). Response properties of long-latency event-related potentials evoked during NREM sleep. *Journal of Sleep Research, 2*, 232–240.

Sallinen, M., Kaartinen, J., & Lyytinen, H. (1997). Precursors of the evoked K-complex in event-related brain potentials in stage 2 sleep. *Electroencephalography and Clinical Neurophysiology, 102*, 363–373.

Sazbon, L., Zagreba, F., Ronen, J., Solzi, P., & Costeff, H. (1990). Course and outcome of patients in vegetative state of nontraumatic aetiology. *Journal of Neurology, Neurosurgery and Psychiatry, 56*(4), 407–409.

Scheffers, M. K., Johnson, R., & Ruchkin, D. S. (1991). P300 in patients with unilateral temporal lobectomies: The effects of reduced stimulus quality. *Psychophysiology, 28*(1), 274–283.

Schiff, N. D., & Plum, F. (2000). The role of arousal and "gating" systems in the neurology of impaired consciousness. *Journal of Clinical Neurophysiology, 17*(5), 438–452.

Schiff, N. D., Ribary, U., Plum, F., & Llinas, R. (1999). Words without minds. *Journal of Cognitive Neuroscience, 11*, 650–656.

Schiff, N. D., Ribary, U., Moreno, D. R., Beattie, B., Kronberg, E., Blasberg, R., et al. (2000). Residual cerebral activity and behavioral fragments can remain in the persistently vegetative brain. *Brain, 125*, 1210–1234.

Shah, M. K., Al-Adawi, S., Dorvlo, A. S., & Burke, C. T. (2004). Functional outcomes following anoxic brain injury: A comparison with traumatic brain injury. *Brain Injury, 18*, 111–117.

Signorino, M., D'Acunto, S., Cercaci, S., Pietropaoli, P., & Angeleri, F. (1997). The P300 in traumatic coma: Conditioning of the oddball paradigm. *Journal of Psychophysiology, 11*, 59–70.

Spencer, K. M., Dien, J., & Donchin, E. (1999). A componential analysis of the ERP elicited by novel events using a dense electrode array. *Psychophysiology, 36*(3), 409–414.

Spencer, K. M., Dien, J., & Donchin, E. (2001). Spatiotemporal analysis of the late ERP responses to deviant stimuli. *Psychophysiology, 38*, 343–358.

Steriade, M. (2000). Corticothalamic resonance, states of vigilance and mentation. *Neuroscience, 101*, 243–276.

Tarkka, I. M., & Stokic, D. S. (1998). Source localization of P300 from oddball single stimulus and omitted-stimulus paradigms. *Brain Topography, 11*(2), 141–151.

Tommasino, C., Grana, C., Lucignani, G., Torri, G., & Fazio, F. (1995). Regional cerebral metabolism of glucose in comatose and vegetative state patients. *Journal of Neurosurgical Anesthesiology, 7*, 109–116.

Tononi, G., & Edelman, G. M. (2000). Schizophrenia and the mechanisms of conscious integration. *Brain Research Reviews, 31*, 391–400.

Van Petten, C. (1995). Words and sentences: Event-related brain potential measures. *Psychophysiology, 32*(6), 511–525.

Verleger, R., Jaskowsky, P., & Wauschkuhn, B. (1994). Suspense and surprise: On the relationship between expectancies and P3. *Psychophysiology, 31*, 359–369.

Walter, G. F. (2000). Diffuse axonal injury: Its role in diffuse brain injury and its significance for severe disability and vegetative state. *Critical Reviews Neurosurgery, 9*, 367–375.

Winter, O., Kok, A., Kenemans, J. L., & Elton, M. (1995). Auditory event-related potentials to deviant stimuli during drowsiness and stage 2 sleep. *Electroencephalography and Clinical Neurophysiology, 96*, 398–412.

Witzke, W., & Schönle, P. W. (1996). Ereigniskorrelierte Potentiale als diagnostisches Mittel in der neurologischen Frührehabilitation. *Neurologische Rehabilitation, 2*, 68–80.

Yamagushi, S., & Knight, R. T. (1991). Anterior and posterior association cortex contributions to the somatosensory P300. *Journal of Neuroscience, 11*(7), 2039–2054.

Yppärilä, H., Karhu, J., Westeren-Punnonen, S., Musialowicz, T., & Partanen, J. (2002). Evidence of auditory processing during postoperative propofol sedation. *Clinical Neurophysiology, 113*, 1357–1364.

Zhang, W. T., Jin, Z., Cui, G. H., Zhang, K. L., Zhang, L., Zeng, Y. W., et al. (2003). Relations between brain network activation and analgesic effect induced by low versus high frequency electrical acupoint stimulation in different subjects: A functional magnetic resonance imaging study. *Brain Research, 982*(2), 168–178.

NEUROPSYCHOLOGICAL REHABILITATION
2005, 15 (3/4), 357–371

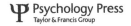

Neurophysiological patterns of vegetative and minimally conscious states

Jean-Michel Guérit

St Luc Hospital, Catholic University of Louvain, and CHIREC, Brussels, Belgium

This paper reviews the possible usefulness of electroencephalogram (EEG) and evoked potential (EP) recording in vegetative and poorly-responsive patients. There is a marked inter-individual EEG and EP variability, which reflects the state heterogeneity. Four clinical applications are described: (1) the identification of primary midbrain dysfunction—and, therefore, a possible reversibility—in post-traumatic states; (2) the identification of the permeability of sensory channels; (3) quantitative follow-up; and (4) individual assessment of cognitive functions and/or consciousness. Regarding this last issue, the loss of primary cortical EPs, although rarely observed, constitutes one major argument against consciousness. Conversely, cognitive EPs definitely proved the persistence of cognitive functions in several vegetative patients. Whether these cognitive functions are conscious or not remains a matter of debate.

INTRODUCTION

From its initial definition as a clinical condition of "wakefulness without awareness" (Jennett & Plum, 1972), it has now become evident that the notion of "vegetative state" encompasses a continuum of situations of more or less extensive brain lesions or dysfunctions whose common denominator is the absence of clinically obvious communication. This led to the wider concept of "minimally conscious state" (Andrews, Murphy, Munday, & Littlewood, 1996). Moreover, besides widespread post-anoxic or post-traumatic brain lesions deeply interfering with cognitive functions, focal brain lesions can also cause decreased communication and so mimic a vegetative state (akinetic mutism,

Correspondence should be sent to Jean-Michel Guérit, Clinique Edith Cavell, rue Edith Cavell 32, B 1180 Brussels, Belgium. Tel: 32 2 340 40 40. Email: jm.guerit@chirec.be

© 2005 Psychology Press Ltd
http://www.tandf.co.uk/journals/pp/09602011.html   DOI:10.1080/09602010443000560

locked-in syndrome), even though cognitive functions are sometimes preserved. Such heterogeneity implies that each vegetative or poorly-responsive patient needs to be individually assessed.

A major advance in the understanding of these situations in individuals came from position emission tomography (PET)-scan studies (Laureys, Berré, & Goldman, 2001; Laureys et al., 2002). These confirmed that the vegetative state was not always consecutive to a global loss of neuronal function but that it could also be due to focal brain lesions or loss of cortico-cortical and/or cortico-thalamic connections. The most dysfunctional brain regions were the parieto-temporal associative cortices, bilaterally. However, despite the fact that functional brain imaging is probably one of the best methods for individual assessment of vegetative cases, it requires patient transportation and, above all, there are few available PET-scan and/or functional magnetic resonance imaging (fMRI) facilities, which makes it hardly conceivable to use these in a routine clinical protocol.

Another way to evaluate non-communicating patients consists of examining brain electrogenesis through electroencephalography (EEG) and/or evoked potentials (EP). Both methods are bedside techniques. These are now routinely and successfully used in acute coma (Guérit et al., 1999a). Surprisingly, there are not many EEG or EP studies in the persistent vegetative state. This can be explained, at least partially, by the technical difficulties raised by EP recording in vegetative patients. Indeed, reliable EP recording requires long periods of relaxation and immobility, which may be hardly obtained in vegetative, non-sedated, patients.

This paper will review the information which can be gained from neurophysiological examination in vegetative and poorly-responsive patients. It will be based both on our own experience and on a review of the literature. After a short reminder of some basics of EEG and EPs, we will briefly describe the main neurophysiological patterns that can be observed in acute coma and show how these evolve from the acute to the chronic stage. Next, we will see to what extent clinical neurophysiology helps provide deeper insight into persisting cognitive functions and/or consciousness in vegetative or poorly-responsive states. We will end up with short statements on the clinical usefulness of EEG and EPs in vegetative or minimally conscious patients.

NEUROPHYSIOLOGIC PATTERNS IN VEGETATIVE AND POORLY-RESPONSIVE PATIENTS

Basics of EEG and EPs

The EEG reflects the neuronal activity of the cerebral cortex and its modulation by the brainstem. It also contains electrical activities coming from deep, sub-cortical structures, but, owing to their large distance to the scalp, their contribution to the scalp EEG is only minor. As a consequence, sub-cortical activities are usually hidden by the cortical electrogenesis. EPs reflect the EEG changes that are induced by sensory stimulation or cognitive processes. Because their amplitude is much lower than that of EEG, their recording requires special signal-analysis techniques (averaging). Averaging allows extracting both cortical and brainstem EP components. However, it takes time, which, as mentioned above, could account for some of the difficulties in recording EPs in vegetative or poorly-responsive cases.

Sensory EPs can be subdivided into "exogenous EPs", which reflect the passive brain reception of sensory inputs, and "endogenous EPs", which reflect the conscious or non-conscious cognitive processing of information. The exogenous EPs that we routinely use in comatose or poorly-responsive patients are the visual (V-), somatosensory, (S-) and brainstem auditory EPs (BAEPs). This combination gives rise to a huge number of neurophysiological parameters, which we summarise by two indices (Guérit, de Tourtchaninoff, Soveges, & Mahieu, 1993): the index of global cortical function (IGCF) and the index of brainstem conduction (IBSC). The IGCF is calculated from VEPs and the cortical components of SEPs and expressed by grades: Grade 0 corresponds to normal IGCF, Grades 1 to 3 to increasing alterations, and Grade 4 to the absence of any cortical EP. The IBSC is calculated from BAEPs and sub-cortical and early cortical SEPs; whenever abnormal, it is qualitatively described in terms of diencephalic, midbrain, pontine or medullar dysfunction. In our practice, cognitive EPs (labelled as "event-related potentials" or ERPs) are obtained through a passive auditory oddball paradigm (Guérit et al., 1999b). The patient is stimulated with two types of auditory stimuli, a frequent (80%) one consisting of lower-frequency (500 Hz) tone bursts and a rare (20%) one consisting of higher frequency (750 Hz) tone bursts. Both types of stimuli give rise to similar exogenous EPs but only the rare ones produce additional activities (mismatch negativity, N2 waves, and the P300 waves—see later), that reflect the cognitive brain reactions to deviance.

Characterisation of EEG and exogenous EPs at the acute stage of coma

By definition, coma is associated with cortical dysfunction, either primary or secondary to alterations of brainstem influences. Therefore, almost all comatose patients display EEG and IGCF alterations. Although some EEG patterns may be more suggestive of anoxic, traumatic, vascular, or metabolic coma, most of these patterns are relatively unspecific of a given aetiology (Chatrian & Turella, 2003). By contrast, the combination of IGCF and IBSC determination gives rise to patterns that are more aetiology-specific (Guérit, 1999).

Anoxic comas. These are associated with IGCF alterations contrasting with normal IBSC ("Pattern 1"). This may be easily explained physiologically by the higher sensitivity of the cerebral cortex to anoxic insults, which contrasts with higher brainstem resistance. Therefore, the prognostic value of this pattern in anoxic coma depends on the degree of IGCF alterations. In the absence of sedative drugs, these are usually homogenous for VEPs and SEPs, whose grades do not differ by more than 1. In our series of anoxic comas, Grades 1, 2, 3, and 4 obtained between the first and the third day after the coma onset were associated with a 65%, 40%, 10%, and 0% probability of good recovery (defined as the possibility to regain some independent life), respectively (Guérit, 1999). In keeping with this, a meta-analysis (Zandbergen et al., 1998) confirmed that the loss of cortical SEPs (i.e., Grade 4) was one of the strongest indicators of no recovery (death or permanent vegetative state). Therefore, we consider it ethically acceptable to waive resuscitation in anoxic patients with Grade 4 at least 12–24 hours after the acute episode. Conversely, as high as 35% of patients with mild IGCF alterations (Grade 1) present with a poor outcome. That is to say that, while the prognostic power of the most severe alterations is very high, milder alterations do not allow drawing any strong conclusion at the acute stage. On the contrary, cognitive EPs are exquisitely sensitive to cortical dysfunction. Therefore, while no definite conclusion may be drawn from their absence, their presence is strongly indicative of a high probability (90% to 95%) of recovery (Fischer et al., 1999; Fischer, Luauté, Adeleine, & Morlet, 2004; Guérit et al., 1999b; Kane, Butler, & Simpson, 2000). This justifies their recording whenever the IGCF are only mildly altered.

Head trauma. By contrast, four different patterns can be associated with head trauma (Guérit, 1999). *Pattern 1* is similar to that observed in brain anoxia. We consider it to reflect diffuse brain oedema or mild diffuse axonal lesions without any repercussion on the brainstem. In Pattern 1, the IGCF grade never exceeds 2. In our experience, this pattern is most often associated with a good prognosis (90% and 80% of good recoveries for Grades 1 and 2, respectively). *Pattern 2* consists of IGCF alterations that are associated with IBSC alterations suggesting midbrain involvement. Contrary to Pattern 1, SEPs are more altered than VEPs, which is explained by the fact that the somatosensory pathways cross the midbrain, contrary to the visual ones. The high midbrain sensitivity to sagittal head deceleration has, indeed, been demonstrated in experimental models (Hume Adams, 1984). The associated IGCF alterations may reflect either hemispheric oedema and/or diffuse axonal lesions, or merely diffuse cortical slowing due to dysfunction of the midbrain ascending reticular activating system (ARAS). Pattern 2 is often associated with a poor clinical examination (decerebrate posturing, i.e., Glasgow coma scale score of 4/15). Its prognosis depends on both the reversibility of the midbrain dysfunction and the extent of associated diffuse axonal injuries, which can be assessed by MRI. Interestingly, recovery of patients with Pattern 2, if any, may intervene after a long period (up to 5 months in our series) during which the patient is considered vegetative. This point will be discussed later. *Pattern 3* consists of the appearance of pontine involvement, which reflects evolving transtentorial herniation, and *Pattern 4* is that of brain death. These two last patterns will not be discussed further, as they lie beyond the scope of this paper.

Transition from the acute to the chronic stage

Figure 1 (top) shows some spontaneous evolutions of the IGCF grades in three illustrative cases of anoxic patients who eventually became permanently vegetative or poorly responsive. Indeed, in most post-anoxic cases, there was an almost systematic trend towards spontaneous IGCF improvement within the first 10 days after coma onset, and towards slower improvement in these patients who could be followed up over a longer period. It is noteworthy that such a trend in anoxic coma has no prognostic value, as none of these patients clinically improved, at least on a rough neurological examination. This observation can be explained by the fact that, at the earliest stage of brain anoxia, abnormalities of cortical electrogenesis result both from reversible neuronal dysfunction and irreversible neuronal destruction (Astrup, Siesjö, & Symon, 1981). From the 10th day, the IGCF only reflects irreversible neuronal destruction, which is the actual prognostically relevant factor. It may thus be concluded that, in anoxic patients, even the mildest grade of IGCF alterations reflects cortical impairment sufficient to preclude clinically obvious cognitive manifestations.

By contrast, no such trend was observed in post-traumatic cases that became permanently vegetative. This difference is likely explainable by the different pathophysiology of traumatic brain damage. In these cases, the neurophysiological pattern obtained at the acute stage would be dominated by the superimposed effects of the diffuse axonal lesions in the sub-cortical hemispheric white matter and/or midbrain, while reversible brain oedema would account for only a small proportion of the neurophysiological changes.

Of utmost interest is the evolution of these patients initially presenting with Pattern 2 who eventually recovered after a variable period during which these were considered as vegetative. Figure 1 (bottom) shows three examples of VEP and SEP evolution in iteratively followed-up patients who recovered after 50, 48, and 38 days, respectively. In all three cases, the SEPs were initially more altered than VEPs, which, as already mentioned, is typical of Pattern 2. Moreover, in all cases, clinical recovery was preceded by that of SEPs, while VEPs remained almost unchanged. The delay between SEP and VEP recovery differed in each patient (between 3 and 15 days). These

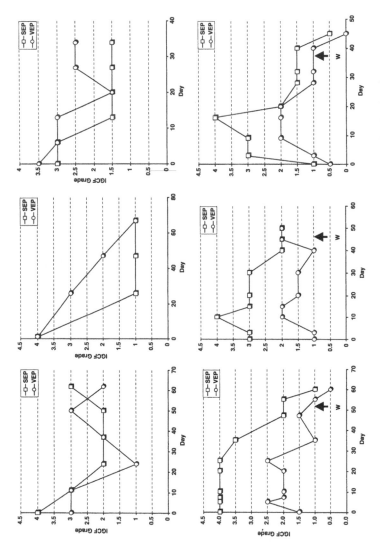

Figure 1. Neurophysiological evolution towards the vegetative state. *Top*: IGCF evolutions of three patients who developed permanent post-anoxic vegetative states. Despite their poor evolution, there was a spontaneous trend toward IGCF recovery in the first 10 days after the acute episode; note also the overall predominance of VEP vs. SEP alterations. *Bottom*: IGCF evolutions of three post-traumatic patients who eventually woke up after 50, 48, and 37 days ("*W*"). SEPs were initially more altered than VEPs and wake-up was preceded by SEP recovery with varying delays

observations emphasise the essential role of midbrain dysfunction in post-traumatic vegetative or poorly-responsive states. It also underlines the fact that some vegetative post-traumatic patients with evidence of midbrain dysfunction can recover. As already mentioned, their evolution actually depends on both the potential reversibility of midbrain dysfunction and the extent of associated diffuse hemispheric axonal lesions, which can be assessed by, and justifies, MRI.

Characterisation of EEG and exogenous EPs in vegetative and poorly-responsive patients

Figure 2 shows the distribution of IGCF grades in our post-traumatic and post-anoxic permanently vegetative or poorly-responsive cases. These are, indeed, extremely variable with some predominance of Grades 1 and 2 in traumatic, and of Grades 2 and 3 in post-anoxic patients. The same holds true for the EEG, whose variability in vegetative patients has been widely recognised (Chatrian & Turella, 2003). There are few patients with Grade 4, but this most likely reflects some bias of our series, due to the rapid waiving of resuscitation in patients exhibiting Grade 4 at the acute stage of anoxic coma. This observation is in keeping with clinical and functional brain imaging data

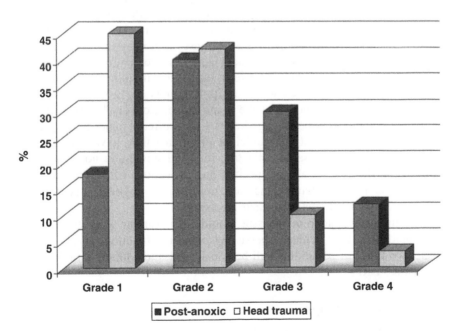

Figure 2. Distribution and variability of IGCF alterations in post-anoxic and post-traumatic vegetative cases (adapted from Guérit, 2001)

(Laureys et al., 2001, 2002) and confirms that the persistent vegetative state may not be considered as a monolithic entity, so that each patient should be considered as a particular case and needs to be individually evaluated.

ASSESSMENT OF COGNITIVE FUNCTIONS AND CONSCIOUSNESS

The variability in the severity of neurophysiological changes in the so-called vegetative states raises the issue of possible cognitive or conscious remnants in some patients. In other words, could clinical neurophysiology identify patients looking at first glance vegetative, but who still exhibit cognitive functions or could even be minimally conscious? This issue has considerable implications, not only in terms of daily patient management, but also from the medico-legal standpoint.

Consciousness assessment in patients who are unable to communicate raises considerable methodological difficulties. Indeed, all current models of consciousness consider that this is subtended by neural networks and that it is consequently impossible to identify any precise neural structure whose destruction would be incompatible with any consciousness remnant. In our opinion, the post-anoxic Grade 4 constitutes the only situation in which one may be sure that the patient has complete loss of consciousness. First, it is incompatible with any perception of the external world. Second, as the primary cortices are more resistant to anoxia than the associative ones, post-anoxic destruction of the primary cortex implies full cortical destruction, irrespective of the brainstem status. As we mentioned previously, even if this situation is relatively rare in our series, it could be encountered more often in these centres where resuscitation is not given up in post-anoxic patients with Grade 4 at the acute stage. Conversely, even if it is likely that patients with persisting Grades 1 to 3 suffered major brain impairment, this does not constitute sufficient proof that they have lost all their cognitive functions; the same holds true for EEG slowing or non-reactivity. Conversely, the EEG is all but specific, and exogenous EPs do not directly assess those brain structures that are involved in cognition, so that no conclusion may be drawn from their presence.

The other way to address this issue would be to examine whether cognitive EPs could positively evidence persisting cognitive functions or consciousness. Two types of paradigms will be considered: the oddball paradigm and "semantic" ERPs.

The oddball paradigm

Three families of peaks are produced by the rare stimuli in the auditory oddball paradigm: the mismatch negativity (MMN), the N2 waves, and the

P300s. The N2 waves did not give rise to any specific study in comatose or vegetative patients, so we will concentrate on the MMN and the P300.

MMN.   The MMN is a negativity that superimposes on the exogenous N100–P200 complex, with latency in the order of 150–200 ms. It may persist in clinically unresponsive patients, both in the acute stage of coma and in the vegetative state (Fischer et al., 1999; Kane et al., 2000; Guérit, 2001). The possibility to get an MMN in poorly-responsive patients was shown to depend on stimulus complexity, as it was more frequently obtained to spectrally rich sounds than pure sinusoidal tones (Kotchoubey et al., 2001). It could also be evoked by spectro-temporal modulations of complex tones in some non-responsive severely brain-injured patients (Jones et al., 2000).

The MMN is considered to reflect automatic detection by the sensory cortex of the physical difference between one stimulus and the preceding one (Näätänen, 1995). However, even if this process most likely constitutes a prerequisite for eventual conscious perception of the stimulus, it is, at this stage of processing, an unconscious one. It is noteworthy that it is normally best obtained when the subject does not pay attention to the auditory stimulus (for example, because he or she is involved in another task). This implies that the MMN evaluates brain functions that are too primitive to provide useful information on possible cognitive remnants. In addition, the MMN is a small component, which may sometimes be hardly obtained in difficult conditions (for example, in the presence of major muscle contamination), so that its absence may not be considered a sufficient argument for consciousness loss. For all these reasons, we do not consider the MMN a good tool for cognitive assessment and, in particular, for awareness assessment in vegetative patients.

P300.   The P300 is the most widely described component in the oddball paradigm (Polich & Kok, 1995 for a review of the main P300 determinants). It is composed of at least two subcomponents, P3a and P3b (Squires, Squires, & Hillyard, 1975). Both components differ in their latencies, with an earlier occurrence for P3a, and their topographies with a frontal predominance for P3a and a parietal one for P3b (Squires et al., 1975). There is good evidence that P3a reflects automatic orientation to the rare stimuli, irrespective of whether the stimuli are eventually consciously perceived or not. Like the MMN, the P3a can sometimes be obtained in passive conditions. For that reason, like the MMN, the presence of P3a may not be considered a sufficient argument for consciousness. On the contrary, P3b is only obtained when subjects actively consider the stimuli as task relevant. There are currently two explaining models of P3b. According to the "updating model", P300 would index brain actions stemming from tasks that are required in the maintenance of working memory when the mental model or context of the stimulus environment is updated (Donchin & Coles, 1988). According to Desmedt (1981) and Verleger (1988), P300 would be related to the "closure of perceptual events", leaving a place for the next event to occur. P3b is a highly non-specific wave whose generators are ill-known and, most probably, multiple and distributed (Baudena, Halgren, Heit, & Clarke, 1995; Halgren et al., 1995a, 1995b). However, the presence of P3b implies that a brain mechanism necessary for that operation which is required for the attribution of significance is intact (Kotchoubey, Lang, Bostanov, & Birbaumer, 2002). Based on P300 recording in normal subjects during forced awakening, Garcia-Larrea and Bastuji (2001) made a step further and proposed that P3b would reflect the transfer of information from "core consciousness" to "extended consciousness", according to the Damasio's model (Damasio, 1999).

Although several authors succeeded in recording what they considered as a P300 in comatose or non-responsive patients (Guérit et al., 1999b; Kotchoubey et al., 2001; Loeper et al., 1998; Mazzini et al., 2001; Marosi et al., 1993; Rappaport, McCandless, Pond, & Kraffl, 1991), there is unfortunately little evidence on the exact nature of this P300 (P3a or P3b). Indeed, the major argument favoring the "P3b" nature of a P300 is that it is only obtained when the stimulus is task-relevant, the proof of which is based on the subject's behavioural response. Hence, by definition, reliable behavioural responses are hardly obtained in unresponsive patients. We tried in some poorly-responsive patients to compare the responses to rare stimuli in so-called "passive" (i.e., without any instruction to the subject) and "active" conditions (by asking the subject mentally to react to the rare stimuli). It should be noted that whether the latter condition is really an "active" one is all but certain, given the absence of behavioural proof of the patient's comprehension. Nevertheless, we demonstrated in some cases (Figure 3) the consistent appearance in the "active" condition of a positive component that was consistently absent in the "passive" one. We consider the ability to modulate cognitive responses by external instructions as an indirect argument favouring some residual perception of the environment, even if a non-specific consequence of an increased level of global arousal cannot formally be ruled out. The other way to prove that the obtained P300 would be a P3b is to look for its parietal predominance. Such parietal predominance could be demonstrated in vegetative or poorly-responsive patients with extremely severe brain injury. Its incidence was higher in post-traumatic cases and depended also on the characteristics of the auditory stimuli, being higher to complex tones than sine tones or vowels (Kotchoubey et al., 2001).

"Semantic" ERPs

In the "semantic oddball paradigm", the subject must mentally count words belonging to a target semantic category interspersed with standard stimuli.

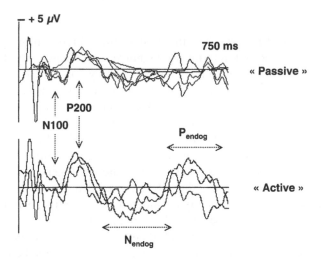

Figure 3. Auditory odd-ball paradigm in a post-traumatic persistent "vegetative" state of 11 years duration. Comparison between responses to rare stimuli in a "passive condition" (no special instruction) (*top*) and an "active condition" (patient instructed mentally to count passive stimuli) (*bottom*). Superimposition of three trials obtained at different days. Exogenous components (N100, P200) are obtained in both conditions. In the "active condition", these are followed by a negative–positive complex (N_{endog}, P_{endog}) (adapted from Guérit, 2001)

Alternate paradigms are the "word pair" paradigm, in which pairs of semantically related words are interspersed with pairs of unrelated words, and the "sentence completion" paradigm, in which sentences with an expected end word are interspersed with sentences with an incongruent end word. Using the two former paradigms, Kotchoubey et al. (2001) found significant P3s in 10/34 severely brain-damaged patients, who were thus capable of semantic processing. In one patient with akinetic mutism, they obtained ERPs with the two former paradigms, but not to sentence completion (Kotchoubey, Schneck, Lang, & Birbaumer, 2003b).

Sentence completion normally produces the N400, whose amplitude is inversely related to the likeness of occurrence of the last word (Hagoort, Brown, & Schwab, 1996; Kutas & Hillyard, 1980). Overall, there are few reports on N400s in the literature, even if some authors (Stemmer, Hild, Witzke, & Schonle, 1996) claimed to have obtained N400s to correct or incorrect proverb completion in vegetative patients. However, due to the stereotyped nature of proverbs, it is unclear whether N400 appearance to wrong end-word actually means reference to its semantic content. The same discussion holds true for ERPs to the patient's own name (Berlad & Pratt, 1995; Folmer & Yingling, 1997; Mazzini et al., 2001).

Summary

Because exogenous EPs just reflect the status of the afferent sensory pathways, they are actually irrelevant in terms for cognitive assessment. Only these post-anoxic vegetative patients who have lost all primary cortical EP components are most likely to have really lost all their cognitive functions and, a fortiori, consciousness. This is because a brain anoxia sufficient to destroy the primary cortex is incompatible with higher cortical activities, which raises the issue of whether these patients might not be considered as dead (Guérit, 2004). However, this holds true only for post-anoxic vegetative states, as the post-traumatic states may be associated with more heterogeneous lesions.

Conversely, there is evidence that ERPs can evidence *cognitive* remnants in some patients who are clinically considered as vegetative. Strictly speaking, these patients should be shifted from the vegetative to the poorly-responsive group. To what extent such demonstration proves *consciousness* remnants is still a matter of debate. One major problem is the heterogeneity of the concept of consciousness and, in particular, the current absence of any model of consciousness that would be straightforwardly amenable to neurophysiological examinations. Even if the MMN or the P3a are likely to reflect processes that are prerequisites for consciousness, their presence does not constitute proof per se of consciousness. Conversely, both their marked intra-individual variability and the technical difficulties which can be encountered in recording these ERPs keep one from drawing any conclusion from their absence. In our opinion, the firm demonstration of a real P3b appearing to careful stimulus manipulation is currently the best method to demonstrate conscious remnants. Indeed, two conditions must be met to get a P3b: a discrimination of the stimulus features which make the oddball, and the need for the subject's task relevance. The N400 and the ERPs to the patient's own name are worth considering too, but more studies are needed to check whether these can really be obtained in some non-responsive patients and in which conditions.

CONCLUSION

The potential usefulness of EEG and EPs in vegetative or poorly-responsive patients is fourfold: prognosis, identification of the best channel for stimulation, quantitative follow up, and assessment of persisting cognitive functions.

First, the *prognosis* of the post-anoxic vegetative state is poor for the second week in patients who do not recover clinically in the absence of sedation. It is mainly determined by clinical examination, and clinical neurophysiology usually does not provide further actually relevant information. By contrast, multimodality EPs can dramatically contribute in identifying those post-traumatic cases whose clinical status is only or mainly a consequence of primary midbrain dysfunction. Whenever there is such suspicion, MRI should be performed to check both the extent of diffuse hemispheric axonal lesions and whether this midbrain dysfunction is the consequence of an irreversible lesion or merely a potentially reversible dysfunction. In the latter hypothesis, the patient must undergo maximal treatment with the hope of possible reversibility.

Second, the actual usefulness of *sensory stimulation* is still a controversial issue and we think it too simplistic to state simply that "it cannot harm the patient" as it is our experience that unsuccessful stimulation sometimes makes nursing teams or families feel unduly guilty. At this respect, exogenous EPs can be of major help in determining "stimulus permeability" and in identifying those patients in whom focal lesions of a given sensory pathway make illusory any attempt to use this channel for stimulation.

Third, one major advantage of clinical neurophysiology is that it can provide quantitative assessment of brain function, which can be helpful for follow-up studies in therapeutic trials.

Fourth, and most important, a major contribution of clinical neurophysiology, in keeping with other imaging studies, has been to prove definitely that the persistent vegetative state is not a monolithic entity, but encompasses a continuum of states. Indeed, ERP recording demonstrates that "vegetative" patients still exhibit cognitive functions and should therefore be considered as poorly responsive rather than vegetative. Whether these cognitive functions are sufficient for consciousness is still a matter of debate. This constitutes a major challenge for further studies.

REFERENCES

Andrews, K., Murphy, L., Munday, R., & Littlewood, C. (1996). Misdiagnosis of the vegetative state: Retrospective study in a rehabilitation unit. *British Medical Journal, 313,* 13–16.

Astrup, J., Siesjö, B., & Symon, L. (1981). Thresholds in cerebral ischemia: The ischemic penumbra zone. *Stroke, 12,* 723–725.

Baudena, P., Halgren, E., Heit, G., & Clarke, J. M. (1995). Intracerebral potentials to rare target and distractors auditory and visual stimuli: III. Frontal cortex. *Electroencephalography and Clinical Neurophysiology, 94,* 251–264.

Berlad, I., & Pratt, H. (1995). P300 in response to the subject's own name. *Electroencephalography and Clinical Neurophysiology, 96,* 472–474.

Chatrian, G. E., & Turella, G. S. (2003). Electrophysiological evaluation of coma, other states of diminished responsiveness, and brain death. In J. S. Ebersole & T. A. Pedley (Eds.), *Current practice of clinical electroencephalography* (pp. 405–462). Philadelphia: Lippincott Williams & Wilkins.

Damasio, A. R. (1999). The feeling of what happens: Body and emotion in the making of consciousness. *French Edition: Le sentiment meme de soi: Corps, emotions, conscience.* Paris: Odile Jacob.

Desmedt, J. E. (1981). P300 in serial tasks: An essential post-decision closure mechanism. *Progress in Brain Research, 54,* 682–686.

Donchin, E., & Coles, M. G. H. (1988). Is the P300 component a manifestation of context updating? *Behavioral and Brain Sciences*, *11*, 357–374.

Fischer, C., Luauté, J., Adeleine, P., & Morlet, D. (2004). Predictive value of sensory and cognitive evoked potentials for awakening from coma. *Neurology*, *63*, 669–673.

Fischer, C., Morlet, D., Bouchet, P., Luaute, J., Jourdan, C., & Salord, F. (1999). Mismatch negativity and late auditory evoked potentials in comatose patients. *Clinical Neurophysiology*, *110*, 1601–1610.

Folmer, R. L., & Yingling, C. D. (1997). Auditory P3 responses to name stimuli. *Brain and Language*, *57*, 306–311.

Garcia-Larrea, L., & Bastuji, H. (2001). Intégration sensorielle, potentiels évoqués et états de vigilance chez le sujet sain. In J. M. Guérit (ed.), *L'évaluation neurophysiologique des comas, de la mort encéphalique et des états végétatifs* (pp. 57–70). Marseille: Editions Solal.

Guérit, J. M. (1999). Medical technology assessment. EEG and EPs in the intensive care unit. *Neurophysiologie Clinique Clinical Neurophysiology*, *29*, 301–317.

Guérit, J. M. (2001). Les potentiels évoqués exogènes et endogènes dans les états végétatifs. In J. M. Guérit (ed.), *L'évaluation neurophysiologique des comas, de la mort encéphalique et des états végétatifs* (pp. 399–410). Marseille: Editions Solal.

Guérit, J. M. (2004). The concept of brain death. In C. Machado & D. A. Shewmon (Eds.), *Brain death and disorders of consciousness* (pp. 15–21). New York: Kluwer Academic/Plenum Publishers.

Guérit, J. M., de Tourtchaninoff, M., Soveges, L., & Mahieu, P. (1993). The prognostic value of three-modality evoked potentials (TMEPs) in anoxic and traumatic comas. *Neurophysiologie Clinique*, *23*, 209–226.

Guérit, J. M., Fischer, C., Facco, E., Tinuper, P., Ronne-Engström, E., & Nuwer, M. (1999a). Standards of clinical practice of EEG and EPs in comatose and other unresponsive states. In G. Deuschl & A. Eisen (eds.), *Recommendations for the practice of clinical neurophysiology (EEG Suppl. 52)* (pp. 117–131). Amsterdam: Elsevier.

Guérit, J. M., Verougstraete, D., de Tourtchaninoff, M., Debatisse, D., & Witdoeckt, C. (1999b). ERPs obtained with the auditory oddball paradigm in coma and altered states of consciousness: Clinical relationships, prognostic value, and origin of components. *Clinical Neurophysiology*, *110*, 1260–1269.

Hagoort, P., Brown, C. M., & Schwaab, T. Y. (1996). Lexical-semantic event-related potential effects in patients with left hemisphere lesion and aphasia and patients with right hemisphere lesions without aphasia. *Brain*, *119*, 627–649.

Halgren, E., Baudena, P., Clarke, J. M., Heit, G., Liégeois, C., Chauvel, P., & Musolino, A. (1995a). Intracerebral potentials to rare target and distractors auditory and visual stimuli: I. Superior temporal plane and parietal lobe. *Electroencephalography and Clinical Neurophysiology*, *94*, 191–220.

Halgren, E., Baudena, P., Clarke, J. M., Heit, G., Marinkovic, K., Devaux, B., Vignal, J. P., & Biraben, A. (1995b). Intracerebral potentials to rare target and distractors auditory and visual stimuli: II. Medial, lateral, and posterior temporal lobe. *Electroencephalography and Clinical Neurophysiology*, *94*, 229–250.

Hume Adams, J. (1984). Head injury. In J. Hume Adams, J. A. N. Corsellis, & L. W. Duchen (Eds.), *Greenfield's neuropathology*, 4th edn, pp. 85–124. London: Edward Arnold.

Jennett, B., & Plum, F. (1972). Persistent vegetative state after brain damage. A syndrome in search of a name. *Lancet*, *1*, 734–737.

Jones, S. J., Vaz-Pato, M., Sprague, L., Stokes, M., Munday, R., & Haque, N. (2000). Auditory evoked potentials to modulation of complex tones in normal subjects and patients with severe brain injury. *Brain*, *123*, 1007–1016.

Kane, N. M., Butler, S. R., & Simpson, T. (2000). Coma outcome prediction using event-related potentials: P3 and mismatch negativity. *Audiology Neuro-otology*, *5*, 186–191.

Kotchoubey, B., Lang, S., Baales, R., Herb, E., Maurer, P., Mezger, G., Schmalohr, D., Bostanov, V., & Birbaumer, N. (2001). Brain potentials in human patients with extremely severe diffuse brain damage. *Neuroscience Letters, 301*, 37–40.

Kotchoubey, B., Lang, S., Bostanov, V., & Birbaumer, N. (2002). Is there a mind? Electrophysiology of unconscious patients. *New Physiological Science, 17*, 38–42.

Kotchoubey, B., Lang, S., Herb, E., Maurer, P., Schmalohr, D., Bostanov, V., & Birbaumer, N. (2003a). Stimulus complexity enhances auditory stimulation in patients with extremely severe brain injuries. *Neuroscience Letters, 352*, 129–132.

Kotchoubey, B., Schneck, M., Lang, S., & Birbaumer, N. (2003b). Event-related brain potentials in a patient with akinetic mutism. *Neurophysiologie Clinique, 33*, 23–30.

Kutas, M., & Hillyard, S. (1980). Event-related brain potentials to semantically inappropriate and surprisingly large words. *Biological Psychology, 11*, 99–116.

Laureys, S., Antoine, S., Boly, M., Elincx, S., Faymonville, M. E., Berré, J., et al. (2002). Brain function in the vegetative state. *Acta Neurologica Belgica, 102*, 177–185.

Laureys, S., Berré, J., & Goldman, S. (2001). Cerebral function in coma, vegetative state, minimally conscious state, locked-in syndrome, and brain death. In J. L. Vincent (Ed.), *2001 Yearbook of intensive care and emergency medicine* (pp. 286–396). Berlin: Springer-Verlag.

Loeper, U., Lindlar, K., Wagner, M., Rockstroh, B., & Schönle, P. E. (1988). ERP and event-related frequency changes in the EEG as indicators of cortical information processing in vegetative state patients. *Journal of Psychophysiology, 12*, 213.

Marosi, M., Prevec, T., Masala, C., Bramanti, P., Giorganni, R., Luef, G., Berek, K., Saltuari, L., & Bramanti, M. (1993). Event-related potentials in vegetative state. *Lancet, 341*, 1473–1474.

Mazzini, L., Zaccala, M., Gareri, F., Giordano, A., & Angelino, E. (2001). Long-latency auditory-evoked potentials in severe traumatic brain injury. *Archives of Physical Medicine and Rehabilitation, 82*, 57–65.

Näätänen, R. (1995). The mismatch negativity: A powerful tool for cognitive neuroscience. *Ear and Hearing, 16*, 6–18.

Polich, J., & Kok, A. (1995). Cognitive and biological determinants of P300: An integrative review. *Biological Psychology, 41*, 103–146.

Rappaport, M., McCandless, K. L., Pond, W., & Kraffl, M. C. (1991). Passive P300 response in traumatic brain injury patients. *Journal of Neuropsychiatry and Cognitive Neurosciences, 3*, 180–185.

Squires, N. K., Squires, K., & Hillyard, S. (1975). Two varieties of long-latency positive waves evoked by unpredictable auditory stimuli in man. *Electroencephalography and Clinical Neurophysiology, 38*, 387–401.

Stemmer, B., Hild, M., Witzke, W., & Schonle, P. W. (1996). Event-related potentials during auditory and visual proverb presentation in non-brain damaged controls and brain-damaged individuals: Results of a pilot study. *Brain and Cognition, 30*, 294–297.

Verleger, R. (1988). Event-related potentials and cognition: A critique of the context-updating hypothesis and an alternative explanation of P3. *Behavioral and Brain Sciences, 11*, 343–356.

Zandbergen, E. G. J., de Haan, R. J., Stoutenbeek, C. P., Koelman, J. H. T. M., & Hijdra, A. (1998). Systematic review of early prediction of poor outcome in anoxic-ischaemic coma. *Lancet, 352*, 1808–1812.

NEUROPSYCHOLOGICAL REHABILITATION
2005, 15 (3/4), 372–380

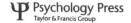

Evoked potentials for the prediction of vegetative state in the acute stage of coma

Catherine Fischer[1] and Jacques Luauté[2]

[1]*Neurologie fonctionnelle, Hôpital Neurologique, Lyon, France,*
[2]*Rééducation neurologique, Hôpital H. Gabrielle, Lyon, France*

For comatose patients in intensive care units, it is important to anticipate their functional outcome as soon and as reliably as possible. Among clinical variables the Glasgow Coma Score (GCS) and the patient's pupil reactivity are the strongest predictive variables. Evoked potentials help to assess objectively brain function. Over the past 20 years, numerous studies have assessed their prognostic utility in terms of awakening from coma. Fewer studies, however, have focused upon the utility of evoked potentials in predicting progression to the vegetative state. In this area evoked potentials appear to have a highly predictive value. In anoxic coma the abolition of somatosensory evoked potentials (SEPs) is related to a poor outcome, defined as death or survival in a vegetative state, with a 100% specificity. Following traumatic brain injury, the predictive value for unfavourable outcome is 98.5% when there are no focal injuries likely to abolish SEP cortical components. In contrast, the presence of event-related evoked potentials, and particularly mismatched negativity (MMN), is a strong predictor of awakening and precludes comatose patients from moving to a permanent vegetative state (PVS).

The development of intensive care treatments has facilitated the survival in recent years of larger numbers of severely brain-damaged patients. In those who enter a persistent vegetative state (defined as a wakeful unconscious state of at least one month duration), the recovery of function will vary from regaining consciousness to remaining unaware in a permanent vegetative

Correspondence should be addressed to: Catherine Fischer, M.D., Neurologie Fonctionnelle, Hôpital Neurologique Lyon, 59 Blvd Pinel, 69677 Bron cedex, France. Email: catherine.fischer@chu-lyon.fr

© 2005 Psychology Press Ltd
http://www.tandf.co.uk/journals/pp/09602011.html   DOI:10.1080/09602010443000434

state (PVS). Indeed, the Multi-Society Task Force on PVS (1994a, 1994b) made a distinction between "persistent" vegetative state, which refers only to a diagnosis with an uncertain future, whereas "permanent" vegetative state implies irreversibility (Multi-Society Task Force on PVS, 1994a, 1994b). Although the mechanisms underlying the progression to a PVS or recovery of consciousness are not fully understood the cause of the brain injury and the site of structural lesions are known to be important (Graham et al., 1995).

The PVS represents the worst possible outcome for the patient's relatives and those who care for them. The condition causes both emotional and moral turmoil; how to adjust to these changes, how to live with them, and importantly how to care for them. Indeed, funding for appropriate care takes time to arrange, there are few specialised centres and these are often expensive. For all these reasons, it would be desirable to know the risk of evolution towards the PVS at the earliest stage following brain injury with the best probability.

Clinical prognostic variables exist but they are not sufficient, especially when the question is whether the patient will progress to a PVS (Luauté et al., 2005). Evoked potentials (EPs) assess the functional state of the brain. Over the past 20 years, numerous studies have investigated the ability of EPs to predict outcome in terms of survival and awakening from coma. Few studies, however, have focused on the ability to predict progression to a PVS. Most studies try to predict poor outcome without any more precise indication regarding PVS. In this text, we will discuss the ability of EPs to predict the progression to a permanent vegetative state when they are recorded in the acute comatose period following brain injury. For each type of EP, we will specify the prognostic utility if such information is accessible. We will distinguish the data regarding anoxic comas and traumatic comas whenever possible.

METHODS

This work is based on a systematic review of the literature and on the analysis of a series of severe comatose patients.

For the systematic review, the main criteria for considering articles were:

1. Type of study: Any type of study investigating the utility of evoked potentials for the prediction of vegetative state in the acute stage of coma.

2. Type of participants: Comatose patients.

3. Type of outcome measures: PVS as defined in 1994, i.e., the outcome assessment must be performed with a delay of more than three months in patients with non-traumatic injuries and more than 12

months in patients with traumatic injuries (Multi-Society Task Force on PVS, 1994a, 1994b).

4. Language: English.

To identify these articles, in addition to personal databases, we carried out searches of electronic databases (MEDLINE between 1966 and 2004). The computerised searches were conducted using combinations of the following descriptors/key words: vegetative state/prediction or prognostic/evoked potentials. Citation-tracking of all primary studies provided an additional search strategy; reference lists from review articles and books identified in the searches were also scanned and then assessed for inclusion.

Patients

Concerning our series of comatose patients, inclusion concerned all comatose patients admitted to an intensive care unit (ICU), between December 1997 and February 2002, with a Glasgow Coma Scale (GCS) score less than 8. The sample totalled 346 patients (213 men and 133 women) aged between 8 and 93 years (mean age: 50.73 $\pm$ 17.9 years) with a GCS score <8 at the time of electrophysiological recording (Glasgow 3–4: 156 cases; Glasgow 5–7: 190 cases). All patients had undergone at least one brain computed tomography (CT) scan or magnetic resonance imaging (MRI). Coma was caused by ischaemic or haemorrhagic stroke syndrome (stroke = 125), traumatic brain injury ($n = 96$), cardiac or respiratory failure (anoxia = 64), complications of tumoural or vascular neurosurgery (neurosurgery = 54), and encephalitis ($n = 7$). The time between coma onset and the recording of EPs ranged between 1–77 days (mean 10.34 $\pm$ 11.4 days). Recordings were performed when the contribution of EPs to prognosis was expected to be useful. Consequently, patients with early progression towards awakening and complete recovery were not recorded and not included in the study. At the time of recording of evoked potentials, no sedative drugs had been administered during the previous 24 hours. Patients were excluded when the aetiology of coma was not clear and when bilaterally abolished brainstem auditory made it impossible to record auditory EPs. No patient in the study had been victim of traumatic cardiac arrest.

Electrophysiological assessment

Brainstem auditory evoked potentials (BAEPs), middle-latency auditory evoked potentials (MLAEPs), N100 and mismatch negativity (MMN) were recorded for all patients. BAEPs and MLAEPs were simultaneously recorded following the technique described previously by Fischer et al. (1994, 1999) and Logi, Fischer, Murri, and Mauguiere (2003).

In case of asymmetry, the better response was chosen for analysis and BAEP results were graded as follows: (1) normal; (2) increase in I–V interval, without any amplitude change; (3) amplitude ratio V/I <0.5 μV; (4) no detectable IV or V waves; and (5) only wave I present. BAEPs were considered as normal for grade 1 and 2; abnormal for grade 3–5. MLAEPs were classified as: (1) normal; (2) isolated delay of Pa latency (Pa $\geq$ 31.6 ms) without Na–Pa amplitude reduction; (3) Na–Pa amplitude <0.3 μV; (4) Na present and Pa absent; and (5) no Na–Pa detected. MLAEPs were considered as normal for grade 1 and 2; abnormal for grade 3–5. MMN and late auditory N100 were recorded in the intensive care unit using the same method as in normal subjects (Fischer et al., 1999). The stimuli were pure tones of 800 Hz, with a level of 80 dB HL delivered binaurally through insert earphones. We used a classical duration paradigm in which 14% of stimuli were deviants with 30 ms duration, including rise and fall time; the duration of the standards being 75 ms.

Outcome measure

A follow-up assessment was performed at one year post-onset. The main outcome measure was the Glasgow Outcome Scale (GOS) as defined by Jennett and Bond in 1975 with five categories: (1) death, (2) vegetative state, (3) severe disability, (4) moderate disability, and (5) good recovery. Since the outcome was judged one year after onset of coma, we could consider patients in vegetative state as permanent according to the definition established by the Multi-Society Task Force on PVS (1994a, 1994b). We also distinguished a group of patients who awoke and then died later on in the follow-up phase, patients defined as "unrelated deaths". We classified as "awoken" at 12 months those patients who, one year after coma onset, were awake with either complete recovery, or moderate or severe disability. Patients in a PVS or whose death was related to the coma were classified as "unawake".

Results, based on this series, concerning the utility of sensory and cognitive evoked potentials for the prediction of awakening and good functional outcome have been published recently (Fischer, Luauté, Adeleine, & Morlet, 2004; Luauté et al., 2005). In the present study we analysed the utility of sensory and event-related potentials (N100 and MMN) regarding the prediction of PVS.

RESULTS AND DISCUSSION

Auditory evoked potentials

BAEPs assess the functional state of subcortical auditory pathways. They assess the eighth cranial nerve, the pons and the lower part of the midbrain.

They have a prognostic value of poor outcome when they are abnormal (Fischer et al., 1999; Guérit, de Tourtchaninoff, Soveges, & Mahieu, 1993). No prognostic value is attached to their normality. BAEPs have no value when it comes to predicting PVS (Multi-Society Task Force on PVS, 1994a, 1994b). It should be noted that only one study provided separate data concerning the prediction of permanent vegetative state with BAEPs (Goodwin, Friedman, & Bellefleur, 1991). In this study, BAEPs were recorded in 41 comatose patients within 72 hours after ICU admission. The aetiology of coma was not detailed. One year post-onset, five patients met the criteria of PVS. Among these five patients, BAEPs recorded initially were considered as normal in two cases and abnormal in the other three.

Middle-latency auditory evoked potentials (MLAEPs) recorded in the 30 msec range evaluate mainly the primary auditory cortex (Yvert et al., 2001). Separate data assessing the predictive value of MLAEPs for PVS are available in one study only (Logi et al., 2003). In this study, 8 out of the 49 post-anoxic comatose patients were in a vegetative state at 3 months post-onset and thus could be considered as permanently vegetative. MLAEPs, recorded in the acute phase were abolished in 13 patients, among whom 12 died and one became permanently vegetative. Among the eight patients who became permanently vegetative, MLAEPs were normal in one case; abnormal with an isolated delay of Pa latency without Na–Pa amplitude reduction in three cases; abnormal with Na–Pa amplitude <0.3 μV in three cases and abolished in one case. These results confer to abolition of MLAEPs a high specificity to predict an evolution towards a PVS.

Somatosensory evoked potentials

Upper limb somatosensory evoked potentials (SEPs) elicited following median nerve stimulation at the wrist assess neural pathways to the somatosensory cortex. They have been widely used in the assessment and prognosis of brain injured patients over the past 20 years and are widely accepted to have a highly predictive utility (Carter & Butt, 2001; Logi et al., 2003; Mauguiere et al., 1999; Robinson, Micklesen, Tirschwell, & Lew, 2003).

Traumatic brain injury.   Following traumatic brain injury the bilateral absence of the primary somatosensory cortical response is associated with a non-awakening prognosis (Cant, Hume, Judson, & Shaw, 1986; Lew et al., 2003; Logi et al., 2003; Robinson et al., 2003).

When Carter and Butt (2001) reviewed 44 studies describing SEPs recorded following severe traumatic brain injury, they found bilaterally absent primary cortical SEP responses carried a positive predictive value for unfavourable outcome of 98.5%. In their review, the bilateral absence of SEPs was accepted if there were no focal lesions (subdural haematomas or epidural haematomas), which would abolish the SEP cortical components, regardless of the subsequent functional progression. In Carter's review the outcomes were collapsed to favourable and unfavourable outcome groups. An unfavourable outcome consisted of the GOS categories of severe disability, vegetative state, or death (PVS was not considered separately). More recently Lew et al. (2003) have performed a study with 22 patients to evaluate the prognostic utility of SEPs and event-related potentials (ERPs). In their study bilateral absence of median nerve SEPs was strongly predictive of the worst functional outcome. SEP responses were absent in five patients. All five patients had poor prognosis (either death or vegetative state) at the 6-month follow-up. In return the prognosis was not better when SEPs were normal ($n = 9$) than when they were abnormal ($n = 8$) (Lew et al., 2003). The specificity and positive predictive value of absent SEPs for predicting death or persistent vegetative state at 6 months after traumatic brain injury was 100%. In summary median nerve SEPs make reliable prediction of persistent vegetative state in severe traumatic brain injury. However, no separate data for PVS are at present available.

Anoxic coma. In 1998, Zandbergen et al. (1998) performed a systematic review of early prediction of poor outcome following anoxic-ischaemic coma. They selected 33 studies describing the results of neurological examination, electroencephalography and SEPs with post-anoxic patients. Fourteen prognostic variables were identified across the studies, three of which had a specificity of 100%: absence of pupillary light reflexes on day 3, absent motor response to pain on day 3, and bilateral absence of early cortical SEPs within the first week. Further studies by Zingler et al. (2003) and Nakabayashi and colleagues have corroborated the specificity of the SEPs (Nakabayashi, Kurokawa, & Yamamoto, 2001). Both studies have found that bilateral loss of SEPs identifies patients who will not regain consciousness with a 100% specificity. A more recent review by Robinson et al. (2003) has also corroborated this finding. Robinson et al. reviewed 41 studies reporting SEPs in comatose patients and subsequent outcomes. Outcomes were categorised as persistent vegetative state or death vs awakening. For each SEP result (normal, abnormal, bilaterally absent), rates of awakening (95% confidence interval) were calculated. The following results were reported for adult hypoxic-ischaemic encephalopathy: absent 0% (0–1%), abnormal 22% (17–26%), normal 52% (48–56%). They concluded that SEPs predict the likelihood of non-awakening from coma with a high level of certainty. Adults in coma from hypoxic-ischaemic encephalopathy with absent SEP responses have <1% chance of awakening.

Event-related potentials

The prognostic utility of ERPs has only been explored in the last few years. However, a number of tests have shown promise. These include the N100 component of the long-latency auditory evoked potential and the P300 and MMN components of an auditory odd-ball paradigm (Fischer et al., 1999, 2004; Guérit et al., 1999; Kane, Butler, & Simpson, 2000; Kane et al., 1996; Lew et al., 2003; Madl et al., 2000). The N100 is elicited in response to broad-band clicks or repetitive tonal sequences and is thought to reflect an orienting response generated within the auditory cortex. The P300 elicited in response to a rare tone occurring among a regular tonal stream is discussed in more detail elsewhere in this special edition and will not be discussed further in this paper. However, in the acute comatose phase it is widely accepted to have less utility than its preceding MMN component. This is because the P300 is generally obtained more effectively in an attentive subject. The MMN, in contrast, is attention-independent and is automatically elicited in response to a deviant sound in a repetitive sequence. The main component of the MMN is generated in the superior temporal plane and is widely thought to reflect a pre-cognitive response generated by comparing the deviant input with a neural memory trace encoding the physical features of the repetitive sound (Naatanen & Alho, 1995; Naatanen & Rinne, 2002).

In our series of 346 comatose patients, 8 were considered in a PVS at one year post-insult. The aetiology of coma was cerebral anoxia ($n = 6$), stroke ($n = 1$), and traumatic brain injury ($n = 1$). The initial assessment of these 8 patients showed that pupils were reactive in 4; GCS was under 4 in 5 patients; BAEPs were normal in the 8 patients; MLAEPs were all abnormal (3 patients showed an isolated delay of Pa latency ≥ 31.6 ms without Na–Pa amplitude reduction; 3 patients showed a Na–Pa amplitude < 0.3 μV and 2 patients had no Na–Pa detected). Late auditory N100 was absent in 7 patients and MMN was absent in the 8 patients. In Table 1 we present the patients' outcome related to the presence/absence of N100 and MMN. It is important to notice that none of the 88 patients who had a MMN present at the early stage of coma progressed to a PVS. Hence, our study showed—for the first time—that the presence of an ERP at the early stage of coma, precisely the MMN, precludes comatose patients from progressing to a PVS.

CONCLUSION

Evoked potentials are useful for objective assessment of brain function in comatose patients. In the early stage of coma they can be recorded for prognosticating further progress towards poor outcome and PVS. From a systematic review of more than 30 studies reporting SEPs in anoxic coma it can be claimed that absent cortical SEPs predict the likelihood of poor outcome

TABLE 1
Outcome of the 346 comatose patients related to the presence/absence of
N100 and MMN

	Death	Unrelated death	PVS	Awakening	Total
N100	35	19	1	143	198
No N100	64	7	7	70	148
Total	99	26	8	213	346
MMN	10	13	0	65	88
No MMN	89	13	8	148	258
Total	99	26	8	213	346

(PVS or death) with a high level of certainty. Adults in coma from hypoxic ischaemic encephalopathy with absent SEPs have less than 1% chance of awakening. Following traumatic brain injury the bilateral absence of SEPs also has a high positive predictive value for a poor outcome but with a less clear-cut threshold and provided that no focal lesions would abolish the SEP cortical components. In contrast, the presence of event-related potentials at any stage of coma and whatever the aetiology, excludes further evolution towards permanent vegetative state. Hence, neurophysiological evaluation of anoxic or traumatic comatose patients should include recording of SEPs and ERPs for the prognostication of PVS.

REFERENCES

Cant, B. R., Hume, A. L., Judson, J. A., & Shaw, N. A. (1986). The assessment of severe head injury by short-latency somatosensory and brain-stem auditory evoked potentials. *Electroencaphalography and Clinical Neurophysiology, 65*(3), 188–195.

Carter, B. G., & Butt, W. (2001). Review of the use of somatosensory evoked potentials in the prediction of outcome after severe brain injury. *Critical Care Medicine, 29*(1), 178–186.

Fischer, C., Bognar, L., Turjman, F., Villanyi, E., & Lapras, C. (1994). Auditory and middle-latency evoked potentials in patients with quadrigeminal plate tumors. *Neurosurgery, 35*, 45–51.

Fischer, C., Luauté, J., Adeleine, P., & Morlet, D. (2004). Predictive value of sensory and cognitive evoked potentials for awakening from coma. *Neurology, 63*(4), 669–673.

Fischer, C., Morlet, D., Bouchet, P., Luauté, J., Jourdan, C., & Salord, F. (1999). Mismatch negativity and late auditory evoked potentials in comatose patients. *Clinical Neurophysiology, 110*(9), 1601–1610.

Goodwin, S. R., Friedman, W. A., & Bellefleur, M. (1991). Is it time to use evoked potentials to predict outcome in comatose children and adults? *Critical Care Medicine, 19*(4), 518–524.

Graham, D. I., Adams, J. H., Nicoll, J. A., Maxwell, W. L., & Gennarelli, T. A. (1995). The nature, distribution and causes of traumatic brain injury. *Brain Pathology, 5*(4), 397–406.

Guérit, J. M., de Tourtchaninoff, M., Soveges, L., & Mahieu, P. (1993). The prognostic value of three-modality evoked potentials (TMEPs) in anoxic and traumatic comas. *Neurophysiologie Clinique, 23*(2–3), 209–226.

Guérit, J. M., Verougstraete, D., de Tourtchaninoff, M., Debatisse, D., & Witdoeckt, C. (1999). ERPs obtained with the auditory oddball paradigm in coma and altered states of consciousness: Clinical relationships, prognostic value, and origin of components. *Clinical Neurophysiology, 110*(7), 1260–1269.

Jennett, B., & Bond, M. (1975). Assessment of outcome after severe brain damage. *Lancet, 1*(7905), 480–484.

Kane, N. M., Butler, S. R., & Simpson, T. (2000). Coma outcome prediction using event-related potentials: P(3) and mismatch negativity. *Audiology & Neuro-Otology, 5*(3–4), 186–191.

Kane, N. M., Curry, S. H., Rowlands, C. A., Manara, A. R., Lewis, T., Moss, T., et al. (1996). Event-related potentials—Neurophysiological tools for predicting emergence and early outcome from traumatic coma. *Intensive Care Medicine, 22*(1), 39–46.

Lew, H. L., Dikmen, S., Slimp, J., Temkin, N., Lee, E. H., Newell, D., & Robinson, L. R. (2003). Use of somatosensory-evoked potentials and cognitive event-related potentials in predicting outcomes of patients with severe traumatic brain injury. *American Journal of Physical Medicine and Rehabilitation, 82*(1), 53–61; 62–54, 80.

Logi, F., Fischer, C., Murri, L., & Mauguiere, F. (2003). The prognostic value of evoked responses from primary somatosensory and auditory cortex in comatose patients. *Clinical Neurophysiology, 114*(9), 1615–1627.

Luauté, J., Fischer, C., Adeleine, P., Morlet, D., Tell, L., & Boisson, D. (2005). Late auditory and cognitive evoked potentials can be useful to predict good functional outcome after coma. *Archives of Physical Medicine and Rehabilitation, 86*, 917–923.

Madl, C., Kramer, L., Domanovits, H., Woolard, R. H., Gervais, H., Gendo, A., et al. (2000). Improved outcome prediction in unconscious cardiac arrest survivors with sensory evoked potentials compared with clinical assessment. *Critical Care Medicine, 28*(3), 721–726.

Mauguiere, F., Allison, T., Babiloni, C., Buchner, H., Eisen, A. A., Goodin, D. S., et al. (1999). Somatosensory evoked potentials. The International Federation of Clinical Neurophysiology. *Electroencaphalography and Clinical Neurophysiology Supplement, 52*, 79–90.

Multi-Society Task Force on PVS. (1994a). Medical aspects of the persistent vegetative state (1). *New England Journal of Medicine, 330*(21), 1499–1508.

Multi-Society Task Force on PVS. (1994b). Medical aspects of the persistent vegetative state (2). *New England Journal of Medicine, 330*(22), 1572–1579.

Naatanen, R., & Alho, K. (1995). Mismatch negativity: A unique measure of sensory processing in audition. *International Journal of Neuroscience, 80*(1–4), 317–337.

Naatanen, R., & Rinne, T. (2002). Electric brain response to sound repetition in humans: An index of long-term-memory–trace formation? *Neuroscience Letters, 318*(1), 49–51.

Nakabayashi, M., Kurokawa, A., & Yamamoto, Y. (2001). Immediate prediction of recovery of consciousness after cardiac arrest. *Intensive Care Medicine, 27*(7), 1210–1214.

Robinson, L. R., Micklesen, P. J., Tirschwell, D. L., & Lew, H. L. (2003). Predictive value of somatosensory evoked potentials for awakening from coma. *Critical Care Medicine, 31*(3), 960–967.

Yvert, B., Crouzeix, A., Bertrand, O., Seither-Preisler, A., & Pantev, C. (2001). Multiple supratemporal sources of magnetic and electric auditory evoked middle latency components in humans. *Cerebral Cortex, 11*(5), 411–423.

Zandbergen, E. G., de Haan, R. J., Stoutenbeek, C. P., Koelman, J. H., & Hijdra, A. (1998). Systematic review of early prediction of poor outcome in anoxic-ischaemic coma. *Lancet, 352*(9143), 1808–1812.

Zingler, V. C., Krumm, B., Bertsch, T., Fassbender, K., & Pohlmann-Eden, B. (2003). Early prediction of neurological outcome after cardiopulmonary resuscitation: A multimodal approach combining neurobiochemical and electrophysiological investigations may provide high prognostic certainty in patients after cardiac arrest. *European Neurology, 49*(2), 79–84.

NEUROPSYCHOLOGICAL REHABILITATION,
2005, 15 (3/4), 381–388

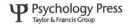

Bispectral analysis of electroencephalogram signals during recovery from coma: Preliminary findings

Caroline Schnakers, Steve Majerus and Steven Laureys

University of Liège, Liège, Belgium

The aim of this study was to investigate the accuracy of bispectral index (BIS), spectral edge frequency (SEF 95%), total power (TOTPOW) and frontal spontaneous electromyography (F-EMG) in monitoring consciousness in severely brain damaged patients. In 29 patients a total of 106 sedation-free and good quality EEG epochs were correlated with the level of consciousness as assessed by means of the Glasgow Liège Scale (GLS) and the Wessex Head Injury Matrix (WHIM). The strongest correlation with behavioural measures of consciousness was observed with BIS recordings. An empirically defined BIS cut-off value of 50 differentiated unconscious patients (coma or vegetative state) from conscious patients (minimally conscious state or emergence from minimally conscious state) with a sensitivity of 75% and specificity of 75%. These preliminary findings are encouraging in the search for electrophysiological correlates of consciousness in severe acute brain damage.

INTRODUCTION

Although the bedside examination is the standard method of measuring neurological function, the electroencephalogram (EEG) is an objective tool that permits continuous and online monitoring of brain function. Traditional EEG measures have also shown their efficacy in predicting outcome after anoxic or traumatic brain damage (Zandbergen et al., 1998). Because

Correspondence should be sent to Steven Laureys, Centre de Recherches du Cyclotron, Sart Tilman, B30, Université de Liège, 4000 Liège, Belgium. Tel: +32 4 366 23 16, Fax: +32 4 366 29 46. Email: steven.laureys@ulg.ac.be

This research was supported by the Fonds National de la Recherche Scientifique (FNRS), and the Centre Hospitalier Universitaire Sart Tilman, Liège, Belgium. Steven Laureys is Research Associate at FNRS and Steve Majerus is post-doctoral Researcher at FNRS.

http://www.tandf.co.uk/journals/pp/09602011.html   DOI:10.1080/09602010443000524

interpretation of the raw EEG signal requires considerable expertise and specialised training, simpler, more standardised measures of brain function are desired. The bispectral index (BIS) of the EEG is an empirical, statistically derived variable that provides information about the interaction of brain cortical and subcortical regions (Rampil, 1998). The BIS was designed as a measure of depth of anaesthesia and sedation. During the development of the monitor, the algorithm used to calculate the BIS was empirically derived and "normalised" on a scale of 0–100. A large number of EEG parameters were examined using statistical (discrimant) analysis to determine which of them provided useful information. Three main parameters were identified, and the BIS is calculated from the weighted sum of these three parameters: BetaRatio (the ratio of the power in the high and low beta ranges; i.e., frequency analysis), SynchFastSlow (calculated from the ratio of the bicoherence in fast and slower frequencies; i.e., bispectral analysis) (Barnett et al., 1971) and the BSR (burst suppression ratio—the proportion of each minute that the EEG is isoelectric; i.e., time domain analysis). Aside from amplifying, digitising and filtering the data, the main precursor step in calculation of the BIS is to apply a pattern recognition algorithm to determine the raw, time domain appearance of the EEG waveform. The weighting for the parameters is determined by this pattern recognition algorithm. In essence if the EEG has an activation appearance, the BIS is mostly determined by the BetaRatio. If the EEG shows signs of burst suppression, then the BIS is mostly determined by the BSR, whereas if the EEG looks compatible with that found during "surgical anaesthesia", then the BIS is mostly determined by SynchFastSlow. The exact weightings used have been determined by correlating the EEG pattern with anaesthetists' clinical impressions of anaesthetic depth. It is important to stress that the BIS has thus only been calibrated for normal, anaesthetised patients, and not for patients with injured brains.

Increasing depth of anaesthesia results in decreasing BIS score. Typically, BIS values range from 40 to 55 during general anaesthesia (for a recent review see Drummond, 2000). It has also been shown to be an index of the degree of sedation during induction and recovery from anaesthesia (Glass et al., 1997) and a measure of the depth of natural sleep (Nieuwenhuijs et al., 2002; Sleigh, Andrzejowski, Steyn-Ross, & Steyn-Ross, 1999). Recently, attempts have been made to assess the usefulness of BIS monitoring in sedated (De Deyne et al., 1998; Simmons, Riker, Prato, & Fraser, 1999) and unsedated (Gilbert et al., 2001) patients in the intensive care unit (ICU). The purpose of the present study is to test the utility of the BIS as an objective index of cerebral function in severely brain damaged patients recovering from coma. Thus, EEG parameters were measured in a population of unsedated ICU patients and correlated with behavioural measures of consciousness. Given the small number of observations, this paper should be viewed as a preliminary record of ongoing research.

MATERIALS AND METHODS

This study was prospectively performed in 29 patients who were comatose on admission to our ICU unit. Only evaluations made when patients had not received sedation were included for analysis. Each data set comprised an EEG measurement and clinical assessments of consciousness. Datasets were generated periodically, two times a week, in test patients during the time from admission at the ICU until hospital discharge. Patients were classified according to internationally established criteria as being in: (1) coma (Plum & Posner, 1983); (2) vegetative state (VS) (Multi-Society Task Force on PVS, 1994); (3) minimally conscious state (MCS), or (4) exit from MCS (Giacino et al., 2002).

The study was approved by the ethics committee of the Medical Faculty of our University and written informed consent was obtained by the patients' family.

Clinical measurements

In this study, we used the Glasgow Liège Scale (GLS; Born et al., 1982) and the Wessex Head Injury Matrix (WHIM; Shiel et al., 2000) as behavioural measurements of consciousness. The GLS combines the Glasgow Coma Scale (GCS) (Teasdale & Jennett, 1974) with a quantified analysis of five brainstem reflexes: fronto-orbicular, vertical oculo-cephalic, pupillary, horizontal oculo-cephalic, and oculo-cardiac (Born et al., 1982). The GLS is calculated as the sum of eye opening, motor response, verbal response, and brainstem reflex subscores and is scored from 3 (worst) to 20 (best) (Laureys, Majerus, & Moonen, 2002). The WHIM score represents the rank order of the most advanced behaviour observed and was designed for the assessment of patients in and emerging from coma and in the vegetative and minimally conscious states. It has been shown to be superior to the GCS and GLS scales for detecting subtle changes in patients emerging from vegetative state and for patients in a minimally conscious state (Majerus & Van der Linden, 2000) and is scored from 1 (worst) to 62 (best) (Schnakers, Majerus, & Laureys, 2004).

EEG measurements

EEG pads were placed in a two-channel referential standard frontal montage after a skin preparation with isopropyl alcohol. Measurement electrodes were placed on the temple and on the centre of the forehead. All leads were connected to a portable EEG monitor (A-2000, Aspect Medical Systems, Newton, USA). Data were sampled at 256 Hz, and high-frequency (70 Hz) and low-frequency (0.3 Hz) filters were used for EEG measurements. The A-2000 monitor provides a continuous output of the raw EEG pattern and divides the raw EEG data, sampled at 256 Hz, into 2 second epochs. At least eight epochs of "clean" EEG data are required to calculate the BIS (the minimum "smoothing period" is 15 seconds). Because sleep is associated with reduced BIS values (Nieuwenhuijs et al., 2002; Sleigh et al., 1999), the EEG monitoring was designed to begin at least 5 minutes after stimulating activities (such as intense auditory and somatosensory stimulation) and lasted 10–45 minutes for each measurement. The following EEG parameters were collected via the RS232 port every 5 seconds and saved on a portable computer for subsequent offline analysis: BIS; spectral edge frequency (SEF 95; the frequency below which 95% of the total EEG power resides); total EEG power (TOTPOW); and frontal spontaneous electromyography (F-EMG; defined as the power in the frequency range 70–110 Hz, assuming that it is not contaminated by external electrical noise, the changes in the power in this waveband probably reflect changes in frontalis muscle activity). Data points were excluded from further analysis under the following circumstances: (1) the electrode impedances were > 10.000 ohm; (2) the A-2000 EEG monitor software indicated that the data were contaminated by gross artefact, such as that caused by eye movement; (3) the F-EMG was ≥ 45 decibels (dB); (4) the signal quality index (SQI), quantified as the percentage of the prior 60 seconds of data that was usable for calculation of EEG spectral variables, was $\leq 80\%$.

Data analysis

All variables were expressed as mean $\pm$ standard deviation of the mean. The two behavioural measures were plotted against each of the EEG variables and the Pearson univariate correlation coefficient calculated. Results were considered significant at $p < .001$.

TABLE 1
Patients' demographic data (mean $\pm$ standard deviation)

Patients	$M \pm SD$
Number of patients	29
Age (years)	61 ± 18
Gender (% female)	38
Non-traumatic aetiology (%)	76
Traumatic aetiology (%)	24
Died (%)	52
First evaluation after admission (days)	5 ± 3
Follow-up (days)	22 ± 16
Number of evaluations per patient	7 ± 4

Note: Non-traumatic cases included anoxic encephalopathy ($n = 9$), cerebrovascular accidents ($n = 10$), encephalitis ($n = 2$), and metabolic encephalopathy ($n = 1$).

RESULTS

The demographic characteristics of the 29 patients enrolled in this study are shown in Table 1. A total of 193 datasets comprising EEG measurements and behavioural evaluations were collected; 38 were excluded because patients had received intravenous sedation within the prior 24 hours; 49 were excluded because EEG data were of sub-optimal quality (see above). Hence, 106 datasets were used for further study. Table 2 summarises the obtained mean behavioural and EEG data. Correlation coefficients between behavioural and EEG assessments are shown in Table 3. BIS most strongly correlated with both GLS and WHIM measurements (Figure 1).

A post-hoc Receiver Operating Characteristic (ROC) analysis (Zweig & Campbell, 1993) showed that at a BIS cut-off value of 50 the sensitivity (i.e., the proportion of unconscious patients who have a BIS below cut-off) was 75% and the specificity (i.e., the proportion of conscious patients who have a BIS above cut-off) also was 75%.

DISCUSSION

The major finding of this study is that BIS significantly correlates with the behavioural evaluation of consciousness as assessed by the GLS or WHIM in brain damaged patients. The easy accessibility of continuous EEG-BIS monitoring makes it a promising alternative to the interpretation of the raw

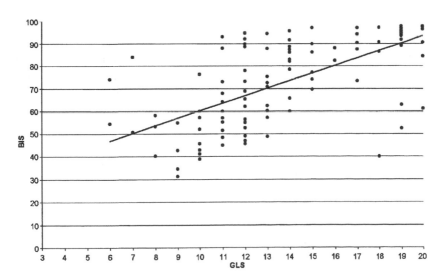

Figure 1. Scatter plot and linear regression between GLS, scores from 3 (brain death) to 20 (best), and BIS, scores from 0 (iso-electrical) to 100 ("fully conscious") ($r = .60$; $p < .001$).

TABLE 2

EEG and behavioural measurements in the different clinical entities

Clinical entity	Number of evaluations	GLS	WHIM	BIS	BIS within-patient variability	SEF 95	TOTPOW	F-EMG
Coma	11	8.6 ± 1.6	5.5 ± 2.3	44.4 ± 12.4	8.0 ± 4.6	6.7 ± 1.6	62.6 ± 4.6	37.2 ± 3.4
VS	32	11.0 ± 1.6	6.7 ± 1.9	63.0 ± 14.7	10.6 ± 4.3	10.0 ± 4.1	60.2 ± 5.0	41.6 ± 6.4
MCS	42	14.7 ± 2.3	23.3 ± 15.8	80.4 ± 14.7	9.0 ± 4.5	11.8 ± 5.3	62.3 ± 4.7	47.3 ± 5.1
Exit from MCS	21	19.2 ± 0.5	57.8 ± 4.0	88.7 ± 13.1	2.8 ± 3.8	25.6 ± 24	58.0 ± 3.4	52.7 ± 12.2

VS = vegetative state, MCS = minimally conscious state, GLS = Glasgow Liège Scale, WHIM = Wessex Head Injury Matrix, BIS = bispectral index (arbitrary values), SEF = 95% spectral edge frequency (in decibels), TOTPOW = total EEG power, F-EMG = frontal spontaneous electromyography (power in the low EMG waveband, 70–110 Hz).

TABLE 3

Univariate correlation coefficients between behavioural and EEG measurements

	BIS	SEF 95	TOTPOW	F-EMG
GLS score	0.60*	0.41**	−0.13†	0.49*
WHIM score	0.57*	0.44**	−0.14†	0.49*
WHIM number of behaviours	0.54*	0.49*	−0.17†	0.54*

*$p < .001$; **$p < .05$; †non-significant.

EEG signal, which requires considerable expertise. The use of EEG parameters in general and of BIS in particular for evaluating levels of consciousness has been a subject of intense investigation in recent years. In several studies, BIS has been shown to significantly correlate with the level of consciousness in anaesthetised patients (for review see Glass et al., 1997). However, many exceptions exist as ketamine and nitrous oxide do not seem to show these correlations with EEG parameters. In a study that examined the relationship between BIS and consciousness in patients receiving propofol, midazolam, or isoflurane anaesthesia, 50% of patients lost consciousness at a BIS of 65 and 95% were unconscious at a BIS of 50 (Glass et al., 1997). When we empirically defined a mean BIS value >50 during the evaluation period as a marker of consciousness, a clinically acceptable sensitivity and specificity of 75% was achieved in the present data sample (i.e., differentiation between *unconscious* comatose or vegetative patients and *conscious* MCS or "exit from MCS" patients).

Our findings highlight the EEG similarities (i.e., gross cortical desynchronisation) of unconscious states such as general anaesthesia, normal deep sleep (stage 3 and 4) and coma or vegetative state. Our data suggest that the BIS is, to a certain degree, a non-specific measure of consciousness, independent of how the loss of consciousness is caused (i.e., respectively pharmacologically, physiologically or pathologically). We observed a progressive increase in BIS values (and to a lesser degree of SEF 95 and F-EMG values) when brain damaged patients go from coma to VS to MCS and finally exit MCS. Although these preliminary findings suggest that BIS is useful to discriminate these different clinical entities encountered at the ICU, the spread of values measured in each clinical entity clearly confirms the importance of expert clinical behavioural evaluation and precludes the use of BIS as an independent infallible "consciousness-meter".

In conclusion, EEG-BIS monitoring obtained from frontal leads seems a useful reflection of consciousness in unsedated severely brain-damaged patients and thus may have a role in the objective monitoring of such patients in the acute and subacute setting. Further research is warranted to better understand the not infrequent false positive and false negative findings and to evaluate whether BIS or related EEG measures (e.g., quantification of complexity or approximate entropy) contain independent prognostic information for comatose and vegetative patients.

REFERENCES

Barnett, T. P., Johnson, L. C., Naitoh, P., Hicks, N., & Nute, C. (1971). Bispectrum analysis of electroencephalogram signals during waking and sleeping. *Science, 172*(981), 401–402.

Born, J. D., Hans, P., Dexters, G., Kalangu, K., Lenelle, J., Milbouw, G., et al. (1982). Practical assessment of brain dysfunction in severe head trauma. *Neurochirurgie, 28*(1), 1–7.

De Deyne, C., Struys, M., Decruyenaere, J., Creupelandt, J., Hoste, E., & Colardyn, F. (1998). Use of continuous bispectral EEG monitoring to assess depth of sedation in ICU patients. *Intensive Care Medicine, 24*(12), 1294–1298.

Drummond, J. C. (2000). Monitoring depth of anesthesia: With emphasis on the application of the bispectral index and the middle latency auditory evoked response to the prevention of recall. *Anesthesiology, 93*(3), 876–882.

Giacino, J. T., Ashwal, S., Childs, N., Cranford, R., Jennett, B., Katz, D. I., et al. (2002). The minimally conscious state: Definition and diagnostic criteria. *Neurology, 58*(3), 349–353.

Gilbert, T. T., Wagner, M. R., Halukurike, V., Paz, H. L., & Garland, A. (2001). Use of bispectral electroencephalogram monitoring to assess neurologic status in unsedated, critically ill patients. *Critical Care Medicine, 29*(10), 1996–2000.

Glass, P. S., Bloom, M., Kearse, L., Rosow, C., Sebel, P., & Manberg, P. (1997). Bispectral analysis measures sedation and memory effects of propofol, midazolam, isoflurane, and alfentanil in healthy volunteers. *Anesthesiology, 86*(4), 836–847.

Laureys, S., Majerus, S., & Moonen, G. (2002). Assessing consciousness in critically ill patients. In J. L. Vincent (Ed.), *2002 Yearbook of intensive care and emergency medicine* (pp. 715–727). Heidelberg: Springer-Verlag.

Majerus, S., & Van der Linden, M. (2000). Wessex Head Injury Matrix and Glasgow/Glasgow-Liège Coma Scale: A validation and comparison study. *Neuropsychological Rehabilitation, 10*(2), 167–184.

Multi-Society Task Force on PVS (1994). Medical aspects of the persistent vegetative state (1). *New England and Journal of Medicine, 330*(21), 1499–1508.

Nieuwenhuijs, D., Coleman, E. L., Douglas, N. J., Drummond, G. B., & Dahan, A. (2002). Bispectral index values and spectral edge frequency at different stages of physiologic sleep. *Anesthesia and Analgesia, 94*(1), 125–129.

Plum, F., & Posner, J. B. (1983). *The diagnosis of stupor and coma* (3rd ed.). Philadelphia: F.A. Davis.

Rampil, I. J. (1998). A primer for EEG signal processing in anesthesia. *Anesthesiology, 89*(4), 980–1002.

Schnakers, C., Majerus, S., & Laureys, S. (2004). Diagnosis and investigation of altered states of consciousness. *Reanimation, 13*, 368–375.

Shiel, A., Horn, S. A., Wilson, B. A., Watson, M. J., Campbell, M. J., & McLellan, D. L. (2000). The Wessex Head Injury Matrix (WHIM) main scale: A preliminary report on a scale to assess and monitor patient recovery after severe head injury. *Clinical Rehabilitation, 14*(4), 408–416.

Simmons, L. E., Riker, R. R., Prato, B. S., & Fraser, G. L. (1999). Assessing sedation during intensive care unit mechanical ventilation with the Bispectral Index and the Sedation-Agitation Scale. *Critical Care Medicine, 27*(8), 1499–1504.

Sleigh, J. W., Andrzejowski, J., Steyn-Ross, A., & Steyn-Ross, M. (1999). The bispectral index: A measure of depth of sleep? *Anesthesia and Analgesia, 88*(3), 659–661.

Teasdale, G., & Jennett, B. (1974). Assessment of coma and impaired consciousness. A practical scale. *Lancet, 2*(7872), 81–84.

Zandbergen, E. G., de Haan, R. J., Stoutenbeek, C. P., Koelman, J. H., & Hijdra, A. (1998). Systematic review of early prediction of poor outcome in anoxic-ischaemic coma. *Lancet, 352*(9143), 1808–1812.

Zweig, M. H., & Campbell, G. (1993). Receiver-operating characteristic (ROC) plots: A fundamental evaluation tool in clinical medicine. *Clinical Chemistry, 39*(4), 561–577.

NEUROPSYCHOLOGICAL REHABILITATION
2005, 15 (3/4), 389–405

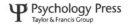

Electrical treatment of reduced consciousness: Experience with coma and Alzheimer's disease

E. B. Cooper[1,2,5], E. J. A. Scherder[3,4], and J. B. Cooper[2,5]

[1]*Department of Neurological Surgery, University of Virginia, Charlottesville, VA, USA*

[2]*Department of Physical Medicine and Rehabilitation, Brody School of Medicine, East Carolina University, Greenville, NC, USA*

[3]*Department of Neuropsychology, Vrije University, Amsterdam, The Netherlands*

[4]*Department of Human Movement Sciences, Rijksuniversiteit Groningen, Groningen, The Netherlands*

[5]*Department of Neurology, Medical College of Virginia, Richmond, VA, USA*

The right median nerve can be stimulated electrically to help arouse the central nervous system for persons with reduced levels of consciousness. The mechanisms of central action include increased cerebral blood flow and raised levels of dopamine. There is 11 years of experience in the USA of using nerve stimulation for acute coma after traumatic brain injury. There is a much longer period of experience by neurosurgeons in Japan with implanted electrodes on the cervical spinal cord for persons in the persistent vegetative state (PVS). But the use of right median nerve electrical stimulation (RMNS) for patients in the *subacute* and *chronic* phases of coma is relatively new. Surface electrical stimulation to treat anoxic brain injury as well as traumatic brain injury is evolving.

Novel applications of electrical stimulation in Amsterdam have produced cognitive behavioural effects in persons with early and mid-stage Alzheimer's disease employing transcutaneous electrical nerve stimulation (TENS). Improvements in short-term memory and speech fluency have also been noted.

Regardless of the aetiology of the coma or reduced level of awareness, electrical stimulation may serve as a catalyst to enhance central nervous system functions. It remains for the standard treatments and modalities to retrain the injured brain emerging from reduced levels of consciousness.

Correspondence should be addressed to: Edwin Cooper, MD, 1001 North Queen Street, Kinston, North Carolina 28501, USA. Tel: (252) 522-5881, Fax: (252) 527-2923. Email: edwincooper@earthlink.net

INTRODUCTION

The right median nerve is a peripheral portal to the central nervous system. The sensory representation of the hand in the cortex is disproportionately large compared to other parts of the body. In the brain stem the ascending reticular activating system (ARAS) maintains the state of wakefulness. The spinoreticular component of the median nerve pathway synapses with neurons of the ARAS (Parent, 1996). Improvement of level of consciousness, whether in persons in acute coma, or those in a chronic vegetative or minimally conscious state, is driven by the electrically induced elevation of dopamine and norepinephrine (Hayashi, 1997; Moriya et al., 2000). Increase in cerebral blood flow, which is measurable shortly after starting the median nerve stimulation (MNS), is another important factor in neurostimulation for re-awakening (Liu et al., 2003).

The right median nerve was chosen as a portal to stimulate the brain stem and cerebrum because increased awareness and a better pattern of speech and abilities to calculate have been observed after right median nerve electrical stimulation (RMNS) (Cooper & Cooper, 2003; Cooper, Jane, Alves, & Cooper, 1999). In the majority of individuals, whether right handed or left handed, Broca's motor/speech planning area is in the left frontotemporal region. Broca's area has been shown to become more active in positron emission tomography (PET) when a subject moves his/her hand, or even contemplates speaking or moving the hand (Montgomery, 1989). This process is also artificially driven by RMNS (Cooper & Cooper, 2003; Spiegel et al., 1999).

EXPERIENCE WITH MEDIAN NERVE ELECTRICAL STIMULATION IN THE USA

Implantation of lower extremity nerve electrodes for treatment of spinal cord injury began in 1972 at the University of Virginia (Cooper, Bunch, & Campa, 1973). In the late 1980s, individuals with quadriplegia triggered their paralysed forearm and hand muscles through voice-activated computerised electrical stimulation (Gersh, 1992). This technique resulted in voluntary hand opening and closing at the Department of Biomedical Engineering at Duke University in Durham, North Carolina. Significant improvement was noted in distal motor abilities in direct response to electrical stimulation (Cooper, Han, & McElhaney, 1988). Proximal voluntary muscle strength in the stimulated arm also improved. But an unexpected result was a crossover effect causing improvement in the strength of the proximal muscles of the unstimulated arm. This observation about intra-cerebral transfer led to the development of median nerve electrical stimulation for coma arousal (Cooper et al., 1999).

Almost two decades ago at Caswell Center in Kinston, North Carolina, a non-ambulatory adult male received surface electrical stimulation to his right forearm for reducing flexor muscle spasticity. The electrical stimulation was performed daily for a period of weeks. Progressive improvements in mental awareness and non-verbal interaction were observed on serial videotapes. There was better postural control of the head and trunk. This unexpected finding of generalised bodily motor improvement after right forearm electrical stimulation for a period of weeks, plus the crossover effect in the quadriplegic population with motor improvement in the non-stimulated upper extremity, led to the postulation that electrical stimulation of the right median nerve causes central nervous system arousal. This theory generated the right median nerve coma stimulation projects at East Carolina University and the University of Virginia in the early 1990s.

Observations have been made in the USA and in Japan in projects for patients with acute and long-term coma states. Progressive improvements that are somewhat predictable regarding eye co-ordination followed by facial, peripheral motor and speech function after several weeks of electrical stimulation have been seen in studies in the USA (Cooper, Jane, Alves, & Cooper, 1999) and Japan (Moriya et al., 1999).

MATERIALS AND METHODS

Multiple MNS studies have been done in the USA at the University of Virginia (Cooper et al., 1999; Peri et al., 2001) and East Carolina University (Cooper & Cooper, 2003). Similar studies have been initiated by neurosurgeons in Japan (Yokoyama, Kamei, & Kanno, 1996) and Taiwan (Liu et al., 2003). Two models of portable battery powered electrical neuromuscular simulators have been utilised (Respond Select and Focus, manufactured by the Empi Corporation). Similar electrical parameters have been standardised for the various studies. These electrical devices provided trains of asymmetric biphasic pulses at an amplitude of 15–20 milliamps with a pulse width of 300 microseconds at 40 Hz for 20 sec/min. The electrical treatment was delivered for 8–12 hours daily with a pair of lubricated one-inch square rubber electrodes placed on the skin over the median nerve. The location was on the palmar side of the right wrist in almost all cases. The number of weeks, or months, of electrical stimulation corresponded directly with the length of time since brain injury to the startup of the electrical treatment.

In acute trauma patients with severe brain injuries producing coma, the electrical stimulation was usually started less than one month post-injury, often in the first week. Glasgow Coma Scales (GCS) scores were 4–8, usually 4–5. In this group of acute patients, usually 2–3 weeks of electrical treatment would be needed. For traumatic brain injury (TBI) coma patients in which the electrical stimulation was started more than one month post-injury, stimulation duration varied widely. Usually a period of several weeks would be needed.

The newer experience of using RMNS in the treatment of patients in the persistent vegetative state or minimally conscious state, shows that longer periods of electrical stimulation measured in months or years would be needed for these more difficult cases.

For children and small adults, a setting of up to 15 milliamps is recommended. Electrical stimulation as high as 20 milliamps has been used in adults in deep coma. This level of stimulation is not usually tolerated by conscious or semi-conscious patients due to the strong tingling and the muscular contraction produced in the right hand. The RMNS is approximately 1.5 times the motor threshold. It produces right thenar apposition and flexion plus flexion of the index and middle fingers. Effects on vital signs are mild. Intracranial pressures usually remain stable. There have been no major complications induced by the peripheral electrical stimulation (Cooper & Kanno, in press).

RESULTS OF ELECTRICAL TREATMENT

Acute stage of TBI coma

In the 1990s, 38 comatose patients with severe closed head injury received right median nerve electrical (or sham) stimulation in a series of pilot studies at the University of Virginia in Charlottesville, Virginia (Cooper et al., 1999; Peri et al., 2001) and the East Carolina University in Greenville, North Carolina (Cooper et al., 1999). Similar RMNS protocols were used at both university medical centres.

There were two pilot studies at the University of Virginia (1994–1995 and 1998–1999). In both studies comatose trauma patients were randomly assigned into electrical treatment or sham treatment groups. The neurobehavioural raters were blinded to the treatment conditions. There were six patients in the first study and 10 patients in the second study. In the earlier study the electrical treatment group had a shorter time in the intensive care unit (Cooper et al., 1999). In the second study the electrically treated comatose patients had a shorter time of endotracheal intubation (Peri et al., 2001).

Coma patients with GCS scores near 8 on the day of injury can be expected to make very functional recoveries with standard treatment. In those cases where the GCS score is 4–5 with decerebrate/decorticate posturing, few can be expected to make good recoveries (Marshall & Marshall, 1996). But with median nerve electrical stimulation, if the patient survives the initial brain injury and other multi-system injuries, the time for awakening from coma is shorter in the electrically stimulated group than in the non-stimulated group. Gradual progress to a functional level is almost twice as frequent in the electrically stimulated group as in the non-stimulated group (Cooper & Kanno, in press).

There were 22 comatose patients treated with electrical stimulation at the medical centre at East Carolina University from 1993 to 1999. Twelve of the

TABLE 1
Twelve GCS-4 Survivor patients treated with early RMNS at ECU

Initials	Age	Sex	Injury year	Glasgow Outcome Scale at ≤ 1 year*
1. C	16	F	1993	Good recovery
2. P	21	M	1994	Severe disability
3. M	22	M	1994	Severe disability
4. C	16	F	1994	Moderate disability
5. A	15	F	1995	Good recovery
6. A	17	F	1995	Good recovery
7. M	26	F	1996	Moderate disability
8. K	19	F	1996	Good recovery
9. K	7	M	1997	Severe disability
10. R	14	M	1997	Severe disability
11. D	21	M	1997	Severe disability
12. E	15	F	1999	Moderate disability

*Cooper and Kanno, in press.

patients were in the Glasgow Coma Scale 4 category. They exhibited decerebrate posturing. These patients were in deep coma for more than a week. It is known that GCS 4 patients have a very poor prognosis (Cooper & Kanno, in press, Marshall & Marshall, 1996).

Therefore in the 12 young deeply comatose patients treated with early RMNS, almost 60% made a satisfactory recovery by one year post-injury (see Table 1).

SELECTED AMERICAN CASES

Two examples of adolescents with very severe traumatic brain injury with diffuse injury and no large haematomas are presented. In both cases, functional neurological survival was not expected.

C, a 16-year-old female, was involved in a motor vehicle accident and sustained a severe closed head injury in 1994. She suffered a basilar skull fracture, cerebrospinal fluid otorrhoea, left facial fracture, and left pelvic fracture. Computerised tomography (CT) scan revealed a left internal capsule contusion, right cerebellar subarachnoid haemorrhage, and blood in the fourth ventricle. Decerebrate posturing was observed and she received a GCS score of 4. She was briefly given electrical stimulation to the right median nerve but intracranial pressures continued to rise. With her extremely poor prognosis, she was expected to die. C was extubated, less than two weeks post-injury. She breathed spontaneously and electrical stimulation was resumed to the right median nerve. Within one week of restarting the electrical neuro-stimulation, she exhibited semi-purposeful movements of her right arm and leg and scored 7 on the GCS.

After a total of two weeks of stimulation, she was out of coma. One month after the injury, C followed simple commands. At two months post-injury C could walk with assistance and could read aloud. Two years later, C talked and walked well. She resumed dancing and driving and graduated from college. For a period of four years, C has been working as a recreation director in a nursing home and most recently at a retirement home (Cooper & Cooper, 2003).

In 2000, a 12-year-old boy, K suffered severe multi-system injuries. A van ran over his body and rested on his head producing severe brain trauma, intra-abdominal injury and multiple extremity fractures plus a compound fracture of the pelvis. On his initial CT scan there was a left frontal contusion, a small amount of subarachnoid haemorrhage in the interpeduncular cistern, and a non-depressed skull fracture of the left parietal bone. There was also a fracture of the left temporal bone. On the follow-up scan two days later, there were several contusions (right frontal and left temporal), increased cerebral oedema with marked effacement of the cortical sulci, and intraventricular haemorrhage. The scan one week post-injury demonstrated diffuse brain swelling and multiple haemorrhagic shear injuries. Haemorrhagic contusions of the left frontal lobe extending into the temporal lobe worsened the prognosis for the return of verbal function. K underwent several abdominal and orthopaedic operations early in his complex hospital course. He remained comatose with elevated intracranial pressures (over 70 mmHg) in spite of two courses of barbiturate therapy. His pupils remained unequal. K's survival was doubtful (Cooper & Cooper, 2003).

Surface electrical stimulation to the left median nerve (his right forearm was in a cast) in the 15 milliamps range was commenced two weeks post-injury. After two weeks of eight hours of daily median nerve stimulation, K began to emerge from his coma. He progressively improved and regained his ability to speak. He could use both of his hands in spite of a right hemiparesis which persisted. Two months post-injury, he was transferred to a rehabilitation centre. Electrical stimulation was resumed, but was switched to the right median nerve to help reduce the right hemiparesis. He continued to improve and was discharged home six weeks later. In schoolwork, he made good grades. Less than three years after the severe TBI system and multi-system injuries, K maintained a "B" average in junior high school. Additionally, he was able to resume some athletic activities, including swimming and ball sports (Cooper & Cooper, in press).

Subacute stage of TBI

J demonstrates the advantage of beginning median nerve electrical stimulation in the first month of coma. J was a 16-year-old girl from southern California whose car was T-boned (side impact) by a truck in 2002. At the scene she had agonal respiration and was unresponsive at GCS 3. In the emergency room at a large community hospital her post-intubation coma score was GCS 4 on the day of the injury. The CT scan showed a large right putaminal haemorrhage and a small amount of blood in the mesencephalon. There was extensive shear injury in left fronto-temporal lobe and corpus callosum. Elevated intracranial pressure (ICP) was treated with mannitol and hyperventilation.

Operations included exploratory laparotomy, splenectomy, and ventriculostomy with monitoring of intracranial pressure, and later tracheostomy and feeding tube insertion. Follow-up brain CT scans on a daily basis showed progressive cerebral oedema and increasing haemorrhage. Two days after the injury there was a 7 mm midline shift. The small haemorrhage in the central mesencephalon was still present. By a week and a half post-injury the swelling and haemorrhage stabilised and gradually decreased. A week later cortical atrophy was observed.

J remained in coma and was decerebrate/decorticate at four weeks post-injury. Bilateral median nerve electrical stimulation (six hours per day for each wrist median nerve stimulation site) was started at five weeks post-injury. She remained in the intensive care unit for her entire two-month hospitalisation. Two weeks after the electrical stimulation was started, she remained left hemiplegic, but could follow commands. After three weeks of electrical treatment she could write, but could not speak. She was transferred to a rehabilitation unit eight weeks post-injury.

Next, J was able to speak in short sentences and communicate by writing. Six weeks post-injury she was able to walk with maximum support but remained left hemiplegic. Three months post-injury she had voluntary control of her left leg when walking. After three months of rehabilitation, she was transferred to a residential rehabilitation facility for an additional three months. She was discharged home to the care of her family in early 2003, eight and a half months post brain injury. She continued to receive outpatient therapies.

Later in the spring of 2003 she graduated from high school on schedule with her class, less than one year post-injury. In the fall of 2003 she was in college taking three courses, achieving "B" grades. She used a manual wheelchair but was able to walk with help and a brace on her left leg. Her left hand remained nonfunctional, flexed at the wrist. She regained good speech, conversing in normal sentences, although her vocal tone was somewhat flat with mild dysarthria (Cooper & Cooper, in press).

Chronic stage of brain injury

Kanno and Okuma, from the Department of Neurosurgery, Fujita Health University, Japan, have reported on the subacute and chronic stages of coma resulting from traumatic and vascular causes (Okuma et al., 2001). The Japanese neurosurgeons were concerned that during the acute and subacute stages that brain atrophy was in progress after the initial brain injury, whether from trauma or anoxic injury. They suggested that even if the aggressive rehabilitation is started at the chronic stage it may be too late to achieve a recovery of brain function because of brain atrophy. Kanno stressed the importance of establishing a new treatment system for patients in the subacute stage (Kanno, 2000; Yamamoto et al., 1997; Yokoyama et al., 1996). Kanno and Okuma discussed median nerve stimulation (MNS) and dorsal column stimulation (DCS) for persistent vegetative state (PVS) produced by trauma, anoxia or other causes. It was their hope that electrical stimulation might stop the progress of the atrophy. (Kanno, 2000; Kanno, Kamei, Yokoyama, 1992).

Kanno and associates have described DCS in Japan. For almost two decades, electrodes have been implanted on the cervical spinal cord of patients in the PVS. All cases were in PVS and had been unconscious for a period of three months or more. In patients who had been in a vegetative state for over a year, improvement was still possible.

Numerous articles in Japan have referred to these patients. There has been a consistent observation of 42% showing clinical improvements (Kanno, Kamei, Yokoyama, 1989). Usually the improvement was in terms of interaction of the patient with the family, the ability to follow simple commands and self-feeding. But PVS adults who were electrically treated with the spinal cord stimulation, did not, in general, regain the ability to walk or talk. In half of the cases the regional blood flow improved. In general, the patients in PVS who showed a positive response to the DCS treatment were younger victims, less than age 40. They were in a vegetative state because of head trauma and not from anoxic injury. The prognosis was better when there was a relatively shorter period of coma prior to therapy. Their CT scans did not show severe damage to the thalamus and did not reveal marked cerebral atrophy. Of the patients who improved, the aetiology of the initial coma was trauma in 75% of the cases. Almost 90% of the improved patients were under age 30. Those over age 50 did not show improvement with the DCS therapy. Kanno observed that cases due to vascular or hypoxic injury rarely improved with the electrical treatment (Kanno et al., 1992).

In northern California, a current case (2004) with anoxic brain injury from cardiac arrest resulting in the persistent vegetative state lasting six months, has commenced daily RMNS. There have been some positive responses noted within the first three months of electrical treatment: better head and trunk posture, tracking with definite eye contact, swallowing (able to take yogurt), and, recently, phonation. K, an adult female, will be the subject of a future article (Davey, 2004).

The relationship between rehabilitation therapy and functional outcomes

In a large multi-centre study in the USA of 491 patients who were enrolled at three major medical centres, brain injury patients who had received acute care and inpatient rehabilitation were analysed regarding outcomes relative to the intensity of rehabilitation therapies. Total therapy hours per day, usually involving speech, occupational, psychological and physical therapy, were calculated. The Functional Independence Measure (FIM) scores were analysed at admission and discharge from the rehabilitation hospitals. Regarding the cognitive outcome, the authors noted, "Examination of cognitive outcomes indicates that therapeutic intensity did not contribute to gains in cognitive ability" (Cifu et al., 2003). Longer length of stay and rehabilitation significantly predicted better motor potential achievement. A better motor score was achieved by greater therapy intensity. The authors concluded, "A multitude of additional treatment factors may be of benefit to outcomes, and additional research is needed to identify those factors. Rehabilitation outcomes research should help guide the development of evidence-based guidelines for rehabilitation" (Cifu et al., 2003).

OBSERVATIONS ABOUT RESPONSES TO RMNS

In the first few days of treatment, mirror movements of the unstimulated left hand may occur. This dynamic crossover effect heralds reactivation of the cerebral hemispheres through the corpus callosum in the electrically stimulated comatose patient. Usually the first simple command that the patient will respond to after one or two weeks of RMNS is a sluggish apposition of the right thumb and index finger. This purposeful right hand response while the brain injured patient still appears to be semi-comatose, demonstrates that the five million electrical pulses delivered to the nervous system in the first 10 days of treatment have been copied and stored in the hard drive of the brain (Cooper & Kanno, in press).

There is a predictable sequence of events that indicates positive response to the median nerve stimulation techniques, both for acute coma patients and long-term patients in the vegetative or minimally conscious state. There should be involuntary contraction of the median innervated muscles of the hand receiving the electrical stimulation. This would include abduction/flexion of the thumb and flexion of mainly the index and middle fingers and slight flexion of the wrist. Depending on the depth of the coma there may be some involuntary or semi-voluntary withdrawal of the whole upper extremity, plus other bodily movements.

The early positive changes observed clinically in electrically stimulated coma and PVS patients would be increased eye movements, followed shortly by some head movements to either side. As the depth of coma/vegetative state lightens, head control and trunk control should improve. Generalised improved skin circulation and increased salivation usually are noted in the first week or two of treatment. Mirror movements may be noted in the unstimulated contralateral hand with slight contractions of that thumb or other hand muscles.

After some basic muscular functions have resumed, there may be changes in facial expression indicating discomfort or attempts to smile. This is followed shortly by groans or phonation. Semi-purposeful hand movements would usually be the next stage. Finally the full awakening to a conscious level may occur. After that there would be considerable variability in the return of cognitive, speech and ambulatory functions. Usually the reawakened coma/PVS patient would be able to eat, but not always able to feed him or herself. In cases that achieve higher neurological function, the ability to talk and walk would be expected to follow.

In previous studies, it was noted that the slope of the timeline of partial neurological recovery is inversely related to the interval of time from the injury to the startup of RMNS. The quality of the functional outcome is influenced by the severity of neurotrauma as diagnosed on early CT scans (Blackman et al., 2003; Eisenberg et al., 1990; Kampfl et al., 1998; Kido et al., 1992; Marshall et al., 1991; Toutant et al., 1984). In severe neurotrauma where the prognosis for brain survival in a functional state is approaching zero, any novel therapeutic intervention that produces better than expected results can be judged by the unexpected change in recovery slope. Professor John Jane (Chairman, Department of Neurological Surgery, University of Virginia), with a long time wealth of neurotrauma research, summarised the challenge of exploring median nerve stimulation: "Very few things do work in this situation and if your techniques make any difference whatsoever, I think it would be well worth it." (J. Jane, 1995, personal communication).

The coma cases presented anecdotally in this paper are examples of electrical treatment where medical expectations for a functional survival had vanished. The improvements noted are doubly validated by the unexpected change in clinical course and the similarity of observations reported from widely separated locations in the USA and Asia. Rigorous proof of the theory that peripheral nerve stimulation influences the function of the injured brain demands larger series of treated/sham treatment comatose subjects. The purpose of this overview is to stimulate such worldwide research.

TENS IN ALZHEIMER'S DISEASE AND ENCEPHALITIS

In a number of studies, transcutaneous electrical nerve stimulation (TENS) was applied to patients in a relatively early stage of Alzheimer's disease (AD) (Scherder, Bouma, & Steen, 1992; 1995; 1998; Scherder & Bouma, 1999; van Dijk, Scherder, Scheltens, & Sergeant, 2002). In those studies, the electric current was applied through two electrodes attached to the trapezius muscle, one electrode on each side of the spinal column, at the level of the first thoracic vertebra. The 30-minutes-a-day application took place during six weeks, followed by a treatment-free period of six weeks. In all studies a control group was included; participants of this group received sham stimulation with the same treatment frequency and treatment time, during the same treatment period. In one recent study, AD patients received RMNS with exactly the same stimulation parameters as described above (Scherder & Van Someren, 2004).

A blinded investigator who did not know whether the patient belonged to the experimental group or the control group, administered a comprehensive neuropsychological test battery, including tests for various memory processes and verbal fluency. In addition, the nursing staff was asked to fill in observation scales and the rest-activity rhythm was measured by means of actigraphy.

Overall, the results indicate that patients who received real TENS treatment showed a statistically significant improvement with respect to nonverbal short-term memory, verbal and nonverbal long-term (recognition) memory, and verbal fluency. Affective behaviour showed *clinically* relevant effects, i.e., patients who were treated with TENS became less depressed, less anxious, and less irritated. Of note is that in two studies the rest-activity rhythm of AD patients, measured by actigraphy, improved. This improvement was reflected in among other things a decrease in nightly restlessness (Scherder, Van Someren, & Swaab, 1999b; Van Someren, Scherder, & Swaab, 1998). Based on data from animal experimental studies (Scherder, Luijpen, & Van Dijk, 2003) the stimulation-parameters frequency, intensity and pulse width were selected in such a way that an optimal activation of the locus coeruleus (LC) and dorsal raphe nucleus (DRN)—brain stem areas which project to the hippocampus (Ezrokhi, Zosimovskii, Korshunov, & Markevich, 1999) and the hypothalamic suprachiasmatic nucleus (SCN) (Legoratti-Sanchez, Guevara-Guzman, & Solano-Flores, 1989)—could be obtained. The biological clock, important for our 24-hour circadian rhythm, is situated in the hypothalamic SCN (Swaab, 2004). Please see next section for more details about possible underlying mechanisms.

The positive effects of TENS in AD patients should be considered with caution. In the first place, the studies were single blind, implying that the person who performed the treatment knew which patients belonged to the experimental group and which patients to the control group; this might have created a bias. Second, the number of participating patients was relatively small in each study, i.e., 8 to 10 patients in each group. In a recent study, a much larger number of AD patients participated (approximately 30 patients in each group) and only a treatment effect on the rest-activity rhythm was observed for those patients who did not take cholinesterase inhibitors (unpublished results). This finding might imply that previous results are based on chance instead of real TENS effects. On the other hand, the group of AD patients in this latter study was quite heterogeneous with respect to the stage of the disease, ranging from relatively early to advanced, and the onset of the disease, much earlier in the latter study compared to the previous studies. Severity and early onset of the disease are two conditions that might reduce treatment efficacy (Cedazo-Minguez & Cowburn, 2001; Ho et al., 2002; Le Bars et al., 2002).

Particularly, the finding that in AD too much activity, for example, during the night, could be inhibited by TENS, was the main reason to apply TENS to two children who showed severe behavioural disinhibition after suffering from herpes simplex encephalitis (HSE). In a 9-year-old girl (Scherder, 1996) and an 11-year-old boy (Scherder et al., 2001), overall affective behaviour as well as nightly restlessness and over-activity by day decreased significantly with the use of TENS. These findings might be less surprising considering that HSE is strongly related to damage of the hippocampus and mamillary complex of the hypothalamus (Kapur et al., 1994), structures that are also affected in AD (Scheltens et al., 1992; Swaab, 2004).

Possible mechanisms underlying the effects of RMNS/TENS

The effects of RMNS in comatose patients and AD patients and the effects of peripheral electrical stimulation applied to the trapezius muscle in AD patients might have two similar mechanisms in which the basal forebrain nucleus basalis of Meynert (NBM) plays a crucial role. The NBM is the origin of the cortical cholinergic system and is important for the level of cortical activity (Dringenberg & Olmstead, 2003) and cognitive processes such as memory (Shinotoh et al., 2003).

The first mechanism concerns the ARAS. The ARAS originates in the brain stem reticular formation, more specifically the LC and the DRN, origins of the noradrenergic and serotonergic neurotransmitter systems, respectively (Kayama & Koyama, 1998). With respect to arousal, the brain stem reticular formation is functionally related to the NBM/cholinergic system (Sauvage & Steckler, 2001). Another area directly connected with the NBM and involved in arousal and attention (Critchley et al., 2003), is the anterior cingulate cortex (ACC). Interestingly, a recent functional magnetic resonance imaging (fMRI) study showed that the ACC is activated by RMNS applied with a painful intensity (Kwan, Crawley, Mikulis, & Davis, 2000). In the studies with comatose patients and patients with AD, the intensity of the stimulation was not nociceptive but high enough to provoke muscular twitches; fMRI studies are needed to examine whether this level of intensity is sufficient to stimulate areas such as the ACC.

A second mechanism that might underlie the effects of peripheral electrical nerve stimulation in coma and AD is related to neurotrophic factors, among which are nerve growth factor (NGF) and brain-derived neurotrophic factor (BDNF). Neurotrophic factors play an important role in neuroplasticity by, among other things, transforming silent synapses into functional ones (Klintsova &

Greenough, 1999). AD is characterised by a reduction of NGF in the NBM whereas the level of NGF in the cerebral cortex is unchanged (Salehi & Swaab, 1999). Interestingly, it has been observed that by exposure to an enriched environment, cerebral NGF is retrogradely transported to the basal forebrain, enhancing its cholinergic activity (Salehi & Swaab 1999). With respect to coma, BDNF might enhance survival of neurons after a hypoglycaemic coma of a short duration (Kokaia, Othberg, Kokaia, & Lindvall, 1994). Interestingly, rats with a transient global ischaemia that were housed in an enriched environment showed increased BDNF levels (Gobbo & O'Mara, 2004). We argue that peripheral electrical stimulation could be considered as a type of enriched environment and could initiate a similar sequence of events (Luijpen et al., 2003).

The juxtaposition of neurological conditions of different aetiologies—young people with traumatic brain injury yielding the spectrum of coma, PVS and the minimally conscious state, next to the progressively plaqued and tangled elderly AD brains—at first does not seem logical. But the final events of cytotoxic concentrations of glutamate released by damaged neurons are reputed to be enemies of both sets of patients who exhibit decreased levels of consciousness (Clausen & Bullock, 2001; Cooper, 1996; Doraiswamy, 2003; Faden, 1996; Greenamyre et al., 1988; Hynd, Scott, & Dodd, 2004). Based on our clinical success with RMNS in some acute coma cases (albeit temporary in mid-stage Alzheimer's disease), we seek a physically effective treatment for the stabilisation of glutamate while increasing the dopamine levels to awaken the damaged brains. Encouraged by unexpected neuroprotective/glutamate results of median nerve stimulation in a new hypoxic rat brain study in Germany (Buitrago et al., 2004), we recommend that future projects explore the commonality of the two neurological maladies of TBI and AD. We hope that common patterns of electrical treatment may ameliorate similar physiological pathways that lead to neural death of the young and old.

CONCLUSION

Over the past two decades independent research projects have focused on electrical treatment of acute coma, persistent vegetative state, Alzheimer's disease and encephalitis. These investigations from the USA, Japan and Europe have yielded unifying theories of cerebral hypo-function that are amenable to novel treatments. Peripheral, spinal and direct brain stimulation improve long-term outcomes of individuals suffering from diffuse neuronal injury.

We present this series of experiences in acute, subacute and chronic coma along with data from Alzheimer's treatment to point out the efficacy of non-invasive peripheral electrical stimulation. The same methodology may be applied to multiple disabling conditions and diseases.

It is encouraging to observe positive effects through peripheral stimulation across three continents with hundreds of varied patients. Right median nerve electrical stimulation remains a simple and effective way to improve the long-term outcomes of patients affected by coma. The same treatment has a positive effect on patients with Alzheimer's disease.

Peripheral electrical stimulation is sufficient to cause clinical improvement. This suggests that neural plasticity is positively influenced by an electrical treatment via an external, non-invasive portal.

We believe that more widespread use of this technique and further investigations will prove beneficial. Improved behavioural and cognitive outcomes have been observed across a wide array of electrical stimulation techniques. Utilisation of inexpensive, safe, and non-invasive techniques such as peripheral electrical stimulation will prove invaluable in the coming years.

REFERENCES

Blackman, J. A., Rice, S. A., Matsumoto, J. A., Conaway, M. R., Elgin, K. M., Patrick, P. D., Farrell, J., Allaire, J. H., & Willson, D. F. (2003). Brain imaging as a predictor of early functional outcome following traumatic brain injury in children, adolescents, and young adults. *Journal of Head Trauma Rehabilitation*, *18*, 493–503.

Buitrago, M., Luft, A., Thakor, N., Blue, M., & Hanley, D. (2004). Effects of somatosensory electrical stimulation on neuronal injury after global hypoxia-ischemia. *Experimental Brain Research*, *158*, 336–344.

Cedazo-Minguez, A., & Cowburn, R. F. (2001). Apolipoprotein E: A major piece in the Alzheimer's disease puzzle. *Journal of Cellular & Molecular Medicine*, *5*, 254–266.

Cifu, D., Kreutzer, J., Kolakowsky-Hayner, S., Marwitz, J., & Englander, J. (2003). The relationship between therapy intensity and rehabilitative outcomes after traumatic brain injury: A multicenter analysis. *Archives of Physical Medicine & Rehabilitation*, *84*, 1441–1448.

Clausen, T., & Bullock, T. (2001). Medical treatment and neuroprotection in traumatic brain injury. *Current Pharmaceutical Design*, *7*, 1517–1532.

Cooper, J. (1996). Actin is a PKC, anchoring protein: Role of this cytoskeletal signaling complex in actin organization, PKC, activation, and intracellular membrane trafficking. *Master's thesis*. East Carolina University Department of Biology, Greenville, NC, USA.

Cooper, E., Bunch, W., & Campa, J. (1973). Effects of chronic human neuromuscular stimulation. *Surgical Forum*, *24*, 477–479.

Cooper, E., & Cooper, J. (2003). Electrical treatment of coma via the median nerve. *Acta Neurochirurgica Supplement*, *87*, 7–10.

Cooper, E., & Cooper, J. (in press). Electrical treatment of comatose teenagers via the median nerve.

Cooper, E., Cooper, J., Alves, W., & Jane, J. (1996). Right median nerve electrical stimulation of comatose patients. *The Society for Treatment of Coma*, unpublished lecture.

Cooper, E., Han, D., & McElhaney, J. (1988). A voice controlled computer system for restoring limited hand functions in quadriplegics. *Proceedings of the American Input Output Systems Applications Conference*, San Francisco, CA.

Cooper, J., Jane, J., Alves, W., & Cooper, E. (1999). Right median nerve electrical stimulation to hasten awakening from coma. *Brain Injury*, *13*, 261–267.

Cooper, E., & Kanno, T. (in press). Electrical treatment of coma.

Critchley, H. D., Mathias, C. J., Josephs, O, O'Doherty, J., Zanini, S., Dewar, B. K., Cipolotti, L., Shallice, T., & Dolan, R. J. (2003). Human cingulate cortex and autonomic control: Converging neuroimaging and clinical relevance. *Brain, 126,* 2139–2152.

Davey, M. (2004). personal communication and patient's website: http://www.saratogahigh. org/shs/departments/staffpages/kabe/kathleenupdate.htm

Doraiswamy, M. (2003). Alzheimer's disease and the glutamate NMDA receptor. *Psychopharmacology Bulletin, 37,* 41–49.

Dringenberg, H. C., & Olmstead, M. C. (2003). Integrated contributions of basal forebrain and thalamus to neocortical activation elicited by pedunculopontine tegmental stimulation in urethane-anesthetized rats. *Neuroscience, 119,* 839–853.

Eisenberg, H., Gary, H., Aldrich, E., Saydjari, C., Turner, B., Foulkes, M., et al. (1990). Initial CT findings in 753 patients with severe head injury. NIH Traumatic Coma Data Bank Report. *Journal of Neurosurgery, 73,* 688–698.

Ezrokhi, V. L., Zosimovskii, V. A., Korshunov, V. A., & Markevich, V. A. (1999). Restoration of decaying long-term potentiation in the hippocampal formation by stimulation of neuromodulatory nuclei in freely moving rats. *Neuroscience, 88,* 741–753.

Faden, A. I. (1996). Pharmacological treatment of central nervous system trauma. *Pharmacology and Toxicology, 78,* 12–17.

Gersh, M. R. (1992). Neuromuscular electrical stimulation in rehabilitation. In S. L. Wolf (Ed.), *Electrotherapy in rehabilitation* (p. 260). Philadelphia, PA: Davis Co.

Gobbo, O. L., & O'Mara, S. M. (2004). Impact of enriched-environment housing on brain-derived neurotrophic factor and on cognitive performance after a transient global ischemia. *Behavioural Brain Research, 152,* 231–241.

Greenamyre, J. T., Maragos, W. F., Albin, R. L., Penney, J. B., & Young, A. B. (1988). Glutamate transmission and toxicity in Alzheimer's disease. *Progress in Neuro-Psychopharmacology & Biological Psychiatry, 12,* 421–430.

Hayashi, N. (1997). Prevention of vegetation after severe head trauma and stroke by combination therapy of cerebral hypothermia and activation of immune-dopaminergic nervous system. *Society for Treatment of Coma, 6,* 133–147.

Ho, G. J., Hansen, L. A., Alford, M. F., Foster, K., Salmon, D. P., Galasko, D. et al., (2002). Age at onset is associated with disease severity in Lewy body variant and Alzheimer's disease. *Neuroreport, 13,* 1825–1828.

Hynd, M. R., Scott, H. L., & Dodd, P. R. (2004). Glutamate-mediated excitotoxicity and neurodegeneration in Alzheimer's disease. *Neurochemistry International, 45,* 583–595.

Kampfl, A., Schmutzhard, E., Franz, G., Pfausier, B., Haring, H. P., Ulmer, H., Felber, S., Golaszewski, S., & Alchner, F. (1998). Prediction of recovery from post-traumatic vegetative state with cerebral magnetic-resonance imaging. *Lancet, 351,* 1763–1767.

Kanno, T. (1995). *Dorsal column stimulation for the persistent vegetative state.* University of Virginia neurosurgery lecture, unpublished.

Kanno, T. (2000). Development of surgical neurorehabilitation. *Society for Treatment of Coma, 9,* 23–24.

Kanno, T., Kamei, Y., & Yokoyama, T. (1989). Effects of dorsal spinal cord stimulation (DCS) on reversibility of neuronal function—experience of treatment for vegetative states. *Pace, 12,* 733–738.

Kanno, T., Kamei, Y., & Yokoyama, T. (1992). Treating the vegetative state with dorsal column stimulation. *Society for Treatment of Coma, 1,* 67–75.

Kapur, N., Barker, S., Burrows, E. H., Ellison, D., Brice, J., Illis, L. S., Scholey, K., Colbourn, C., Wilson, B., & Loates, M. (1994). Herpes simplex encephalitis: Long term magnetic resonance imaging and neuropsychological profile. *Journal of Neurology, Neurosurgery & Psychiatry, 57,* 1334–1342.

Kayama, Y., & Koyama, Y. (1998). Brainstem neural mechanisms of sleep and wakefulness. *European Urology, 33,* 12–15.

Kido, D., Cox, C., Hamill, R., Rothenberg, B., & Woolf, P. (1992). Traumatic brain injuries: Predictive usefulness of CT. *Radiology, 182,* 777–781.

Klintsova, A. Y., & Greenough, W. T. (1999). Synaptic plasticity in cortical systems. *Current Opinions in Neurobiology, 9,* 203–208.

Kokaia, Z., Othberg, A., Kokaia, M., & Lindvall, O. (1994). BDNF makes cultured dentate granule cells more resistant to hypoglycaemic damage. *Neuroreport, 5,* 1241–1244.

Kwan, C. L., Crawley, A. P., Mikulis, D. J., & Davis, K. D. (2000). An fMRI study of the anterior cingulate cortex and surrounding medial wall activations evoked by noxious cutaneous heat and cold stimuli. *Pain, 85,* 359–374.

Le Bars, P. L., Velasco, F. M., Ferguson, J. M., Dessain, E. C., Kieser, M., & Hoerr, R. (2002). Influence of the severity of cognitive impairment on the effect of the Ginkgo biloba extract EGb 761 in Alzheimer's disease. *Neuropsychobiology, 45,* 19–26.

Legoratti-Sanchez, M. O., Guevara-Guzman, R., & Solano-Flores, L. P. (1989). Electrophysiological evidences of bidirectional communication between the locus coeruleus and the suprachiasmatic nucleus. *Brain Research Bulletin, 23,* 283–288.

Liu, J. T., Wang, C. H., Chou, I. C., Sun, S. S., Koa, C. H., & Cooper, E. (2003). Regaining consciousness for prolonged comatose patients with right median nerve stimulation. *Acta Neurochir Suppl, 87,* 11–14.

Luijpen, M. W., Scherder, E. J. A., Van Someren, E. J. W., Swaab, D. F., & Sergeant, J. A. (2003). Non-pharmacological interventions in cognitively impaired and demented patients—a comparison with cholinesterase inhibitors. *Reviews in the Neurosciences, 14,* 343–368.

Marshall, L., Marshall, S., Klauber, M., Eisenberg, H., & Jane, J. (1991). A new classification of head injury based on computerized tomography. *Journal of Neurosurgery, 75,* S14–S20.

Marshall, F., & Marshall, S. (1996). Outcome prediction in severe head injury. In R. Wilkins & S., Rengachary, (Eds.), *Neurosurgery* (pp. 2717–2722). New York: McGraw-Hill.

Montgomery, G. (1989). The mind in motion. *Discover, 10,* 58–68.

Moriya, T., Hayashi, N., Sakurai, A., Utagawa, A., Kobayashi, Y., Yajima, K. et al. (2000). Usefulness of median nerve stimulation in patients with severe traumatic brain injury determined on the basis of changes in cerebrospinal fluid dopamine. *Society for Treatment of Coma, 9,* 159–161.

Moriya, T., Hayashi, N., Utagawa, A. et al. (1999). Median nerve stimulation method for severe brain damage, with its clinical improvement. *Society for Treatment of Coma, 8,* 111–114.

Okuma, I., Kaitou, T., Hayashi, J., Funahashi, M., & Kanno, T. (2001). Electrical stimulation therapy for prolonged consciousness disturbance. *Society for Treatment of Coma, 10,* 67–71.

Parent, A. (1996). Spinal cords: Fiber tracts; Medulla. In P. Coryell, L. Napora, & R. Adin (Eds.), *Carpenter's human neuroanatomy* (pp. 381–383, 435). Baltimore, MD: Williams & Wilkins.

Peri, C., Shaffrey, M., Farace, E., Cooper, E., Cooper, J., & Jane, J. (2001). Pilot study of electrical stimulation on median nerve in comatose severe brain injured patients 3-months outcome. *Brain Injury, 15,* 903–910.

Salehi, A., & Swaab, D. F. (1999). Diminished neuronal metabolic activity in Alzheimer's disease. *Journal of Neural Transmission, 106,* 955–986.

Sauvage, M., & Steckler, T. (2001). Detection of corticotrophin-releasing hormone receptor 1 immunoreactivity in cholinergic, dopaminergic and noradrenergic neurons of the murine basal forebrain and brainstem nuclei—potential implication for arousal and attention. *Neuroscience, 104,* 643–652.

Scheltens, P. H., Leys, D., Barkhof, F., Huglo, D., Weinstein, H. C., Vermersch, P., Kuiper, M., Steinling, M., Wolters E. C. H., & Valk, J. (1992). Atrophy of medial temporal lobes on MRI in 'probable' Alzheimer's disease and normal ageing: Diagnostic value and neuropsychological correlates. *Journal of Neurology, Neurosurgery & Psychiatry, 55,* 967–972.

Scherder, E. J. A. (1996). Transcutaneous electrical nerve stimulation in severe viral encephalitis. A case study. *Children's Hospital Quarterly, 8*(4), 187–191.

Scherder, E. J. A., & Bouma, A. (1999). Effects of transcutaneous electrical nerve stimulation on memory and behaviour may be stage-dependent. *Biological Psychiatry, 45*, 743–749.

Scherder, E. J. A., Bouma, A., & Steen, L. (1992). Influence of transcutaneous electrical nerve stimulation on memory in patients with dementia of the Alzheimer type. *Journal of Clinical & Experimental Neuropsychology, 14*, 951–960.

Scherder, E. J. A., Bouma, A., & Steen, A. M. (1995). Effects of short-term transcutaneous electrical nerve stimulation on memory and affective behaviour in patients with probable Alzheimer's disease. *Behavioural Brain Research, 67*, 211–219.

Scherder, E. J. A., Bouma, A., & Steen, A. M. (1998). Effects of 'isolated' transcutaneous electrical nerve stimulation on memory and affective behaviour in patients with probable Alzheimer's disease. *Biological Psychiatry, 43*, 417–424.

Scherder, E. J. A., Luijpen, M. W., & van Dijk, K. R. A. (2003). Activation of the dorsal raphe nucleus and locus coeruleus by transcutaneous electrical nerve stimulation in Alzheimer's disease: A reconsideration of stimulation-parameters derived from animal studies. *Chinese Journal of Physiology, 46*, 143–150.

Scherder, E. J. A., Van Deursen, S., Van Manen, S. R., Ferenschild, K., Simis, R., & Vuijk, P. J. (2001). Effects of TENS and methylphenidate in tuberculous meningo-encephalitis. *Brain Injury, 15*, 545–558.

Scherder, E. J. A., & Van Someren, E. J. W. (2004). *Effects of right median nerve stimulation on memory in Alzheimer's disease. A randomized controlled intervention study.* Manuscript submitted for publication.

Scherder, E. J. A., Van Someren, E. J. W., & Swaab, D. F. (1999). Transcutaneous electrical nerve stimulation (TENS) improves the rest-activity rhythm in midstage Alzheimer's disease. *Behavioural Brain Research, 101*, 105–107.

Shinotoh, H., Fukushi, K., Nagatsuka, S., Tanaka, N., Aotsuka, A., Ota, T., Namba, H., Tanada, S., & Irie, T. (2003). The amygdala and Alzheimer's disease: Positron emission tomography study of the cholinergic system. *Annals of the New York Academy of Sciences, 985*, 411–419.

Spiegel, J., Tintera, J., Gawehn, J., Stoeter, P., & Treede, R. (1999). Functional MRI of human primary somatosensory and motor cortex during median nerve stimulation. *Clinical Neurophysiology, 110*, 47–52.

Swaab, D. F. (2004). Neuropathology of the human hypothalamus and adjacent structures. Part 2. In M. J. Aminoss, S. Boller, & D. F. Swaab (Eds.), *Handbook of clinical neurology* (Vol. 80). Amsterdam: Elsevier Science.

Toutant, S., Klauber, M., Marshall, L., Toole, B., Bowers, S., Seeling, J. et al. (1984). Absent or compressed basal cisterns on first CT scan: Ominous predictors of outcome in severe head injury. *Journal of Neurosurgery, 61*, 691–694.

van Dijk, K. R. A., Scherder, E. J. A., Scheltens, P., & Sergeant, J. A. (2002). Effects of transcutaneous electrical nerve stimulation (TENS) on non-pain related cognitive and behavioural functioning. *Reviews in the Neurosciences, 13*, 257–270.

Van Someren, E. J. W., Scherder, E. J., & Swaab, D. F. (1998). Transcutaneous electrical nerve stimulation (TENS) improves circadian rhythm disturbances in Alzheimer disease. *Alzheimer's Disease & Associated Disorders, 12*, 114–118.

Yamamoto, K., Sugita, S., Ishikowa, K., Morimitsu, H., Shimamoto, H., & Shigemori, M. (1997). A case of persistent vegetative state treated with median nerve stimulation. *Society for Treatment of Coma, 6*, 117–121.

Yokoyama, T., Kamei, Y., & Kanno, T. (1996). Right median nerve stimulation for comatose patients. *Society for Treatment of Coma, 5*, 117–125.

NEUROPSYCHOLOGICAL REHABILITATION
2005, 15 (3/4), 406–413

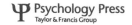

Deep brain stimulation therapy for the vegetative state

Takamitsu Yamamoto and Yoichi Katayama

Nihon University School of Medicine, Itabashi-ku, Japan

Twenty-one cases of a vegetative state (VS) caused by various kinds of brain damage were evaluated neurologically and electrophysiologically three months after brain injury. These cases were treated by deep brain stimulation (DBS) therapy, and followed up for over 10 years. The mesencephalic reticular formation was selected as a target in two cases, and the thalamic centre median-parafascicular (CM-pf) complex was selected as a target in the other 19 cases. Eight of the 21 patients emerged from the VS, and became able to obey verbal commands. However, they remained in a bedridden state except for one case. DBS therapy may be useful for allowing patients to emerge from a VS, if the candidates are selected according to appropriate neurophysiological criteria. A special neurorehabilitation system may be necessary for emergence from the bedridden state in the treatment of VS patients. Further, DBS therapy is expected to provide a useful method in minimally conscious state (MCS) patients to achieve consistent discernible behavioural evidence of consciousness, and emergence from the bedridden state.

INTRODUCTION

As a result of progress in emergency treatment, many patients who would have died previously now recover. Although many lives are saved, the number of patients in a vegetative state (VS) is increasing. The Multi-Society Task Force on PVS (1994a, 1994b) summarised the medical

*Correspondence should be addressed to: Takamitsu Yamamoto M.D., Ph.D., Department of Neurological Surgery and Division of Applied System Neuroscience, Nihon University School of Medicine, 30-1 Ohyaguchi Kamimachi, Itabashi-ku, Tokyo 173-8610, Japan. Fax: 81-3-3554-0425. Email: nusmyama@med.nihon-u.ac.jp

The present work was supported by grants from the Ministry of Science and Culture (Grant No. 12307029 and 15209047) and from the Ministry of Education, Culture, Sports, Science, and Technology for the promotion of the industry–university collaboration at Nihon University, Japan.

aspects of the VS. They provided a statement that the VS is a clinical condition of complete unawareness of the self and the environment, accompanied by sleep–wake cycles, with either complete or partial preservation of hypothalamic and brainstem autonomic function. In addition, patients in the VS show no evidence of sustained, reproducible, purposeful, or voluntary behavioural responses to visual, auditory, tactile, or noxious stimuli; show no evidence of language comprehension or expression; have bowel and bladder incontinence; and have variably preserved cranial nerve and spinal reflexes. On the other hand, the definition and diagnostic criteria of the minimally conscious state (MCS) were reported in 2002 (Giacino et al., 2002). The MCS is characterised by inconsistent but clearly discernible behavioural evidence of consciousness and can be distinguished from coma and the VS by documenting the presence of specific behavioural features that are not found in either of these latter conditions. Retrospectively, our cases were classified as VS and MCS according to the above statements.

However, there are various grades of severity and various stages leading to various outcomes, even if the patient displays neurological signs identical to the VS (Katayama et al., 1991; Tsubokawa et al., 1990a; Tsubokawa, Yamamoto, & Katayama, 1990b; Yamamoto et al., 2001, 2003). We evaluated patients in the VS by an electrophysiological approach, and compared the results of the examination with the long-term prognosis. As a result, we found that, even if the symptoms are similar from a neurological point of view, the degree of brain injury varies to a considerable degree. Also, there will be a considerable number of patients who may not be able to recover spontaneously, but who can be saved from the VS by means of appropriate treatment (Katayama et al., 1991; Tsubokawa et al., 1990a, 1990b; Yamamoto et al., 2001, 2003). We report the long-term follow-up results of deep brain stimulation (DBS) therapy in comparison with the findings of electrophysiological evaluations in VS patients. In addition, the long-term effects of DBS therapy for the MCS are assessed comparatively.

METHODS

Materials

Retrospectively, our cases were classified as VS (21 cases) and MCS (5 cases) according to the above statements on the VS and MCS. These cases were evaluated neurologically and electrophysiologically at 3 months after brain injury. They received DBS therapy mainly between 3 and 6 months after brain injury, and only one VS case received it at 8 months after brain injury. We followed up these cases for a period of over 10 years and examined their long-term functional recovery. The ages of the VS patients ranged from 19 to 75 years (mean = 44.0), and the cause of the initial coma were head injury (9 cases), cerebrovascular accident (9 cases), and anoxia (3 cases). The ages of the MCS patients ranged from 18 to 47 years (mean = 33.5), and the cause of the initial coma were head injury (3 cases) and cerebrovascular accident (2 cases).

Electrophysiological evaluations

The electrophysiological evaluations included assessments of the auditory brainstem response (ABR), somatosensory evoked potential (SEP), pain-related P250 and continuous electro-encephalogram (EEG) frequency analysis (Katayama et al., 1991; Tsubokawa et al., 1990b). The EEG was monitored continuously for at least 48 hours at the bedside, and also displayed as a compressed spectral array. We classified the continuous EEG frequency analysis into three types: (1) no desynchronisation pattern: changes of peak frequency were present only in the alpha and lower frequencies, and not in the higher frequencies; (2) slight desynchronisation pattern: desynchronisation was present but did not appear frequently; the duration was short, being under 10% of the time course, and the power of the high frequency was low; and (3) desynchronisation pattern: desynchronisation (a change to low amplitude and high frequency) appeared frequently, and the increase in the high frequency power was obvious at desynchronisation. The ABR recordings were classified into three patterns: (1) no response; (2) prolonged latency of the Vth wave; and (3) normal recordings. Prolonged latency of the Vth wave meant that the I–V wave latency was over two standard deviations longer than in normal cases. The SEP recordings, on the well-preserved side in cases where laterality was present, were classified into three patterns: (1) no N20; (2) prolonged N20; and (3) normal N20. Prolonged latency of N20 meant that the Erb-N20 latency was over two standard deviations longer than in normal cases recorded at our hospital. The pain-related P250 recordings were classified into three patterns: (1) no P250; (2) P250 recorded with under 7 μV; and (3) P250 recorded with over 7 μV.

Deep brain stimulation therapy

Chronic DBS was applied using a chronically implanted flexible wire electrode inserted by stereotactic surgery under local anaesthesia. As target points for the VS patients, the mesencephalic reticular formation (2 cases) and the CM-pf complex (19 cases) were selected, while the CM-pf complex (5 cases) was selected for the MCS patients. The features of the stimulation at the given targets were such that the patients presented strong arousal responses which were observed immediately at the start of stimulation. The patients opened their eyes with dilated pupils, the mouth sometimes also opened widely with meaningless vocalisations, and a slight increase in systemic blood pressure was observed during the stimulation. Moreover, some cases revealed slight movements of the extremities, and the EEG showed desynchronisation during the DBS stimulation. Stimulation was given every 2–3 hours during the daytime, and was continued for 30 min at one session. The frequency of the stimulation was mostly fixed at 25 Hz, and the intensity was decided according to the responses of each individual patient, being at slightly higher than the threshold for inducing an arousal response. To apply the chronic DBS, we employed a chronically implanted flexible electrode (3380, Medtronic Co.) and a transmitter-receiver system (3470 and 3425, Medtronic Co.). The target point in the mesencephalic reticular formation was the nucleus cuneiformis, which is located in the dorsal part of the nucleus ruber and ventral part of the deep layer of the superior colliculus. The CM-pf complex (P, 7–9; L, 5–6; H, 0–1) was selected as the stimulating point in the non-specific thalamic nucleus (see Figure 1).

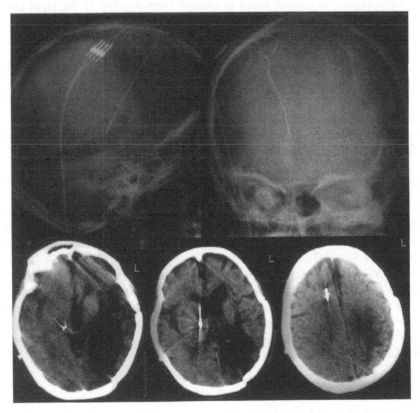

Figure 1. CM-pf complex stimulation therapy for VS. The skull X-P (upper) and axial CT scans (lower) indicate the location of the DBS electrode

RESULTS

Effects of DBS for the VS

The main feature of the present stimulation therapy was that the patients presented strong arousal responses as mentioned earlier, which were observed immediately at the start of stimulation. Although the intensity of the arousal responses differed in each case, such arousal responses were seen in all 21 cases and had no relation to emergence or non-emergence from the VS. We defined emergence from the VS as when the VS patient became able to obey our orders or to show an apparent yes by nodding. Eight of the 21 cases emerged from the VS, and could communicate with some speech or other responses, but needed some assistance with their everyday life in bed. Even after long-term rehabilitation, their state of being bedridden remained unchanged in seven of these eight cases. The other case became able to live in a wheelchair. The remaining 13 cases were unable to communicate at all and failed to emerge from the VS. In the eight cases that emerged from the VS following DBS therapy, the Vth wave of the ABR and N20 of the SEP were recorded even with a prolonged latency; continuous EEG frequency analysis demonstrated a desynchronisation pattern or slight desynchronisation pattern; and the pain-related P250 was recorded with an amplitude of over 7 μV. As regards the initial cause of the coma, the cases in whom treatment was effective had suffered brain damage through head injury or cerebrovascular accident, while the three cases of anoxia caused by cardiac arrest were among those in whom treatment was ineffective (Yamamoto et al., 2001, 2003).

Survival period after DBS

A total period of over 10 years follow-up has passed for all 21 DBS cases together, with 4 cases surviving for over 10 years. The survival rate among the 21 cases after the DBS therapy was: 21 cases (100%) at 1 year; 16 cases (76%) at 2 years; 12 cases (57%) at 3 years; 10 cases (48%) at 4 years; 6 cases (29%) at 5 years; 5 cases (24%) at 6 years; 5 cases (24%) at 7 years; 5 cases (24%) at 8 years; 5 cases (24%) at 9 years; and 4 cases (19%) at 10 years. The difference in survival period between the group which recovered ($n = 8$) and the non-recovering group ($n = 13$) was significant ($p < .05$) at over approximately 6 years survival. The causes of death were: infectious disease ($n = 15$), ileus ($n = 1$), and cancer ($n = 1$) (Yamamoto et al., 2003).

Effect of DBS for the MCS

All of the 5 cases of MCS displayed inconsistent behavioural evidence of consciousness before DBS therapy, and they became able to communicate with definite behavioural responses after the DBS. Four cases emerged from the bedridden state, and were able to enjoy life in their own home. The other case still remained in a bedridden state. Electrophysiological evaluations of these 5 cases revealed the following: the Vth wave of the ABR and N20 of the SEP were recorded even with a prolonged latency; continuous EEG frequency analysis demonstrated a desynchronisation pattern; and the pain-related P250 was recorded with an amplitude of over 7 μV.

DISCUSSION

Selection of the stimulation point

DBS can be effective for achieving emergence from the VS, and an assessment of the possibility of recovery can be made before application of the treatment by checking the patient's neurological status and undertaking electrophysiological evaluations at three months after the initial insult. DBS applied to the mesencephalic reticular formation or CM-pf complex can exert a strong arousal response and elicit marked increases in regional cerebral blood flow and regional cerebral metabolic rate of oxygen (Tsubokawa et al., 1990a,b). In the VS, cerebrocortical functions are more disturbed than brainstem functions, and the relationship between the brainstem and cerebral cortex is important for maintaining consciousness. On this basis, we mainly selected the CM-pf complex for DBS therapy. Electrical stimulation of the CM-pf complex is known to induce incremental recruiting and an augmentory response of the EEG with low-frequency stimulation, and EEG desynchronisation with high-frequency stimulation (Dempsey & Morison, 1942; Jasper, 1955). Luthi and McCormick (1998) have pointed out the importance of the low-threshold calcium spike and H-current in the waxing and waning of the EEG induced by CM-pf complex stimulation.

The DBS therapy for the VS was not sufficiently effective to allow all cases to emerge from the VS. We stress that chronic DBS therapy may be useful for enabling patients to emerge from the VS, if the candidates are selected according to appropriate electrophysiological criteria. These criteria meant that the Vth wave of the ABR and N20 of the SEP were recorded even with a prolonged latency; continuous EEG frequency analysis demonstrated a desynchronisation pattern; or slight desynchronisation pattern; and the pain-related P250 was recorded with an amplitude of over 7 μV. The eight cases that did emerge from the VS were all in a bedridden state for a long period of time, and only one patient recovered sufficiently to live in a wheelchair. In addition to the DBS therapy, we consider that not only the usual rehabilitation care such as physiotherapy but also a special neurorehabilitation programme may be necessary for the treatment of patients in VS.

Selection of the stimulation method

We have usually applied chronic spinal cord stimulation (SCS) for treatment of the MCS and not of the VS. For spinal cord stimulation, PISCES or Quad electrodes (Medtronic Co.) were inserted into the spinal epidural space under fluoroscopy, and stimulation was applied to the upper cervical spinal region. The frequency of stimulation was 5–25 Hz. The stimulation was applied with the minimum stimulation intensity that produced motor responses, and the frequency was selected to induce a motor twitch in each case.

In fact, we have applied DBS for treatment of the MCS in only five cases. In comparison with the VS patients, the MCS patients showed remarkable functional recovery, emerged from the bedridden state, became able to speak correctly, and to enjoy life in their own home. Clinical application of DBS therapy for the MCS is expected to accelerate recovery from this state. In our experience, SCS is also effective for MCS patients. However, there are several points of difference between DBS of the CM-pf complex and SCS. Stimulation of the CM-pf complex can induce a strong arousal response immediately after the start of stimulation; however, SCS cannot induce such a strong arousal response. In neural activation studies employing near infrared spectroscopy (NIRS), stimulation of the CM-pf complex has been shown to elicit marked and long-lasting increases in total haemoglobin and oxy-haemoglobin at the cerebral cortex as compared to SCS.

Time period after the onset of brain injury

We have in practice classified patients into the VS or MCS three months after the onset of brain injury, since most of the spontaneous recovery occurs within the first three months. When we assess the effects of each of the treatments, the most important factor is the time period from the onset of brain injury. The VS diagnosed at one month, three months, or six months after the onset of brain injury constitutes a set of quite different states, and quite different long-term follow-up results tend to be observed. We should therefore stress the time period after the onset of brain injury, when we discuss the long-term follow-up results. We can employ DBS and SCS for treatment of the VS and MCS, and the indications should be considered in the light of neurological and electrophysiological examinations. Not only the classification of the neurological state such as VS or MCS, but also the time period after the onset of brain injury need be taken into account in the treatment of such patients.

REFERENCES

Dempsey, E. W. A., & Morison, R. S. (1942). A study of thalamocortical relation. *American Journal of Physiology, 135,* 291–292.

Giacino, J. T., Ashwal, S., Childs, N., Cranford, R., Jennett, B., Katz, D. I. et al. (2002). The minimally conscious state: Definition and diagnostic criteria. *Neurology, 58*, 349–353.

Jasper, H. H., Naquet, R., & King, L. E. (1955). Thalamocortical recruiting responses in sensory receiving areas in the cat. *Electroencephalography and Clinical Neurophysiology, 7*, 99–114.

Katayama, Y., Tsubokawa, T., Yamamoto, T., Hirayama, T., Miyazaki, S., & Koyama, S. (1991). Characterization and modification of brain activity with deep brain stimulation in a persistent vegetative state. *Pacing and Clinical Electrophysiology, 14*, 116–121.

Luthi A., & McCormick, D. A. (1998). H-current: Properties of a neuronal and network pacemaker. *Neuron, 21*, 9–12.

Multi-Society Task Force on PVS (1994a). Medical aspects of the persistent vegetative state. (Part 1). *New England Journal of Medicine, 330*, 1499–1508.

Multi-Society Task Force on PVS (1994b). Medical aspects of the persistent vegetative state. (Part 2). *New England Journal of Medicine, 330*, 1572–1579.

Tsubokawa, T., Yamamoto, Y., Katayama, Y., Hirayama, T., Maejima, S., & Moriya, T. (1990a). Deep brain stimulation in a persistent vegetative state: Follow-up results and criteria for selection of candidates. *Brain Injury, 4*, 315–327.

Tsubokawa, T., Yamamoto, Y., & Katayama, Y. (1990b). Prediction of the outcome of prolonged coma caused by brain damage. *Brain Injury, 4*, 329–337.

Yamamoto, T., Katayama, Y., Oshima, H., Fukaya, C., Kawamata, T., & Tsubokawa, T. (2001). Deep brain stimulation therapy for a persistent vegetative state. *Acta Neurochirurgica, 79*(Suppl), 79–82.

Yamamoto, T., Katayama, Y., Kobayashi, K., Kasai, M., Oshima, H., & Fukaya, C. (2003). DBS therapy for a persistent vegetative state: Ten years follow-up results. *Acta Neurochirurgica, 87*(Suppl), 15–18.

NEUROPSYCHOLOGICAL REHABILITATION
2005, 15 (3/4), 414–427

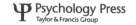

Levodopa treatment for patients in persistent vegetative or minimally conscious states

Wakoto Matsuda[1], Yoji Komatsu[2], Kiyoyuki Yanaka[3], and Akira Matsumura[3]

[1]*Graduate School of Medicine, University of Kyoto, Kyoto, Japan;*
[2]*Tsukuba Medical Centre Hospital, Ibaraki, Japan;*
[3]*Institute of Clinical Medicine, Ibaraki, Japan*

The persistent vegetative state (PVS) and the minimally conscious state (MCS) are conditions of altered consciousness after severe brain damage due to a variety of pathologies. However, the specific pathophysiological mechanisms and a therapeutic strategy for intervention have not as yet been established. We review previous reports of levodopa treatment for patients in PVS, MCS, or other mental disorders, and have focused on five representative cases: four of PVS and one of MCS after severe brain injury. In summary, our review suggests the effectiveness of levodopa treatment is probably dependent upon the following criteria: (1) Diagnosis of PVS or MCS as distinct from other related conditions, (2) Concomitant symptoms of parkinsonism, and (3) Concomitant neuroradiological findings of high intensity lesions in the dopaminergic pathway on T2 weighted MRI.

The apparent success of levodopa in the five cases described may reflect a specific subgroup of PVS and MCS patients, where the administration of levodopa is effective. However, we should not regard PVS or MCS as a single entity, since levodopa is unlikely to be effective in all cases. Therapeutic strategies should aim to identify the key pathophysiological mechanism for each patient and target interventions accordingly.

Correspondence should be sent to Dr Wakoto Matsuda, Department of Morphological Brain Science, Graduate School of Medicine, University of Kyoto, Konoe-cho, Yoshida, Sakyo-ku, Kyoto, 606-8501, Japan. Tel: +81-75-753-4331, Fax: +81-75-753-4340. Email: wako@mua.biglobe.ne.jp

The authors are very grateful for the support and valuable comment of Dr Tatsuya Koeda.

INTRODUCTION

Persistent vegetative state (PVS) is a condition of patients with severe brain damage in whom coma has progressed to a state of wakefulness without detectable awareness. In this state, there is an absence of any adaptive response to the external environment, and an absence of any evidence of a functioning mind, which is either receiving or projecting information (Jennett & Plum, 1972; Zeman, 1997). In contrast, the minimally conscious state (MCS) is characterised by inconsistent, but clearly discernible behavioural evidence of awareness (Giacino et al., 2002). Although recent neuropathological and neuroradiological studies have revealed common structural abnormalities including diffuse axonal injury (DAI) and damage to the dorsolateral aspect of the rostral brainstem and the thalamus (Adams, Graham, & Jennett, 2000; Kampfl et al., 1998a; Uzan ct al., 2003), thc complctc pathophysiology of PVS and MCS remains unclear. Consequently, a defined therapeutic strategy has yet to be established. In this article, we review published case reports of PVS and MCS patients who underwent dopaminergic treatment, summarise the clinical characteristics of the patients in whom levodopa treatment was effective, and discuss the criteria for and best application of this treatment.

DOPAMINERGIC TREATMENT FOR UNCONSCIOUS PATIENTS

There are reports of recovery from PVS, MCS and other mental disorders with the administration of levodopa and/or other dopaminergic agents (such as amantadine, bromocriptine) in post-encephalitic disease (Sacks, Kohl, Messeloff, & Schwartz, 1972), hepatic coma (Abramsky & Goldschmidt, 1974; Fisher & Baldessarini, 1971; Parkes, Sharpstone, & Williams, 1970), post-operative akinetic mutism (Ross & Stewart, 1981), degenerative disease (Horiguchi, Inami, & Shoda, 1990), and severe brain injury (Fukushima et al., 1972; Higashi et al., 1977; Koeda & Takeshita, 1998; Kraus & Maki, 1997a,b; Lal, Merbtiz, & Grip, 1988; Haig & Ruess, 1990; Matsuda et al., 2003; van Woerkom, Minderhoud, Gottschal, & Nicolai, 1982; Zafonte, Watanabe, & Mann, 1998; Passler & Riggs, 2001).

However, in these previous reports, the terms "vegetative" or "minimally conscious" were not always applied according to the widely accepted criteria in the report of the Multi-Society Task Force on PVS (1994) and more recently the guidelines of the Royal College of Physicians (1996, 2003). Hence, the therapeutic benefit from dopaminergic treatment has been considered equivocal.

CLINICAL, NEURORADIOLOGICAL, AND
ELECTROPHYSIOLOGICAL CHARACTERISTICS

In this review, the term persistent vegetative state (PVS) refers to vegetative state that has continued for four weeks or more. Among the previous reports, we selected four cases classified as PVS and one case of MCS, according to the recent international criteria (Giacino et al., 2002; Royal College of Physicians, 2003). These cases were treated with levodopa after severe brain injury, and all showed rapid recovery from PVS or MCS. The term "recovery" used here was defined as the emergence from PVS or MCS and the patient's ability to communicate or use objects functionally, which refers to a remarkable improvement of motor disturbances and the ability to obey simple verbal commands correctly (see below). Moreover, the emergence from MCS is based on functional interactive communication and/or use of two different objects (Giacino et al., 2002). The clinical characteristics and neuroradiological data relating to these patients are summarised in Table 1.

Clinical and neurological features

Clinical course and diagnosis.   All the cases in Table 1 suffered a closed head injury in a traffic accident. They were comatose on arrival (Glasgow Coma Scale, GCS, score 3–6). Computed tomography (CT) revealed evidence of cerebral bleeds across the five cases. Cases 2, 3 and 4 underwent haematoma evacuation and decompression craniotomy on admission. Four of the five cases (cases 1, 3, 4, and 5) remained unresponsive to simple verbal commands at the start of the investigation. Only case 2 recognised family members, and responded to her name; however, she was unable to speak or move. The physical conditions of these patients were good in general, but they were bedridden and their condition remained unchanged for 3–22 months. Four of the five cases (cases 1, 3, 4, and 5) were diagnosed PVS, and one (case 2) was likely MCS.

Underlying parkinsonism and response to levodopa.   Further neurological examination revealed post-traumatic parkinsonian features (tremor, rigidity, or akinesia) in all these cases. In particular, rigidity/spasticity and akinesia were observed in all these patients. In three of the five cases (cases 3, 4, and 5), the parkinsonian symptoms were predominantly in unilateral extremities.

After the start of levodopa treatment, these symptoms were reduced and all cases displayed rapid recovery from PVS or MCS in 4 days–1.5 months. In case 1, five days after the start of the levodopa treatment, the patient said his mother's name. A few days after this, he lifted an object, wiped his face and pointed to an object on command. After several months, he showed continued

TABLE 1

Clinical characteristics, neuroradiological findings, and levodopa treatment of five representative cases

Case	Author	Age/sex	Origin	GCS	Diagnosis/chronic state	Duration of PVS/MCS	OR Tremour	Rigidity	Akinesia	Predominant extremities of symptoms	CT/MRI findings	Medication/starting dose (mg/day)	Recovery after the start of treatment	EEG after treatment	Continuance of treatment
1	Haig & Ruess, 1990	24/M	TA	3?	CTN, IFT, PVS	6 months	–	+? (Spasticity)	+	?	thalamus, temporal lobe	LD/CD, 100/10*2	5 days	?	D
2	Koeda & Takeshita, 1998	7/F	TA	4	DAI, t-ICH, CTN, MCS	22 months +[#]	+	+	+	bil.	bil. CP, bil. PL, CC, parietal lobe	LD, 50*1 (2 mg/kg)	1.5 months	Undone	D+C (restarted)
3	Matsuda et al., 1999, 2003	14/M	TA	4	DAI, lt.SDH, PVS	3 months	+	+	+	lt.	lt. DLM	LD/BZ, 100/25*2	20 days	Improved[#]	D
4	Matsuda et al., 1999, 2003	27/M	TA	4	DAI, rt.EDH, PVS	12 months	+	–	+	rt.	rt. CP, lt. DLM	LD, 450 LD/BZ, 100/25*3	25 days	Improved[#]	C
5	Matsuda et al., 1999, 2003	51/M	TA	6	DAI, t-SAH, PVS	7 months	–	–	+	rt.	rt. CP, lt. DLM (disappeared)[#]	LD/CD, 100/10*3	4 days	Improved	C

bil = bilateral; BZ = benserazide; C = continuance; CC = corpus callosum; CD = carbidopa; CP = cerebral peduncle; CTN = contusion; D = discontinuance; DAI = diffuse axonal injury; DLM = dorsolateral midbrain; EDH = epidural hematoma; GCS = Glasgow Coma Scale; IFT = infarction; LD = levodopa; lt = left; MCS = minimally conscious state; OR = operation; PL = pallidum; PVS = persistent vegetative state; rt = right; TA = traffic accident; t-ICH = traumatic intracerebral hemorrhage; t-SAH = traumatic subarachnoid hemorrhage; y = years; # = 'unpublished data' physical and cognitive progress. He propelled a manual wheelchair, and was independent in shaving, face washing, feeding, and use of urinal. He obtained equivalent vocabulary skills to age 10, and lived at home with family (Haig & Ruess, 1990). In case 2, about one and a half months after starting of the treatment, rigidity gradually decreased. The patient could maintain a sitting position for five minutes and roll over by herself without any help. As a result, she became able to write almost all Japanese characters and communicate by writing letters (Koeda & Takeshita, 1998). In case 3, 20 days after the start of treatment, rigidity/spasticity was reduced and the patient was able to obey simple verbal commands. Three months after the start of the treatment, he was able to walk while supporting himself with parallel bars, and had obtained the equivalent intelligence of an elementary school child. One year after the trauma, he was able to walk to high school by himself. In case 4, 25 days after the start of treatment, the levodopa prescription was changed to levodopa/benserazide. After this, the patient gradually began to respond to his family and the nurses by blinking his eyes. He improved enough to be able to express yes/no, and thereafter by operating a simple electronic signal with his hand. Ten months after the start of the treatment, he began to use a word processor to express his thoughts. In case 5, four days after starting treatment, akinesia and rigidity were reduced and the patient was able to obey simple verbal commands. Two months after starting treatment, he was able to say his name and address correctly (Matsuda et al., 2003).

These rapid ameliorations following levodopa treatment seem to be significant. Additionally, in underlying parkinsonian symptoms, the right/left predominant symptomatic patterns in some cases may be valuable findings for the evaluation of akinesia, rigidity/spasticity in the differentiation from contractures due to long-term disuse of extremities.

Neuroradiological features

Predicting factors for recovery.   In four of the five cases (cases 2, 3, 4, and 5), magnetic resonance imaging (MRI) revealed diffuse axonal injury (DAI) involving the cerebral peduncle, dorsolateral midbrain, pallidum, or corpus callosum (Table 1 and Figure 1). In previous reports, recovery from brainstem injury has been shown to be closely dependent on the extent of the injury (Kampfl et al., 1998b; Matsumura et al., 1993; Shibata, Matsumura, Meguro, & Narushima, 2000). Consequently, high intensity lesions on T2 weighted MRI of the cerebral peduncle or dorsolateral midbrain are highly significant predictors of non-recovery (Kampfl et al., 1998b). Similarly, unilateral abnormalities in the brainstem are considered to be a prospective sign for good recovery, and bilateral brainstem damage a sign for poor recovery, even in cases with similar initial GCS scores (Matsumura et al., 1993).

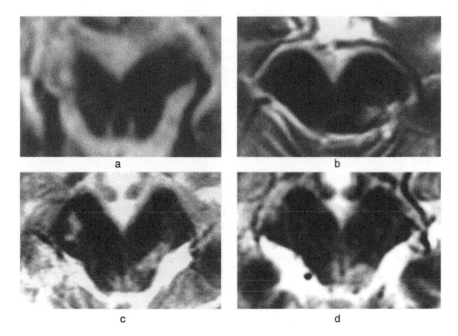

Figure 1. (a) High intensity lesions in the right cerebral peduncle on T2 weighted magnetic resonance imaging in case 2. (b) High intensity lesions in the dorsolateral midbrain in case 3. (c) High intensity lesions in the right cerebral peduncle and the left dorsolateral midbrain in case 4. (d) High intensity lesions in the right cerebral peduncle and the left dorsolateral midbrain in case 5. (Figure 1a: *Brain Development, 20* (1998) 124–126; Figure 1b, c, d: *Journal of Neurology, Neurosurgery, and Psychiatry,* 74 (2003) 1571–1573. Adapted and reproduced with permission from Elsevier Science and BMJ Publishing Group, respectively.)

Other reports have suggested that deep dorsal injuries in the brainstem tend to be associated with a poor prognosis (Shibata et al., 2000). It has also been suggested that the response to dopaminergic drugs is less predictable in patients with DAI (Jankovic, 1994). Hence, the MRI findings in four of the cases detailed here, predicted the patients would actually have a poor response to levodopa, but they showed rapid remarkable improvement. The recovery of these cases implies a significant efficacy of levodopa treatment, at least in certain cases (Koeda & Takeshita, 1998; Yoshikawa, Oda, & Koeda, 1999; Matsuda et al., 2003).

Pathophysiological signs on MRI findings.   Cases 3, 4, and 5 exhibited high intensity lesions in the dorsolateral midbrain on T2 weighted MRI. Cases 2, 4, and 5 exhibited high intensity lesions in the cerebral peduncle, which might involve the substantia nigra or ventral tegmental area. These MRI findings implied that their midbrains might have been injured by direct "tentorial compression" (Jellinger et al., 2004) and have caused *contra coup* injuries, rather than those of Kernohan notch (Evans, Gacinovic, Costa, & Lees, 2004) because of the anatomical distribution of the lesions. These injuries might be induced by translatory or rotatory acceleration when the cranium was struck at a point along its sagittal axis, or by posterolateral damage (Jellinger et al., 2004).

Correlations between parkinsonian symptoms and MRI findings. In the period of the high-definition CT and MRI era, there appear occasional reports documenting the relationship between post-traumatic parkinsonian symptoms and certain CT or MRI findings (Bhatt et al., 2000; Doder et al., 1999; Evans et al., 2004; Krauss et al., 1995; Nayernouri, 1985), and MRI findings of a patient with post-traumatic tremor without parkinsonism (Zijlmans et al., 2002). Among these previous reports, we selected nine cases which are summarised in Table 2. In all of the nine cases, tremor, rigidity, and/or akinesia were observed. Evidence of abnormal intensity (density) lesions in the substantia nigra, subpallidum, subthalamic nucleus, or striatum were also observed in these reports. In eight of the nine cases, the substantia nigra was implicated on imaging, whereas in two of the nine cases the striatum was implicated. In four of the six cases in which the treatments were described, the symptoms were responsive to dopaminergic agents.

Consequently, these reports may also support a correlation between parkinsonism and MRI findings.

Recommended timing of scanning. For the time being it is clear that MRI findings, particularly in the acute stage (within weeks or one month), are useful for evaluating primary brain damage, because high intensity lesions on the T2 weighted image detected in the acute stage occasionally disappear in just a few weeks (Matsumura et al., 1993). Indeed, high intensity lesions in the midbrain of case 5 had disappeared in two months (unpublished data), although those of cases 3 and 4 were still detected after three months (Matsuda et al., 2003). Thus, neuroradiological evaluation by MRI should be taken in the acute stage whenever possible.

Electrophysiological features

In the period before CT and MRI, the electroencephalogram (EEG) was considered a useful device to help evaluate the efficacy of levodopa treatment. In a small number of reports, the EEG delta or theta wave activity was found to be attenuated and replaced by an increase in alpha activity after the administration of levodopa. There are, however, few distinctive features in the EEG record that are able to predict the efficacy of levodopa before the start of the

TABLE 2

Correlations between post-traumatic parkinsonian symptoms and CT/MRI findings in the previous reports

Case	Author	Age/sex	Origin	Diagnosis	Tremour	Rigidity	Akinesia	CT/MRI findings	Dopaminergic treatment	Supplementation
1	Nayernouri, 1985	37/M	Hitting (violence)	DAI?	–	+	+	SN	Responsive (LD/CD)	
2	Krauss et al., 1995	23/M	?	DAI	+	?	?	SN	?	
3	Krauss et al., 1995	37/M	?	DAI	+	?	?	SN	?	
4	Doder et al., 1999	36/M	TA	?	+	+	+	Striatum	Unresponsive (LD/CD)	
5	Bhatt et al., 2000	46/M	TA	t-ICH	+	+	+	SN, striatum	Responsive (LD/CD)	
6	Bhatt et al., 2000	39/M	TA	DAI?	+	+	+	SN	Responsive (LD/CD)	
7	Bhatt et al., 2000	35/M	TA	CTN	– ?	+	+	SN, subpallidum	?	
8	Evans et al., 2004	27/M	Hitting (fall)	SDH	+	+	+	SN	Responsive (BCP, LD/CD)	Parkinsonism due to Kernohan notch
9	Zijlmans et al., 2002	19/M	TA	?	+	–	–	SN, STN	Unresponsive (LD/CD)	Not regarded as parkinsonism

BCP = Bromocriptine; CD = carbidopa; CTN = contusion; DAI = diffuse axonal injury; LD = levodopa; SN = substantia nigra; STN = subthalamic nucleus; TA = traffic accident; t-ICH = traumatic intracerebral hemorrhage; t-SAH = traumatic subarachnoid hemorrhage; y = years; # = 'unpublished data'

421

treatment (Abramsky & Goldschmidt, 1974; Higashi et al., 1977; Parkes et al., 1970).

In the five cases examined in this review, three showed improvement on EEG (cases 3, 4: unpublished data; case 5: Matsuda et al., 1999), but there were no distinctive findings compared with the above reports. Thus, conventional EEG findings cannot be utilised as predictors of recovery, but are useful for an evaluation of the effectiveness of treatment.

LEVODOPA AND OTHER DOPAMINERGIC TREATMENT

Selection of agent, dosage, and frequency of dosing

Levodopa treatment was recommended for relief of rigidity/spasticity in all the cases while the patients were in the chronic stage after severe brain injury (Table 1). The selected dopaminergic agents were levodopa (cases 2, 4), levodopa/carbidopa (cases 1, 5), and levodopa/benserazide (cases 3, 4). In the adult cases (Cases 1, 3, 4, and 5), the starting dose of levodopa was 450 mg a day; levodopa/carbidopa 100/10 mg two or three times a day; levodopa/benserazide 100/25 mg two or three times a day, respectively. In the pediatric case (case 2), levodopa was administered as 50 mg (2 mg/kg) a day. Dosages were increased step by step with close observation of clinical progress. These medications did not produce harmful side effects in any of the cases.

In general, levodopa is converted by an aromatic amino acid decarboxylase (AADC) to dopamine in the dopaminergic nerve terminals. However, because AADC also resides in peripheral tissues, a significant fraction of the levodopa decarboxylated into dopamine produces nausea and other untoward side effects (Nestler, Hyman, & Malenka, 2001). Thus, levodopa typically is better coadministered with an AADC inhibitor such as carbidopa or benserazide.

Drug dependence, decompensation, and withdrawal

One serious problem is that some patients with long-lasting PVS/MCS show dependence on levodopa or progressive decompensation in the course of levodopa treatment. In the cases of this review, one case (case 2) showed recovery from MCS and the levodopa treatment was discontinued, but it was restarted after one month because of the exacerbation of rigidity (unpublished data). However, not all of the patients require permanent medication. Recovery from PVS was observed in two cases (cases 1, 3) after several days of treatment and these effects were sustained even after the levodopa treatment was discontinued.

Indeed, some patients apparently only need levodopa as a trigger agent to interrupt the vicious cycle of exhaustion to neurotransmitters. However, deciding which cases fall into this category is very difficult at this point, and the withdrawal of levodopa involves other side effects and ethical problems in any event (Jellinger et al., 2004).

Other dopaminergic agents

In addition to levodopa treatment, there are other reports of treatment using dopaminergic agents such as amantadine, bromocriptine, and methylphenidate (Daly & Love, 1958; Horiguchi et al., 1990; Passler & Riggs, 2001; Ross & Stewart, 1981; Zafonte et al., 1998).

Amantadine acts both pre- and post-synaptically by increasing dopamine release into extracellular pools by blocking reuptake and by facilitating the synthesis of dopamine. Bromocriptine is a direct agonist of dopamine receptor, which acts post-synaptically. A patient with akinetic mutism after surgical removal of a tumour from the anterior hypothalamus involving the medial forebrain bundle responded to treatment with bromocriptine but not to levodopa/carbidopa or methylphenidate (Ross & Stewart, 1981). Methylphenidate is a nonspecific pre-synaptic catecholamine mimetic, which reverses the reticular activating system. Akinetic mutism after surgical removal of a fourth ventricular astrocytoma was reversed by methylphenidate (Daly & Love, 1958). In contrast, levodopa acts pre-synaptically as a precursor of dopamine and norepinephrine. In the six cases in Table 2 with post-traumatic parkinsonian symptoms, two (cases 4, 9) were unresponsive to levodopa treatment. In both cases, the dopaminergic pathways were damaged post-synaptically (in the striatum; case 4), or damaged in the subthalamic nucleus, which compensated for substantia nigra lesions, resulting in preventing the onset of a Parkinson syndrome (case 9).

It follows from these pharmacological considerations that efficacy of levodopa and neuroradiological findings in the five cases in Table 1 may imply incomplete (mosaic) damage in the pre-synaptic dopaminergic pathways such as the substantia nigra or the ventral tegmental area. Consequently, dopaminergic agents should be selected rationally depending upon anatomical structures and neurotransmitter systems of each individual.

CRITERIA FOR LEVODOPA TREATMENT AND ITS APPLICATION

Several observations in the foregoing review have suggested criteria for the probable effectiveness of levodopa treatment in patients after severe brain injury.

Criteria for recommendation of levodopa treatment

The main points for recommending levodopa treatment are:

1. A diagnosis of PVS or MCS, as distinct from other related conditions such as coma, brain death, and locked-in syndrome.

2. Concomitant symptoms of parkinsonism (particularly with unilateral predominant rigidity/spasticity and akinesia).

3. Concomitant neuroradiological findings of high intensity lesions in the dopaminergic pathway on T2 weighted MRI (particularly in the acute stage).

Application and withdrawal of levodopa treatment

With levodopa treatment, a coadministration of levodopa and an AADC inhibitor is recommended. Levodopa with AADC inhibitor should be started with a low dosage (e.g., levodopa/carbidopa 100/10 mg twice a day, or levodopa/benserazide 100/25 mg twice a day for adult patients). The dosage and frequency of dosing should be increased step by step under close observation of clinical progress, including the development of any side effects. When there are harmful side effects, or no efficacy observed for several months despite maximum dose, or no change of mental status, reduction or discontinuance of levodopa treatment should be considered, with particular care not to induce other side effects such as malignant syndrome.

Other dopaminergic agents

Even if the levodopa treatment is ineffective, other dopaminergic agents or the combined use of levodopa and these agents may be effective. In particular, damage to the pre-synaptic dopaminergic pathways and/or intact post-synaptic dopaminergic pathways, other dopaminergic agents which act post-synaptically (such as amantadine or bromocriptine) may be effective. Once again, selection of medication should depend upon the anatomical structures and neurotransmitter systems of the patients.

CLOSING REMARKS

The neuroradiological impairments and clinical characteristics in the five cases reviewed in Table 1 imply that the dopaminergic pathways were selectively damaged by DAI, probably due to tentorial compression. Injuries to these anatomical structures are known to cause defects in the nigrostriatal (A9), mesocortical, or mesolimbic systems (A10).

Neither parkinsonian symptoms nor brainstem lesions are typical of PVS or MCS patients in general. Moreover, levodopa is often ineffective for post-traumatic parkinsonism with DAI (Jankovic, 1994). Therefore, the successful cases examined in this review may reflect a specific subgroup of PVS or MCS patients. The causes of PVS or MCS include a variety of pathological triggers, such as traumatic brain injury, hypoxic damage, cerebrovascular injury, infection, toxins, poisoning, degenerative disease, tumours, and congenital or developmental disorders (Giacino et al., 2002; Multi-Society Task Force on PVS, 1994; Royal College of Physicians, 2003). Thus, the clinical concept of PVS or MCS makes each a "syndrome", and the terms "vegetative" or "minimally conscious" simply describe observed behaviour, without necessarily implying any specific pathology. Quite simply, these syndromes should not be considered to be unitary entities. When determining the best treatment for PVS or MCS patients, the anatomical and physiological mechanisms particular to each case are crucial (Kotchoubey, 2004; Matsuda, Komatsu, Yanaka, & Matsumura, 2004).

There may be some patients in any group of patients with PVS or MCS after severe brain injury in whom the dopaminergic pathways may have been selectively damaged. Similarly, other individuals with damage to other neural systems are to be found among PVS or MCS patients, and such individuals may respond to other treatment better suited to their particular condition.

In conclusion, it is important to recognise parkinsonian symptoms and minimal neuroradiological findings because such individuals may respond to levodopa or alternative treatment. These five cases illustrate how important it is to identify the key pathophysiological mechanism for each PVS or MCS patient and thus devise the most appropriate therapeutic strategy for them.

REFERENCES

Abramsky, O., & Goldschmidt, Z. (1974). Treatment and prevention of acute hepatic encephalopathy by intravenous levodopa. *Surgery, 75,* 188–193.

Adams, J. H., Graham, D. I., & Jennett, B. (2000). The neuropathology of the vegetative state after an acute brain insult. *Brain, 123,* 1327–1338.

Bhatt, M., Desai, J., Mankodi, A., Elias, M., & Wadia, N. (2000). Posttraumatic akinetic-rigid syndrome resembling Parkinson's disease: A report on three patients. *Movement Disorders, 15,* 313–317.

Daly, D. D., & Love, J. G. (1958). Akinetic mutism. *Neurology, 8,* 238–242.

Doder, M., Jahanshahi, M., Turjanski, N., Moseley, I. F., & Lees, A. J. (1999). Parkinson's syndrome after closed head injury: A single case report. *Journal of Neurology, Neurosurgery, and Psychiatry, 66,* 380–385.

Evans, A. H., Gacinovic, S., Costa, D. C., & Lees, A. J. (2004). Parkinsonism due to Kernohan notch: Clinical, structural, and functional imaging correlates. *Neurology, 62,* 2333–2334.

Fischer, J. E., & Baldessarini, R. J. (1971). False neurotransmitters and hepatic failure. *Lancet,* *2,* 75–80.

Fukushima, T., Uchiyama, S., Hori, T., Yoshimatsu, N., Ishijima, B., Manaka, S., Sekino, H., & Hirakawa, K. (1972). L-DOPA treatment in patients with consciousness and mental disturbances. *Brain and Nerve, 24,* 1673–1678 [in Japanese].

Giacino, J. T., Ashwal, S., Childs, N., Cranford, R., Jennett, B., Katz, D. I., Kelly, J. P., Rosenberg, J. H., Whyte, J., Zafonte, R. D., & Zasler, N. D. (2002). The minimally conscious state: Definition and diagnostic criteria. *Neurology, 58,* 349–353.

Haig, A. J., & Ruess, J. M. (1990). Recovery from vegetative state of six-months' duration associated with Sinemet (levodopa/carbidopa). *Archives of Physical Medicine and Rehabilitation, 71,* 1081–1083.

Higashi, K., Sakata, Y., Hatano, M., Abiko, S., Ihara, K., Katayama, S., Wakuta, Y., Okamura, T., Ueda. H., Zenke, M., & Aoki, H. (1977). Epidemiological studies on patients with a persistent vegetative state. *Journal of Neurology, Neurosurgery, and Psychiatry, 40,* 876–885.

Horiguchi, J., Inami, Y., & Shoda, T. (1990). Effects of long-term amantadine treatment on clinical symptoms and EEG of a patient in a vegetative state. *Clinical Neuropharmacology, 13,* 84–88.

Jankovic, J. (1994). Post-traumatic movement disorders: Central and peripheral mechanisms. *Neurology, 44,* 2006–2014.

Jellinger, K. A., Matsuda, W., Komatsu, Y., Matsumura, A., & Yanaka, K. (2004). Parkinsonism and persistent vegetative state after head injury. *Journal of Neurology, Neurosurgery, and Psychiatry, 75,* 1082–1083 [Corresponding letter and author's reply].

Jennett, B., & Plum, F. (1972). Persistent vegetative state after brain damage: A syndrome in search of a name. *Lancet, 1,* 734–737.

Kampfl, A., Franz, G., Aichner, F., Pfausler, B., Haring, H. P., Felber, S., Luz, G., Schocke, M., & Schmutzhard, E. (1998a). The persistent vegetative state after closed head injury: Clinical and magnetic resonance imaging findings in 42 patients. *Journal of Neurosurgery, 88,* 809–816.

Kampfl, A., Schmutzhard, E., Franz, G., Pfausler, B., Haring, H.-P., Ulmer, H., Felber, S., Golaszewski, S., & Aichner, F. (1998b). Prediction of recovery from post-traumatic vegetative state with cerebral magnetic-resonance imaging. *Lancet, 351,* 1763–1767.

Koeda, T., & Takeshita, K. (1998). A case report of remarkable improvement of motor disturbances with L-dopa in a patient with post-diffuse axonal injury. *Brain and Development, 20,* 124–126.

Kotchoubey, B. (2004). Persistent vegetative state: Should we generalize? *Journal of Neurology, Neurosurgery, and Psychiatry,* (http://jnnp.bmjjournals.com/cgi/eletters/74/11/1571#122). [Electronic letter, 21 April]

Kraus, M. F., & Maki, P. M. (1997a). Effect of amantadine hydrochloride on symptoms of frontal lobe dysfunction in brain injury: Case studies and review. *Journal of Neuropsychiatry and Clinical Neurosciences, 9,* 222–230.

Kraus, M. F., & Maki, P. (1997b). The combined use of amantadine and l-dopa/carbidopa in the treatment of chronic brain injury. *Brain Injury, 11,* 455–460.

Krauss, J. K., Wakhloo, A. K., Nobbe, F., Tränkle, R., Mundinger, F., & Seeger, W. (1995). Lesions of dentatothalamic pathways in severe post-traumatic tremor. *Neurological Research, 17,* 409–416.

Lal, S., Merbtiz, C. P., & Grip, J. C. (1988). Modification of function in head-injured patients with Sinemet. *Brain Injury, 2,* 225–233.

Matsuda, W., Komatsu, Y., Yanaka, K., & Matsumura, A. (2004). Persistent vegetative state after severe head injury: We should not generalize. *Journal of Neurology, Neurosurgery, and Psychiatry,* (http://jnnp.bmjjournals.com/cgi/eletters/74/11/1571#139). [Electronic letter, 17 June]

Matsuda, W., Matsumura, A., Komatsu, Y., Yanaka, K., & Nose, T. (2003). Awakenings from persistent vegetative state: Report of three cases with parkinsonism and brain stem lesions on MRI. *Journal of Neurology, Neurosurgery, and Psychiatry, 74*, 1571–1573.

Matsuda, W., Sugimoto, K., Sato, N., Watanabe, T., Yanaka, K., Matsumura, A., & Nose, T. (1999). A case of primary brain-stem injury recovered from persistent vegetative state after L-dopa administration. *Brain and Nerve, 51*, 1071–1074 [in Japanese].

Matsumura, A., Mitsui, I., Ayuzawa, S., Takeuchi, S., & Nose, T. (1993). Prediction of the reversibility of the brain stem dysfunction in head injury patients. In N. Nakamura, T. Hashimoto, & M. Yasue (eds.), *Recent advances in neurotraumatology* (pp. 192–195). Tokyo, Japan: Springer-Verlag.

Multi-Society Task Force on PVS (1994). Medical aspects of the persistent vegetative state. *New England Journal of Medicine, 330*, 1499–1508, 1572–1579.

Nayernouri, T. (1985). Posttraumatic parkinsonism. *Surgical Neurology, 24*, 263–264.

Nestler, E. J., Hyman, S. E., & Malenka, R. C. (2001). *Molecular neuropharmacology: A foundation for clinical neuroscience.* USA: McGraw-Hill.

Parkes, J. D., Sharpstone, P., & Williams, R. (1970). Levodopa in hepatic coma. *Lancet, 2*, 1341–1343.

Passler, M. A., & Riggs, R. V. (2001). Positive outcomes in traumatic brain injury–vegetative state: Patients treated with bromocriptine. *Archives of Physical Medicine and Rehabilitation, 82*, 311–315.

Ross, E. D., & Stewart, R. M. (1981). Akinetic mutism from hypothalamic damage: Successful treatment with dopamine agonists. *Neurology, 31*, 1435–1439.

Royal College of Physicians (1996). The permanent vegetative state. Review by a working group convened by the Royal College of Physicians and endorsed by the Conference of Medical Royal Colleges and their faculties of the United Kingdom. *Journal of the Royal College of Physicians of London, 30*, 119–121.

Royal College of Physicians (2003). The vegetative state: Guidance on diagnosis and management. *Clinical Medicine, 3*, 249–254.

Sacks, O. W., Kohl, M. S., Messeloff, C. R. & Schwartz, W. F. (1972). Effects of levodopa in parkinsonian patients with dementia. *Neurology, 22*, 516–519.

Shibata, Y., Matsumura, A., Meguro, K., & Narushima, K. (2000). Differentiation of mechanism and prognosis of traumatic brain stem lesions detected by magnetic resonance imaging in the acute stage. *Clinical Neurology and Neurosurgery, 102*, 124–128.

Uzan, M., Albayram, S., Dashti, S. G. R., Aydin, S., Hanci, M., & Kuday, C. (2003). Thalamic proton magnetic resonance spectroscopy in vegetative state induced by traumatic brain injury. *Journal of Neurology, Neurosurgery, and Psychiatry, 74*, 33–38.

van Woerkom, T. C. A. M., Minderhoud, J. M., Gottschal, T., & Nicolai, G. (1982). Neurotransmitters in the treatment of patients with severe head injuries. *European Neurology, 21*, 227–234.

Yoshikawa, H., Oda, Y., & Koeda, T. (1999). Remarkable improvement of severe diffuse axonal injury without L-dopa treatment. *Brain and Development, 21*, 140–141 [Corresponding letter and author's reply].

Zafonte, R. D., Watanabe, T., & Mann, N. R. (1998). Amantadine: A potential treatment for the minimally conscious state. *Brain Injury, 12*, 617–621.

Zeman, A. (1997). Persistent vegetative state. *Lancet, 350*, 795–799.

Zijlmans, J., Booij, J., Valk, J., Lees, A., & Horstink, M. (2002). Posttraumatic tremor without parkinsonism in a patient with complete contralateral loss of the nigrostriatal pathway. *Movement Disorders, 17*, 1086–1088.

NEUROPSYCHOLOGICAL REHABILITATION
2005, 15 (3/4), 428–430

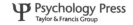

Psychology Press
Taylor & Francis Group

Part III: Behavioural assessment and rehabilitation techniques

Foreword by Barbara A. Wilson

Traditionally, neuropsychologists have had little involvement with people who are in coma or who are vegetative or who are in the minimally responsive state. This is a field where the medical profession, nurses, physiotherapists, occupational therapists and speech and language therapists have been the prime movers. Until fairly recently most neuropsychologists have entered the scene only when patients have recovered consciousness. In the past few years, however, an increasing number of psychologists have become involved in the assessment and management of patients in states of reduced awareness. The very first special issue of this journal focused on coma and the persistent vegetative state (1993) and was edited by two psychologists, Tom McMillan and Sarah Wilson. At least four other clinical psychologists made contributions, which were among the earliest publications from their profession in this specialised field.

However, neuropsychologists have always been involved in assessment and these are skills we can transfer to the management of low awareness patients. Improvements in the functioning of such patients are often very small and gradual, and can easily be missed if one is not looking for them or not monitoring the situation very closely. If hospital and nursing home staff believe that patients are showing no change over weeks or months, they may become disillusioned and poorly motivated. Good measures to identify change can influence clinical practice. One such measure is the Wessex Head Injury Matrix (WHIM; Shiel et al., 2000) and the measure used in the paper by Shiel and Wilson in this issue. The WHIM was developed following observations of 88 patients recovering from severe traumatic brain injury, and was a joint project between two psychologists, a physiotherapist, an occupational therapist and a neurologist/medical rehabilitation specialist. Psychologists have also been influential in behavioural observational studies, and this has indeed been the basis of the WHIM.

Continuing with the theme of detailed behavioural observations, neuro-psychologists have contributed to decision making in complex cases. It is not easy, for example, to differentiate between people who are vegetative and people who are minimally conscious (Andrews, Murphy, Munday, & Littlewood, 1996; Childs, Mercer, & Childs, 1993) yet decisions are made (at least in the UK) on whether or not to remove food and water on the basis of this distinction. Thus if people are vegetative, courts may allow removal of food and water whereas if people are minimally conscious removal is not allowed. Neuropsychologists can help distinguish between the two. McMillan (1997) describes a young woman who was thought to be vegetative but when carefully observed showed evidence of cognition. A further assessment of the same woman a few days later (Shiel & Wilson, 1998) confirmed McMillan's findings. This was in contrast to medical opinion at the time. One of the main reasons for the difference of opinion was that the psychological observations had taken place over two days rather than a half hour or so and systematic trials were conducted to comple-ment the observational data.

One of the main changes in neuropsychological rehabilitation over the past two decades has been the recognition that rehabilitation starts in intensive care. Even though patients in the vegetative or the minimally conscious state cannot be involved in the negotiation of their long-term goals (and such involvement reflects another major change in the past two decades), we can still set appropriate goals for our patients and we can involve the families in the negotiation process so this is yet another area where clinical neuropsychologists have a part to play. For a further discussion of goal setting with low awareness patients see Shiel (2003) and Wilson, Herbert, and Shiel (2003).

It would seem therefore that there are at least four reasons why neuro-psychologists should be part of the multidisciplinary team involved in the care of low awareness patients: namely, in the assessment of the behavioural repertoire of these patients; in the careful observation of change; in helping to make decisions about the diagnosis; and in the early goal setting and other treatment with health care staff and families. We cannot function efficiently, however, if we work in isolation. We need to recognise the contributions of the medical profession, nurses, therapists, radiographers, dietitians, physiol-ogists and other professions contributing to good clinical care and research. This special issue reflects the cross-disciplinary nature of this field as can be seen by the papers in this issue. We have papers concerned with the assess-ment of the behavioural repertoire of low awareness patients and with change over time; there is some discussion of differential diagnosis; and there are papers concerned with treatment issues, for example, the use of assistive technology, the value of music therapy, the consideration of the psychological needs of patients, families and health care professionals and the management of conflicts between staff and family members of low awareness patients. A particularly exciting aspect of this special issue is that contributions come from a variety of different professional groups. Psychologists are well represented along with therapists, nurses and medical doctors and others, thus reflecting the genuinely multidisciplinary nature of this field of work.

REFERENCES

Andrews, K., Murphy, L., Munday, R., & Littlewood, C. (1996). Misdiagnosis of the vegetative state—Retrospective study in a rehabilitation unit. *British Medical Journal, 313*, 13–16.

Childs, N. L., Mercer, W. N., & Childs, H. W. (1993). Accuracy of diagnosis of persistent vegetative state. *Neurology, 43*, 1465–1467.

McMillan, T. (1997). Neuropsychological assessment after extremely severe head injury in a case of life or death. *Brain Injury, 11*, 483–490.

McMillan, T. M., & Wilson, S. L. (Eds.) (1993). Coma and the persistent vegetative state [Special issue]. *Neuropsychological Rehabilitation, 3*, 97–212.

Shiel, A., & Wilson, B. A. (1998). Assessment after extremely severe head injury in a case of life or death: Further support for McMillan. *Brain Injury, 12*, 809–816.

Shiel, A., Wilson, B.A., McLellan, D. L., Horn, S., & Watson, M. (2000). *The Wessex Head Injury Matrix (WHIM)*. Bury St Edmunds, UK: Thames Valley Test Company.

Shiel, A. (2003). Rehabilitation of people in states of reduced awareness. In B. A. Wilson (Ed.), *Neuropsychological rehabilitation: Theory and practice* (pp. 253–269). Lisse, NL: Swets and Zeitlinger.

Wilson, B. A., Herbert, C. M., & Shiel, A. (2003). *Behavioural approaches in neuropsychological rehabilitation* (pp. 33–48). Hove, UK: Psychology Press.

PART III: ORGANIZATION OF PAPERS

1. Behavioural assessment tools
F. C. Wilson et al.; Rappaport; Kalmar & Giacino

2. Rehabilitation
Andrews; Reimer & LeNavenec; Elliott & Walker; Shiel & B. A. Wilson; Munday; Naudé & Hughes; Magee; Finch; Crawford & Beaumont

NEUROPSYCHOLOGICAL REHABILITATION
2005, 15 (3/4), 431–441

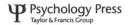

Vegetative and minimally conscious states: Serial assessment approaches in diagnosis and management

F. Colin Wilson[1], Lorraine E. Graham[1], and Tina Watson[2]

[1]*Green Park Health Care Trust, Belfast, UK*
[2]*Thompson House Hospital, Lisburn, UK*

Assessment of vegetative (VS) and minimally conscious state (MCS) patients presents clinicians with inherent difficulties (Royal College of Physicians, 2003) in terms of the reliable detection of potential signs of awareness given that all current assessment tools rely on observed behaviour. Recently developed measures such as SMART (Gill-Thwaites & Munday, 1999) and WHIM (Shiel et al., 2000), employing structured operational defined behavioural observations can facilitate the serial assessment of patient awareness, progress and appropriate goal setting particularly as one-off bedside assessments are more likely to be inaccurate. The use of sensitive tailored approaches involving experienced multidisciplinary teams is strongly advocated (Royal College of Physicians and British Society of Rehabilitation Medicine, 2003), notwithstanding clinicians should carefully consider potential confounding clinical factors, which may deleteriously influence patient arousal or ability to respond. Finally, areas for future development and recommendations regarding multidisciplinary assessment approaches with VS and MCS patients are outlined.

INTRODUCTION

Recent Royal College of Physicians (RCP) and British Society of Rehabilitation Medicine (BSRM) consensus guidelines (Turner-Stokes, 2003) in relation to vegetative and minimally conscious state(s) highlight the

---

Correspondence should be sent to Dr F. Colin Wilson, Consultant Clinical Neuropsychologist, Forster Green Hospital and Joss Cardwell Centre, Green Park Health Care Trust, 401 Holywood Road, Belfast, BT4 2LS, UK. Tel: +44 (28) 90768878, Fax: +44 (28) 90760313. Email: f.colinwilson@btopenworld.com

---

© 2005 Psychology Press Ltd
http://www.tandf.co.uk/journals/pp/09602011.html   DOI:10.1080/09602010543000091

importance, where doubt exists, of establishing a patient's level of "awareness and interaction". These guidelines suggest that assessment of such patients "should be undertaken by a team with specialist experience of profound brain injury" (p. 34). Consensus guidance on vegetative state (VS) and minimally conscious state (MCS) has been the subject of various working parties (Giacino et al., 1997, 2002; International Working Party on Vegetative State, 1996; Multi-Society Task Force on PVS, 1994; Royal College of Physicians, 1996, 2003) over the last decade.

Essentially, for a definitive diagnosis of vegetative state, lack of any evidence of awareness of self and/or the environment across serial assessment(s) and setting(s) would be warranted. Cartlidge (2001) helpfully defines "consciousness" as characterised by "an awareness of self and environment and an ability to respond to environmental factors", with two prerequisite components—sufficient arousal and self-awareness. However it is now recognised that frequent misdiagnosis among individuals with profound brain injury, i.e., individuals in locked-in syndrome or with profound physical and cognitive disability does occur (Andrews, Murphy, Munday, & Littlewood, 1996; Childs, Mercer, & Childs, 1993; Wilson, Harpur, Watson, & Morrow, 2002). Given that at least some VS patients present with isolated behavioural fragments (Schiff et al., 2002) not normally associated with VS, highlights the inherent difficulties associated with accurate diagnosis. For clinicians and families of individuals in states of profound brain injury, the spectre of misdiagnosis and hence sub-optimal management can be an ongoing source of worry or distress. Undoubtedly, no other diagnosis within the field of neurological rehabilitation carries with it such a vast range of clinical, medico-legal, ethical, philosophical, moral and religious implications than those of VS or MCS. Before discussing recent developments in the area of VS and MCS assessment, it is appropriate to outline current diagnostic definitions.

The Multi-Society Task Force on PVS (1994) provides the following consensus definition of vegetative state: (1) no evidence of awareness of self or environment and an inability to interact with others; (2) no evidence of sustained, reproducible, purposeful, or voluntary behavioural responses to visual, auditory, tactile or noxious stimuli; (3) no evidence of language comprehension or expression; (4) intermittent wakefulness manifested by the presence of sleep–wake cycles; (5) sufficiently preserved hypothalmic and brainstem autonomic functioning to permit survival in the presence of adequate medical and nursing care; (6) bowel and bladder incontinence; and (7) variably preserved cranial nerve reflexes (pupilary, oculocephalic, corneal, vestibulo-ocular, and gag) and spinal reflexes. Of the seven defining criteria, three are defined as the absence of evidence of gross cognitive functioning (awareness, responses, language comprehension, or expression). These criteria highlight the need to carefully define the *absence* of evidence of cognitive functioning (awareness of self or environment) in this patient group and to standardise assessment approaches. Interestingly, recent neuropathological findings have highlighted the possible critical role of thalami damage in VS patients. Adams, Graham, and Jennett (2000) studied 49 former patients (35 following traumatic brain injury, TBI), who remained vegetative until death between 1 month and 8 years after brain injury, indicated common (71%) grades 2 and 3 diffuse axonal injury in TBI cases. In addition, in traumatic cases, the thalamus was abnormal in 96% of cases surviving over 3 months and in all non-traumatic cases examined. Adams et al. also observed structurally normal cerebral cortex, cerebellum and brainstem in both TBI and non-TBI cases.

More recently, the American Academy of Neurology, in an attempt to define MCS has recommended the following consensus-based criteria (Giacino et al., 2002): Patients in MCS can demonstrate inconsistent but nevertheless discernible evidence of consciousness. The consensus-based definition indicates that MCS patients have limited but discernible awareness of self or environment. Diagnostic criteria are met, if, on a reproducible or sustained basis, one or more of the following occurs: (1) following simple commands, (2) gestural or verbal yes/no responses (independent of response accuracy), (3) intelligible verbalisation and (4) purposeful behaviour that occurs in response to relevant environmental stimuli (appropriate smiling or crying, vocalisations or meaningful gestures in direct response to the language content of questions, reaching objects with object accommodation or pursuit eye movement or sustained fixation in direct response to moving or salient stimuli). In addition, preliminary evidence suggests that at least some MCS patients may be able to process familiar voices and respond, at least at a cortical level to emotional stimuli (Bekinschtein et al., 2004). The Aspen Consensus Conference (Giacino et al., 1997) agreed that it is likely that a border zone exists between VS and MCS and it is possible that sustained visual pursuit eye movements may represent one of the first signs of emergence from VS (Multi-Society Task Force on PVS, 1994).

Since the previous special issue of *Neuropsychological Rehabilitation* dedicated to vegetative state, over a decade ago, a number of valuable assessment measures for the assessment of patients emerging from coma or in states of low awareness have been developed. Previously adopted measures such as Rancho Los Amigos Scale (Malkmus, Booth, & Kodimer, 1980), Coma/Near Coma (CNC) Scale (Rappaport, Dougherty, Devon, & Kelting, 1992), Coma Recovery Scale (Giacino, Kezmarsky, DeLuca, & Cicerone, 1991) and Western Neuro Sensory Stimulation Profile (WNSSP: Ansell & Keenan, 1989) have been joined by other measures such as the Sensory Stimulation Assessment Measure (SSAM: Rader & Ellis, 1994), Coma Exit Chart (Freeman, 1996), Sensory Modality Assessment and Rehabilitation Technique (SMART: Gill-Thwaites, 1997), Preliminary Neuropsychological

Battery (PNB: Cossa et al., 1999), Putney Auditory Comprehension Screening Test (PACST: Beaumont, Majoribanks, Flury, & Lintern, 2002) and Wessex Head Injury Matrix (WHIM: Shiel et al., 2000) among others.

The Royal College of Physicians (2003) has recently advocated the use of structured observations and specific measures such as SMART and WHIM. Our clinical experience that will be outlined later (Wilson et al., 2002; 2003) would also endorse this position. This paper will discuss clinical factors pertinent to accurate assessment in the context of experienced multi-disciplinary teams, review recent developments in terms of VS and MCS assessment measures, particularly SMART and WHIM, and highlight areas for future development.

CONFOUNDING FACTORS IN CLINICAL ASSESSMENT

Prior to patient assessment, the following factors should always be considered. The cause of the condition should be established. As far as is possible hydration, oxygenation, blood pressure and the blood glucose level should be normalised. Potentially treatable problems such as sepsis and raised intracranial pressure should be addressed. In addition, any confounding metabolic conditions such as hyper or hyponatraemia, hypercalcaemia and hypothyroidism must be considered and excluded. Due consideration should also be given to the discontinuation of sedatives, muscle relaxants, antipsychotics and anti-convulsant medications (Ledingham & Warrell, 2000; Royal College of Physicians, 2003).

Toxic-metabolic and drug mediated sedative effects can potentially mask a patient's ability to respond and hence a patient's observed level of awareness. Indeed, Strens, Mazibrada, Duncan, and Greenwood (2004) described two patients where the effects of medication had probably confounded the *reliable* assessment of arousal and awareness. In each patient, deemed "unaware" at 3 months post-injury, the use of large doses of anti-epileptic, anti-spastic and sedative agents may have contributed to suppressed "awareness" which, when withdrawn, permitted a more accurate assessment of awareness. On re-assessment, at 8 months post-injury (patient 1 was minimally aware) and patient 2, at 6 months post-injury was able to communicate using a keyboard and respond accurately to yes/no questions despite remaining aphasic. However it is also possible that the effects of certain types of medication may have a facilitator influence on the clinician's ability to elicit meaningful responses, Matsuda et al. (2003) presented three cases of vegetative state with parkinsonian features (asymmetrical rigidity, akinesia or tremor) after severe traumatic brain injury. Magnetic resonance imaging indicated brain-stem injury. Each patient showed neurological improvement (at 3, 7, and 12 months post-injury) following levodopa administration, although earlier case studies found a more limited benefit from levodopa (Haig & Ruess, 1990; Higashi et al., 1978). Finally, current diagnostic assessments depend on observed behaviour and therefore sensory deficits, motor dysfunction or diminished drive may result in a potential underestimation of a patient's cognitive capacity (Giacino et al., 2002).

RECENT DEVELOPMENTS IN VS AND MCS ASSESSMENT

Sensory Modality Assessment and Rehabilitation Technique (SMART: Gill-Thwaites & Munday, 1999) was designed as both an assessment and treatment tool, which is conducted over a 12–14 week period, and includes 3 weeks of assessment, 8 weeks of treatment and a further 3-week review assessment period. SMART was specifically designed to identify signs of awareness in patients diagnosed in VS and has both formal and informal components. The informal components include a Communication and Lifestyle history questionnaire as well as information from staff and family (SMART "informs"). The formal components include a structured and graded assessment of sensory capabilities (visual, auditory, tactile, olfactory, and gustatory), wakefulness, basic motor functioning and communicative ability as well as time-sampled behavioural observations prior to the 10 SMART assessment sessions, which each last 30–40 minutes, during the baseline period (up to a maximum of 3 weeks). A common 5-point hierarchical scale is employed across each of the eight assessment domains. Patient responses are rated from no response (Level 1) through withdrawal response (Level 3) to a differentiating response (Level 5). Based on these observational criteria, if a consistent response (Level 5) is detected in any modality (except wakefulness) on at least five consecutive occasions, then awareness of self or immediate environment has been observed indicating emergence from VS. In addition, meaningful patient responses permit clinicians to devise an individual stimulation programme. If patients demonstrate a statistically reliable response over the course of intervention sessions, then the programme is upgraded accordingly.

An earlier study involving 30 patients (Gill-Thwaites, 1997) indicated that SMART–Rancho Los Amigos equivalent scores were significant higher than those derived from WNSSP and referring physicians' ratings. A previous study by Sarah Wilson and colleagues (Wilson, Powell, Brock, & Thwaites, 1996) observed that VS patients may show different rates of change/improvement across different assessed domains. Wilson et al. (1996) advocated that the active involvement of family, friends and other team members was important in order to elicit a patient's "best" response. Gill-Thwaites and Munday (2001) provide data on 60 patients (50% with hypoxic/anoxic injury and 35% following TBI) who were admitted to the profound brain injury unit, Royal Hospital for Neurodisability (London). Intra-observer reliability studies indicated no significant differences in terms of SMART total scores between two experienced assessors. In addition, test–retest reliability of SMART total scores was in excess of 0.95 and the SMART–Rancho Los Amigos equivalent scores were also within the "highly acceptable" range (0.80).

Wessex Head Injury Matrix (WHIM: Shiel et al., 2000) is a hierarchical behavioural scale developed using a paired comparison technique, to monitor operational defined changes from coma through to emergence from post-traumatic amnesia (PTA) in patients following severe head injury. Behaviours can be observed to occur either spontaneously or elicited in response to naturally occurring or specifically presented stimulation. The WHIM scale provides scope for repeated observations across time and context and may be employed to gauge consistency of patient response (Shiel et al., 2000) or establish treatment goals (Shiel et al., 2004). Majerus, Van Der Linden, and Shiel (2000) reported excellent test–retest reliability and good inter-rater reliability, with good concurrent validity between WHIM and Glasgow Coma Scale (GCS). Comparison between WHIM and both GCS and Glasgow Leige Scale (GLS) highlighted that WHIM was a more sensitive indicator of emergence from coma or VS than either GCS or GLS. Majerus et al. (2000) observed that WHIM hierarchical scale order was generally confirmed in those in coma following either traumatic brain injury or stroke. It is possible that WHIM scale items (15–47) could be employed to provide the basis for observational evidence of entry to and emergence from MCS.

Observational studies of VS and MCS patients following severe traumatic brain injury as well as severe hypoxic insult, beyond the traditional timeframe of post-acute rehabilitation, have broadly confirmed WHIM sensitivity and scale item order (Wilson et al., 2002, 2003). Shiel et al. (2004) argue that, particularly for those patients where appropriate serial assessment is not undertaken, subtle changes in awareness may go unobserved. Indeed Shiel et al. reported that environmental manipulations such as postural changes can affect the number of observed/elicited behaviours and highlight that assessment should be carried out at different times of day and across different environmental conditions. Barbara Wilson and colleagues (Wilson, Herbert, & Shiel, 2003) argue that the use of WHIM and SMART are not mutually incompatible, while SMART can be employed with VS patients and has a lower floor level than WHIM. Nevertheless, when patients reach ceiling on SMART, it may be appropriate to employ WHIM up to emergence from post-traumatic amnesia. Notwithstanding, following careful serial re-assessment using sensitive measures, if no response to visual, auditory, tactile or noxious stimuli suggesting volition or conscious purpose and no evidence of language comprehension or meaningful expression is observed, then a more definitive diagnosis of VS is possible having excluded possible confounding clinical factors. While, to date, the use of refined assessment tools such as SMART and WHIM have been advocated only where doubt exists in terms of clinical diagnosis (Royal College of Physicians and British Society of Rehabilitation Medicine, 2003). The use of these measures, given the possibility of misdiagnosis, although time-consuming, should be considered as a matter of course particularly if after the patient emerges from coma, no further evolution in awareness on bedside assessment is observed.

ASSESSMENT APPROACHES FOR FURTHER DEVELOPMENT

Behavioural observation techniques such as stimulus-response observations and event recording can also be employed in the assessment of VS and MCS patients. For clinicians designing such assessment procedures, it is important to devise clear "a priori" criteria in order to operationally define the "nature" of definite patient responses and thus obtain an objective behavioural record. The specific designed procedure should, as a minimum, ensure a level of statistical reliability regarding observations. Given most basic "cognitive" assessments require a consistent yes/no response, the use of the binomial test to rule out performance at or below chance levels is appropriate (for details, see Siegel and Castellan, 1988, pp. 38–40). McMillan (1996), McMillan and Herbert (2000) as well as Shiel and Wilson (1998) provide some guidance to clinicians in terms of appropriate assessment domains (autobiographical information, general knowledge, new learning, mood, current awareness and future life choices), which may be included, depending on the reliability of patient responses in a structured assessment of patient awareness. Practically, it is important to use short, simple, repeated counterbalanced probe questions as well as giving due consideration to the impact of fatigue or other deleterious influences, which may suppress patient arousal and ability to respond.

The Putney Auditory Comprehension Screening Test (PACST: Beaumont et al., 2002) was developed at the Royal Hospital for Neurodisability. Although not specifically designed to assess patients in MCS, it may nevertheless be suitable particularly for those patients with severe/profound physical disability and impaired vision (Beaumont et al., 2002). As PACST seeks to establish the reliability of a patient's "yes" and "no" responses by whatever means to a series of 60 increasingly complicated verbally presented questions, it would seem to have some potential as an appropriate assessment tool of emergence from MCS (i.e., above chance performance). A bedside test battery developed in Italy, specifically for use with minimally responsive patients (Preliminary Neuropsychological Battery, PNB: Cossa et al., 1999) also shows some promise. The PNB employs a forced choice paradigm, which requires patients to indicate "yes" or "no" to 60 visual stimuli (geometric figures, letters, words, digits). It would therefore be possible, the authors argue, to distinguish between patients performing at or below chance level from those who are capable of making consistent responses. However the possibility of profound visual loss or marked visual disturbances in VS and MCS is considered high (Andrews et al., 1996; Whyte & DiPasquale, 1995) and, as such, due caution in the use of this battery is warranted especially as intact cortico-visual functioning cannot be assured.

DISCUSSION

Undoubtedly, particular care should be taken when undertaking assessments with VS or MCS patients, as early one-off examinations may create what Andrews (1993) termed a "self-fulfilling prophesy", i.e., those who are deemed to have a poor chance of recovery are not treated aggressively. Clearly, good multidisciplinary teamwork, involving professionals with sufficient expertise is required to reliably establish appropriate diagnosis and formulate clinical management plans with VS patients (Andrews et al., 1996; Wilson et al., 2002). The need for systematic longer-term case review has also been highlighted especially in the light of the possibility of emergence from VS or MCS (Andrews et al., 1996; Childs & Mercer, 1996; Levin et al., 1991; Wilson et al., 2002), late functional recovery (McMillan & Herbert, 2000, 2004) and potential life or death consequences for VS or MCS patients (McMillan, 1996; Shiel & Wilson, 1998).

In recent years, within the UK at least, occupational therapists, speech and language therapists and clinical neuropsychologists have become increasingly involved in the assessment and management of VS and MCS patients. The contribution and expertise of these groups of professionals in supporting and refining diagnostic assessments of patients in VS or MCS has been recognised (Andrews et al., 1996; Royal College of Physicians, 2003). This review has highlighted the value of repeated serial assessment tools such as SMART (Gill-Thwaites & Munday, 2001) and WHIM (Shiel et al., 2000) in working with VS and MCS patients.

Finally, with the increasing involvement of various groups of professionals, the need to devise clear and standardised interdisciplinary working practices, assessment, and management approaches would seem timely (Wilson et al., 2002). In the interim, at the very least, interdisciplinary teams should employ standardised behavioural observational approaches with appropriate reliability and statistical controls as part of working practice with patients and actively seek to involve relatives in their assessment(s) as far as possible (Royal College of Physicians, 2003).

REFERENCES

Adams, J. H., Graham, D. I., & Jennett, B. (2000). The neuropathology of the vegetative state after an acute brain insult. *Brain, 123*(7), 1327–1338.

Andrews, K. (1993). Should PVS patients be treated. *Neuropsychological Rehabilitation, 3,* 109–119.

Andrews, K., Murphy, L., Munday, R., & Littlewood, C. (1996). Misdiagnosis of the vegetative state: Retrospective study in a rehabilitation unit. *British Medical Journal, 313,* 13–16.

Ansell, B. J., & Keenan, M. A. (1989). The Western Neuro Sensory Stimulation Profile: A tool for assessing slow to recover head injured patients. *Archives of Physical Medicine and Rehabilitation, 70,* 104–108.

Beaumont, J. G., Majoribanks, J., Flury, S., & Lintern, T. (2002). *Putney Auditory Comprehension Screening Test (PACST).* Bury St. Edmunds, UK: Thames Valley Test Company.

Bekinschtein, T., Niklison, J., Sigman, L., Manes, F., Leiguarda, R., Armony, J., Owen, A., Carpintiero, S., & Olmos, L. (2004). Emotion processing in the minimally conscious state. *Journal of Neurology, Neurosurgery and Psychiatry, 75,* 788.

Cartlidge, N. (2001). States related to or confused with coma. *Journal of Neurology, Neurosurgery and Psychiatry, 71,* (Suppl. 1), 18–19.

Childs, N. L., & Mercer, W. N. (1996). Late improvement in consciousness after post-traumatic vegetative state. *New England Journal of Medicine, 334,* 24–25.

Childs, N. L., Mercer, W. N., & Childs, H. W. (1993). Accuracy of diagnosis of persistent vegetative state. *Neurology, 43,* 1465–1467.

Cossa, F. M., Fabiani, M., Farinato, A., Laiacona, M., & Capitani, E. (1999). The 'preliminary neuropsychological battery'. An instrument to grade the cognitive level of minimally responsive patients. *Brain Injury, 13*(8), 583–592.

Freeman, E. A. (1996). The Coma Exit Chart: Assessing the patient in prolonged coma and the vegetative state. *Brain Injury, 10,* 615–624.

Giacino, J. T., Ashwal, S., Childs, N., Cranford, R., Jennett, B., Katz, D. I., et al. (2002). The minimally conscious state: Definition and diagnostic criteria. *Neurology, 58,* 349–353.

Giacino, J. T., Kezmarsky, M. A., DeLuca, J., & Cicerone, K. D. (1991). Monitoring rate of recovery to predict outcome in minimally-responsive patients. *Archives of Physical Medicine and Rehabilitation, 72,* 897–901.

Giacino, J. T., Zasler, N. D., Katz, D. I., Kelly, J. P., Rosenberg, J. H., & Filley, C. M. (1997). Development of practice guidelines for assessment and management of the vegetative and minimally conscious states. *Journal of Head Trauma Rehabilitation, 12,* 79–89.

Gill-Thwaites, H. (1997). The Sensory Modality Assessment Rehabilitation Technique: A tool for the assessment and treatment of patients with severe brain injury in a vegetative state. *Brain Injury, 11,* 723–734.

Gill-Thwaites, H., & Munday, R. (1999). The Sensory Modality Assessment and Rehabilitation Technique (SMART): A comprehensive and integrated assessment and treatment protocol for the vegetative state and minimally responsive patient. *Neuropsychological Rehabilitation, 9,* 305–320.

Gill-Thwaites, H., & Munday, R. (2001). *Sensory Modality Assessment and Rehabilitation Technique (SMART): A tool for the assessment and treatment of the brain damaged patient in a vegetative or minimally conscious state.* London: Occupational Therapy Department, Royal Hospital for Neurodisability.

Haig, A. J., & Ruess, J. M. (1990). Recovery from vegetative state of six months' duration associated with Sinemet (levodopa/carbidopa). *Archives of Physical Medicine and Rehabilitation, 71,* 1081–1083.

Higashi, K., Hatano, M., Abiko, S., Fukuda, Y., Noda, S., Yamashita, T., & Kaku, R. (1978). Clinical analysis of patients recovered from persistent vegetative state, with special emphasis on the therapeutic and prophylactic effects of L-dopa. *Brain Nerve, 30*, 27–35 [in Japanese].

International working party report on the vegetative state (1996). *Report on the vegetative state.* London: Royal Hospital for Neurodisability.

Ledingham, J. G. G., & Warrell, D. A. (2000). *Concise Oxford Textbook of Medicine* (pp. 1284–1286). Oxford: Oxford University Press.

Levin, H. S., Saydjari, C., Eisenberg, H. M., Foulkes, M., Marshall, L. F., Ruff, R. M., et al. (1991). Vegetative state after closed head injury: A traumatic coma data bank report. *Archives of Neurology, 48*, 580–585.

Majerus, S., Van Der Linden, M., & Shiel, A. (2000). Wessex Head Injury Matrix and Glasgow/Glasgow-Liege coma scale. A validation and comparison study. *Neuropsychological Rehabilitation, 10*, 167–184.

Malkmus, D., Booth, B., & Kodimer, C. (1980). *Rehabilitation of the head injured adult: Comprehensive cognitive management.* Downey, CA: Professional Staff Association of Rancho Los Amigos Hospital.

Matsuda, W., Komatsu, Y., Matsumara, A., Yanaka, K., & Nose, T. (2003). Awakenings from persistent vegetative state: Report of three cases with Parkinsonism and brain stem lesions on MRI. *Journal of Neurology, Neurosurgery and Psychiatry, 74*, 1571–1573.

McMillan, T. M. (1996). Neuropsychological assessment after extremely severe head injury in a case of life or death. *Brain Injury, 11*, 483–490.

McMillan, T. M., & Herbert, C. M. (2000). Neuropsychological assessment of a potential "euthanasia" case: A 5-year follow up. *Brain Injury, 14*(2), 197–203.

McMillan, T. M., & Herbert, C. M. (2004). Further recovery in a potential treatment withdrawal case 10 years after brain injury. *Brain Injury, 18*(9), 935–940.

Multi-Society Task Force on PVS. (1994). Medical aspects of the persistent vegetative state: First of two parts. *New England Journal of Medicine, 330*, 1499–1508.

Rader, M. A., & Ellis, D. W. (1994). The Sensory Stimulation Assessment Measure (SSAM): A tool for early evaluation of severely brain injured patients. *Brain Injury, 8*, 309–321.

Rappaport, M. D., Dougherty, B. A., Devon, L., & Kelting, B. A. (1992). Evaluation of coma and vegetative states. *Archives of Physical Medicine and Rehabilitation, 73*, 628–634.

Royal College of Physicians (1996). *The permanent vegetative state.* [A Working Party Report]. London: Royal College of Physicians.

Royal College of Physicians (2003). *The vegetative state: Guidance on diagnosis and management.* [A report of a working party]. London: Royal College of Physicians.

Schiff, N. D., Ribary, U., Moreno, D. R., Beattie, B., Kronberg, E., Blasberg, R., Giacino, J., McCagg, C., Fins, J. J., Llinas, R., & Plum, F. (2002). Residual cerebral activity and behavioural fragments can remain in the persistently vegetative brain. *Brain, 125*(6), 1210–1234.

Shiel, A., & Wilson, B. A. (1998). Assessment after extremely severe head injury in a case of life or death: Further support for McMillan. *Brain Injury, 12*, 809–816.

Shiel, A., Wilson, B. A., Elliott, L. E., Foley, J., Menon, D., & Pickard, J. D. (2004). *Approaches to assessment and rehabilitation of people in states of reduced awareness.* Paper presented at Symposium on Neuropsychological Rehabilitation 12–13th July, Ayers Rock, Australia.

Shiel, A., Wilson, B. A., McLellan, L., Horn, S., & Watson, M. (2000). *The Wessex Head Injury Matrix (WHIM).* Bury St. Edmunds, UK: Thames Valley Test Company.

Siegal, S., & Castellan, N. J. (1988). *Non-parametric statistics for the behavioural sciences* (2nd ed.). London: McGraw-Hill.

Strens, L. H., Mazibrada, G., Duncan, J. S., & Greenwood, R. (2004). Misdiagnosing the vegetative state after severe brain injury: The influence of medication. *Brain Injury, 18*(2), 213–218.

Turners-Stokes, L. (Ed.). (2003). *Rehabilitation following acquired brain injury: National clinical guidelines*. London: Royal College of Physicians and British Society of Rehabilitation Medicine.

Whyte, J., & DiPasquale, M. C. (1995). Assessment of vision and visual attention in minimally responsive brain injured patients. *Archives of Physical Medicine and Rehabilitation, 76*, 804–810.

Wilson, B. A., Herbert, C. M., & Shiel, A. (2003). *Behavioural approaches in neuropsychological rehabilitation: Optimising rehabilitation procedures*. Hove, UK: Psychology Press.

Wilson, F. C., Harpur, J., Watson, T., & Morrow, J. I. (2002). Vegetative state and minimally responsive patients—Regional survey, long-term case outcomes and service recommendations. *NeuroRehabilitation, 17*, 231–236.

Wilson, F. C., Harpur, J., Watson, T., & Morrow, J. I. (2003). Adult survivors of severe cerebral hypoxia—case series survey and comparative analysis. *NeuroRehabilitation, 18*, 291–298.

Wilson, S. L., Powell, G. E., Brock, D., & Thwaites, H. (1996). Vegetative state and response to sensory stimulation: An analysis of twenty-four cases. *Brain Injury, 10*, 807–818.

NEUROPSYCHOLOGICAL REHABILITATION
2005, 15 (3/4), 442–453

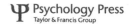

The Disability Rating and Coma/Near-Coma scales in evaluating severe head injury

Maurice Rappaport

San Jose, CA, USA

The Disability Rating (DR) and Coma/Near-Coma (C/NC) scales for evaluating severe head injury are described. Scales are related to patient status, course and outcome and also underlying electroneurophysiological dysfunction. They lend themselves to high inter-rater reliability with brief training and can be completed in minutes, conserving staff time and energy.

Outcomes after severe head injury usually fall into at least five general categories: good recovery; partial recovery; vegetative state with modest recovery; marked vegetative state with minimal recovery; and death. The Disability Rating (DR) and Coma/Near-Coma (C/NC) scales were developed after rehabilitation staff in long-term facilities reported seeing changes in patients in vegetative states but had no systematic way of charting changes or knowing the significance of the changes observed.

The DR scale is shown in Appendix 1, the C/NC scale in Appendix 2. It was found that scores on these scales correlated with a patient's physical and mental condition, monitored progress or lack of progress over time and predicted outcome, even when evaluations took place many months after initial injury. Scores were also correlated with electroneurophysiological measures of brain function. (Rappaport, 1996; Rappaport, Hall, & Hopkins, 1997, 1981b; Rappaport, Hall, Hopkins, & Belleza, 1982; Rappaport, Maloney, & Ortega, 1985; Rappaport, Herrero Bache, & Rappaport, 1989; Rappaport, Hemmerle, & Rappaport, 1990; Rappaport, Dougherty, & Kelting, 1992; Rappaport, & Clifford, 1994).

Details on method of scoring and the relationship between actual scores and the current and future clinical status of patients is described in the articles referred to above.

Correspondence should be addressed to Maurice Rappaport, 1185 McKendrie Street, San Jose, CA 95126-1407, USA. Tel: 408-985-9825, Fax: 408-248-3051, Email: rappapor@ix.netcom.com

© 2005 Psychology Press Ltd
http://www.tandf.co.uk/journals/pp/09602011.html   DOI:10.1080/09602010443000335

The DR scale (revised 8/87) rates patients on four categories: Arousability, Awareness and Responsivity; Cognitive Ability For Self-Care; Dependence On Others; and Psychosocial Adaptability. There are 10 disability categories ranging from no disability to death with the range of scores specified for each category of disability. Scores range between 0 and 30 with the higher scores reflecting greater disability. This order of rating was established since staff find it easier to rate level of disability rather than level of wellness as used in the Glasgow Outcome Scale (Jennett, Snoek, & Bond, 1981). The DR scale is reported as more sensitive than the Glasgow scale (Hall, Cope, & Rappaport, 1985).

The C/NC scale is used whenever the DR score is greater then 21 (Extremely Severe Disability). The C/NC categories include: Moderate Coma; Marked Coma; and Extreme Coma where the definition of these states is included on the form. The increased sensitivity of the C/NC scale shows low level changes that are not apparent on the DR scale.

Both the DR and C/NC scales help identify patients who are likely to benefit from on going long-term rehabilitation therapy. It provides a rationale for selecting and supporting long-term intensive rehabilitation therapy for some severe head injury patients. One study that followed severe head injury patients for up to 10 years demonstrated this long-term outcome relationship (Rappaport et al., 1989). Other studies have also demonstrated that the DR scale can predict length of hospitalisation and discharge status of individuals who have had head injuries or cerebrovascular accidents (Eliason & Topp, 1984). Further comparisons of the advantages of the DR scale in monitoring recovery from severe head injury have been reported by Gouvier, Blanton, LaPorte, and Nepomuceno, (1987), Fryer and Haffey (1987), Hall, Hamilton, Gordon, and Zasler (1983), Rappaport et al. (1992), Fleming (1994), and Giacino and Zasler (1995). Both the DR and C/NC scales are correlated significantly with brain dysfunction as reflected in abnormal cortical and subcortical electroencephalographic evoked potential patterns (Rappaport, Hall, & Hopkins, 1981a; Rappaport et al., 1985; Rappaport, 1986, 1996).

In general, as cited by the the the Center for Outcome Measurement in Brain Injury (COMBI, 2000), the relative benefits compared to other scales include: proven reliability and validity; ability to be scored through interview with individual or family members; score times ranging between 30 seconds and 30 minutes where additional efforts must be employed to obtain information from family and available staff directly or through telephone interviews; and expertise in the field not needed to obtain accurate assessments.

Inter-rater reliability in using these scales is quite high after brief training. ($r > .90$) Training consists of two raters independently rating several patients and then comparing and discussing score differences and making compromise adjustments. Once trained in this fashion reliable scores can be obtained subsequently using only one trained rater. Time to complete a rating takes a matter of a few minutes, making this type of approach economical in terms of time and energy.

The DR and C/NC scales take their place among many other scales discussed in this special issue that are helpful in evaluating, following and predicting outcome in patients who have sustained severe brain injury whether due to trauma, anoxia, infection or other disabling events.

REFERENCES

COMBI (2000). *Santa Clara Valley Medical Center*. Retrieved from tbisci@tbi-sci.org, Editor, Jerry Wright.

Eliason, M. R., & Topp, B. W. (1984). Predictive validity of Rappaport's Disability Rating Scale in subjects with acute brain dysfunction. *Physical Therapy, 64*, 1357–1360.

Fleming, J. F. (1994). Prognosis of rehabilitation outcome in head injury using the disability rating scale. *Archives of Physical Medicine and Rehabilitation, 75*, 156–162.

Fryer, L. J., & Haffey, W. J. (1987). Cognitive rehabilitation and community readptation: Outcomes from two program models. *Journal of Head Trauma Rehabilitation, 2*(3), 51–63.

Giacino, J. T., & Zasler, N. D. (1995). Outcome after severe traumatic brain injury: Coma, the vegetative state and the minimally responsive state. *Journal of Head Trauma Rehabilitation, 10*(1), 40–56.

Goodin, D. S., Starr, A., & Chippendale, T. (1983). Sequential changes in the P3 component of the auditory evoked potential in confusional states and dementing illnesses. *Neurology, 33*, 1215–1218.

Gouvier, W. D., Blanton, M. A., LaPorte, K., & Nepomuceno, M. D. (1987). Reliability and validity of the Disability Rating Scale and the levels of cognitive functioning scale in monitoring recovery from severe head injury. *Archives of Physical Medicine and Rehabilitation, 68*, 94–97.

Hall, K., Cope, N., & Rappaport, M. (1985). Glasgow Outcome Scale and Disability Rating Scale: Comparative usefulness in following recovery in traumatic brain injury. *Archives of Physical Medicine and Rehabilitation, 66*, 35–37.

Hall, K., Hamilton, B. B., Gordon, W. A., & Zasler, N. D. (1993). Characteristics and comparisons of functional assessment indices: Disability Rating Scale, Functional Independence Measure, and Functional Assessment Measure. *Journal of Head Trauma Rehabilitation, 8*(2), 60–74.

Jennett, B., Snoek, J., & Bond, M. R. (1981). Disability after severe head injury: Obsevations on use of Glasgow Outcome Scale. *Journal of Neurology, Neurosurgery, and Psychiatry, 44*, 258–293.

Rappaport, M. (1986). Brain evoked potentials in coma and the vegetative state. *Journal of Head Trauma Rehabilitation, 1*, 15–29.

Rappaport, M. (1996). Electrophysiological Assessment. In L. J. Horn & N. D. Zasler (Eds.), *Medical rehabilitation of traumatic brain injury* (pp. 271–316). Philadelphia, PA: Hanley & Belfus, Inc.

Rappaport, M., & Clifford, J. O. (1994). Comparison of passive P300 brain evoked potentials in normal and severely traumatically brain injured patients. *Journal of Head Trauma Rehabilitation, 9*, 94–104.

Rappaport, M., Dougherty, A., & Kelting, D. L. (1992). Evaluation of coma and vegetative states. *Archives of Physical Medicine and Rehabilitation, 73*, 628–634.

Rappaport, M., Hall, K., & Hopkins, K. (1977). Evoked potentials and disability in brain damaged patients. *Archives of Physical Medicine and Rehabilitation, 58*, 333–338.

Rappaport, M., Hall, K., & Hopkins, K. (1981a). Evoked potentials and head injury: 1. Rating of evoked potential abnormality. *Clinical EEG (electroencephalography)*, *12*(4), 154–166.

Rappaport, M., Hall, K., Hopkins, K., & Belleza, T. (1982). Disability Rating Scale for severe head trauma: Coma to community. *Archives of Physical Medicine and Rehabilitation, 63*, 118–123.

Rappaport, M., Hemmerle, A., & Rappaport, M. L. (1990). Intermediate and long latency SEPs in relation to clinical disability in traumatic brain injury patients. *Clinical EEG (electroencephalography), 21*(4), 188–191.

Rappaport, M., Herrero Bache, C., & Rappaport, M. L. (1989). Head injury outcome: Up to ten years later. *Archives of Physical Medicine and Rehabilitation, 70*, 885–892.

Rappaport, M., Hopkins, K., & Hall, K. (1981b). Evoked potentials and head injury: 2. Clinical applications. *Clinical EEG (electroencephalography), 122*(4), 167–176.

Rappaport, M., McCandless, K. L., & Pond, W. (1991). Passive P300 response in brain injury patients. *Journal of Neuropsychiatry and Clinical Neurosciences, 3*, 180–185.

Rappaport, M., Maloney, J. R., & Ortega, H. (1985). Survival in young children after drowning: Brain evoked potentials as outcome predictors. *Clinical EEG (electroencephalography), 16*(4), 183–191.

Scranton, J., Fogel, M., & Erdman, W. (1970). Evaluation of functional levels of patients during and following rehabilitation. *Achives of Physical Medicine and Rehabilitation, 51*, 1–21.

Teasdale, G. M., & Jennett, B. (1974). Assessment of coma and impaired consciousness: A practical scale. *Lancet, 2*, 81–84.

APPENDIX 1

Disability Rating Scale (Rappaport et al., 1982)

Disability Rating Scale (DRS)

Name:_____ Sex ___ DOB _____ Brain Injury Date_____

Cause of Injury:

___ MVA/MCA* ____ Head Trauma** ____ Infection ____ Stroke ____ Anoxia ____ Metabolic ____ Drowning

___ Developmental (congenital) ____ Degenerative ____ Other (specify) _____

* MVA = motor vehicle accident; MCA = motorcycle accident. *Circle one*
** Gun shot, blunt instrument, blow to head, fall etc.
Scale for gauging general level of disability from "none" to "Extreme Vegetative State"

Category	Item	Instructions	Score
Arousability, awareness and responsivity[1]	Eye opening ☐	0 = spontaneous 1 = to speech 2 = to pain 3 = none	
	Communication ability ☐	0 = oriented 1 = confused 2 = inappropriate 3 = incomprehensible 4 = none	
	Motor response ☐	0 = obeying 1 = localizing 2 = withdrawing 3 = flexing 4 = extending 5 = none	
Cognitive ability for self care activities	Feeding ☐	0 = complete 1 = partial 2 = minimal 3 = none	
	Toileting ☐	0 = complete 1 = partial 2 = minimal 3 = none	
	Grooming ☐	0 = complete 1 = partial 2 = minimal 3 = none	
Dependence on others[2]	Level of functioning ☐	0 = completely independent 1 = independent in special environment 2 = mildly dependent 3 = moderately dependent 4 = markedly dependent 5 = totally dependent	
Psychosocial adaptability	"Employability" ☐	0 = not restricted 1 = selected jobs 2 = sheltered workshop (non-competitive) 3 = not employable	
		Total DR Score	

[1]*Modified from Teasdale & Jennett (1974)*
[2]*Modified from Scranton et al. (1970)*

APPENDIX 1 (Contd.)

Eye opening

  0 Spontaneous
  1 To speech
  2 To pain
  3 None

Communication ability: Either verbal, writing or letter board or sign (viz. eye blink, head, nod, etc)

  0 Oriented
  1 Confused
  2 Inappropriate
  3 Incomprehensible
  4 None

Best motor response

  0 Obeying
  1 Localizing
  2 Withdrawing
  3 Flexing
  4 Extending
  5 None

[a]needs limited assistance (non-resident helper)
[b]needs moderate assistance (person in home)
[c]needs assistance with all major activities at all times
[d]24 hour nursing care required

Cognitive ability: For feeding, toileting, grooming (Does patient know how and when? Ignore motor disability)

  0 Complete
  1 Partial
  2 Minimal
  3 None

Level of functioning: (Consider both physical and cognitive disability)

  0 Completely independent
  1 Independent in special environment
  2 Mildly dependent[a]
  3 Moderately dependent[b]
  4 Markedly dependent[c]
  5 Totally dependent[d]

"Employability": (As a full-time worker homemaker or student)

  0 Not restricted
  1 Selected jobs, competitive
  2 Sheltered workshop, not competitive
  3 Not employable

Disability Categories

Total DR Score	Level of disability
0	None
1	Mild
2–3	Partial
4–6	Moderate
7–11	Moderately severe
12–16	Severe
17–21	Extremely severe
22–24	Vegetative state
25–29	Extreme vegetative state

DRS INSTRUCTIONS

Item definitions

Eye opening

0: *Spontaneous*: eyes open with sleep/wake rhythms indicating active arousal mechanisms; does not assume awareness.

1: *To speech and/or sensory stimulation*: a response to any verbal approach, whether spoken or shouted, not necessarily the command to open the eyes. Also, response to touch, mild pressure.

2: *To pain*: tested by a painful stimulus. Standard painful stimulus is the application of pressure across index fingernail of best side with wood of a pencil; for quadriplegics pinch nose tip and rate as 0, 1, 2 or 5.

3: *None*: no eye opening even to painful stimulation.

Best communication ability

(If patient cannot use voice because of tracheostomy or is aphasic or dysarthric or has vocal cord paralysis or voice dysfunction then estimate patient's best response and enter note under comments.)

0: *Oriented*: implies awareness of self and the environment. Patient able to tell you (a) who he is; (b) where he is: (c) why he is there; (d) year; (e) season; (f) month; (g) day; (h) time of day.

1: *Confused*: attention can be held and patient responds to questions but responses are delayed and/or indicate varying degrees of disorientation and confusion.

2: *Inappropriate*: intelligible articulation but speech is used only in an exclamatory or random way (such as shouting and swearing); no sustained communication exchange is possible.

3: *Incomprehensible*: moaning, groaning or sounds without recognisable words; no consistent communication signs.

4: *None*: no sounds or communication signs from patient.

Best motor response

0: *Obeying*: obeying command to move finger on best side. If no response or not suitable try another command such as "move lips", "blink eyes", etc. Do not include grasp or other reflex responses.

1: *Localising*: a painful stimulus at more than one site causes a limb to move (even slightly) in an attempt to remove it. It is a deliberate motor act to move away from or remove the source of noxious stimulation. If there is doubt as to whether withdrawal or localisation has occurred after three or four painful stimulations, rate as localisation. Standard painful stimulus is the application of pressure across index fingernail of best side with wood of a pencil; for quadriplegics pinch nose tip and rate as 0, 1, 2 or 5.

2: *Withdrawing*: any generalised movement away from a noxious stimulus that is more than a simple reflex response.

3: *Flexing*: painful stimulation results in either flexion at the elbow, rapid withdrawal with abduction of the shoulder or a slow withdrawal with adduction of the shoulder.

If there is confusion between flexing and withdrawing, then use pin prick on hands, then face.

4: *Extending*: painful stimulation results in extension of the limb.

5: *None*: no response can be elicited. Usually associated with hypotonia. Exclude spinal transection as an explanation of lack of response: be satisfied that an adequate stimulus has been applied.

Cognitive ability for feeding, toileting and grooming

Rate each of the three functions separately. For each function answer the question, "Does the patient show awareness of how and when to perform each specified activity?" Ignore motor disabilities that interfere with carrying out a function. (This is rated under Level of functioning described below.) Rate best response for toileting based on bowel and bladder behaviour. Grooming refers to bathing, washing, brushing of teeth, shaving, combing or brushing of hair and dressing.

0: *Complete*: continuously shows awareness that patient knows how to feed, toilet or groom self and can convey unambiguous information that patient knows when this activity should occur.

1: *Partial*: intermittently shows awareness that patient knows how to feed, toilet or groom self and or can intermittently convey reasonably clear information that patient knows when the activity should occur.

2: *Minimal*: shows in a primitive way how to feed, toilet or groom self and/or shows infrequently by certain signs, sounds or activities that patient is vaguely aware when the activity should occur.

3: *None*: shows virtually no awareness at any time that patient knows how to feed, toilet or groom self and cannot convey information by signs, sounds, or activity that patient knows when the activity should occur.

Level of functioning

0: *Completely independent*: able to live as patient wishes, requiring no restriction due to physical, mental, emotional or social problems.

1: *Independent in special environment*: capable of functioning independently when needed requirements are met (mechanical aids).

2: *Mildly dependent*: able to care for most of own needs but requires limited assistance due to physical, cognitive and/or emotional problems (e.g., needs non-resident helper).

3: *Moderately dependent*: able to care for self partially but needs another person at all times.

4: *Markedly dependent*: needs help with all major activities and the assistance of another person at all times.

5: *Totally dependent*: not able to assist in own care and requires 24-hour nursing care.

Employability

The psychosocial adaptability or employability item takes into account overall cognitive and physical ability to be an employee, homemaker or student. This determination should take into account considerations such as the following: (1) able to understand, remember and follow instructions; (2) can plan and carry out tasks at least at the level of an office clerk or in simple routine, repetitive industrial situations or can do school assignments; (3) ability to remain oriented, relevant and appropriate in work and other psychosocial situations; (4) ability to get to and from work or shopping centres using private or public transportation effectively; (5) ability to deal with number concepts; (6) ability to make purchases and handle simple money exchange problems; (7) ability to keep track of time schedules and appointments.

0: *Not restricted*: can compete in the open market for a relatively wide range of jobs commensurate with existing skills; or can initiate, plan, execute and assume responsibilities associated with homemaking; or can understand and carry out most age-relevant school assignments.

1: *Selected jobs, competitive*: can compete in a limited job market for a relatively narrow range of jobs because of limitations of the type described above and/or because of some physical limitations; or can initiate, plan, execute and assume many but not all responsibilities associated with homemaking; or can understand and carry out many but not all school assignments.

2: *Sheltered workshop, non-competitive*: cannot compete successfully in job market because of limitations described above and/or because of moderate or severe physical limitations; or cannot without major assistance initiate, plan, execute and assume responsibilities for homemaking; or cannot understand and carry out even relatively simple school assignments without assistance.

3: *Not employable*: completely unemployable because of extreme psychosocial limitations of the type described above; or completely unable to initiate, plan, execute and assume any responsibilities associated with homemaking; or cannot understand or carry out any school assignments.

INSTRUCTIONS

Place date of rating at top of column. Place appropriate rating next to each of the eight items listed. Add eight ratings to obtain total DR score.

APPENDIX 2

Rappaport Coma/Near-Coma Scale (Rappaport et al., 1992)

(For patients with a Disability Rating (DR) score >21, i.e., Vegetative State)

(Complete form twice a day for 3 days then weekly for 3 weeks; every two weeks thereafter if DR score >21. If DR <21 follow monthly with DR scores)

NAME _____ SEX _____ DATE OF BIRTH _____ TYPE OF INJURY:MVA _____ STROKE _____ DR _____

DATE OF INJURY / ILLNESS _____ DATE OF ADMISSION _____ HEAD INJURY _____ ANOXIA _____ DATE _____

FACILITY _____ RATER _____ OTHER (describe) _____ TIME _____

Parameter	Stim #	Stimulus	# of trails	Response measure	Score options	Score criteria			
AUDITORY*	1	Bell ringing 5 sec. At 10 sec intervals	3	Eye opening, or orientation towards sound	0 / 2 / 4	3X / 1 or 2X / No response			
COMMAND RESPONSIVITY with priming **	2	Request patient to open or close eyes, mouth, or move finger, hard or leg	3	Response to command	0 / 2 / 4	Responds to command 2 or 3X / Tentative or inconsistent 1X, / No response			
VISUAL with priming** Must be able to open eyes; if not score 4 for each stimulus situation (items 3, 4, 5) and check here ___***___	3	Light flashes (1/sec. X5) in front; slightly left, right and up & down each trial	5	Fixation or avoidance	0 / 2 / 4	Sustained fixation or avoidance 3X / Partial fixation 1 or 2X / No response			
	4	Tell patient "Look at me"; move face 20" away from side to side	5	Fixation & tracking	0 / 2 / 4	Sustained tracking (for at least 3X) / Partial tracking 1 or 2X / No tracking			
THREAT	5	Quickly move hand forward to within 1–3" of eyes	3	Eye blink	0 / 2 / 4	3 blinks / 1 or 2 blinks / No blinks			
OLFACTORY (block tracheostomy 3D5secs. If present)	6	Ammonia capsule/bottle 1" under nose for about 2 seconds	3	Withdrawal (w/d) or other response linked to stimulus	0 / 2 / 4	Responds 2 or 3X quickly / Slowed/partial w/d; grimacing 1X / No w/d or grimacing			

(Continued overleaf)

451

APPENDIX 2 (Cont.)

Category	No.	Stimulus		Response tested	Score	Score criteria
TACTILE	7	Shoulder tap—Tap shoulder briskly 3X without speaking to patient; each side	3	Head or eye orientation or shoulder movement to tap	0 2 4	Orients toward tap 2 or 3X Partially orients 1X No orienting or response
	8	Nasal swab (each nostril; entrance only—do not penetrate deeply)	3	Withdrawal or eye blink or mouth twitch	0 2 4	Clear, quick (w/in 2 sec.) 2 or 3X Delayed or partial response 1X No response
PAIN (Allow up to 10 sec. For response) If spinal cord injury check here ___ and go to stimulis 10	9	Firm pinch finger tip; pressure of wood pencil across nail; each side	3	See Score criteria	0 2 4	Withdrawal 2 or 3X Gen. agita/non-specific movement 1X No response
	10	Robust ear pinch/pull X3; each side	3	Withdrawal or other response linked to stimulus	0 2 4	Responds 2 or 3X Gen. agita/non-specific movement 1X No response
VOCALISATION (assuming no tracheostomy) If tracheostomy present do not score but check here ___	11	None. (Score best response)	—	See Score criteria	0 2 4	Spontaneous words Non-verbal vocalis. (moan, groan) No sounds

Total CNC Score (add scores)	A
Number of items scored	B
Average CNC Score (A / B)	C
Coma/Near-Coma Level (0-4)	D

COMMENTS: (Include important changes in physical condition such as infection, pneumonia, hydrocephalus, seizures, further trauma, etc.)

* If possible use brain stem auditory evoked response (BAER) test at 80 db nHL to establish ability to hear in at least one ear.

** Whether or not patient appears receptive to speech, speak encouragingly and supportively for about 30 sec. to help establish awareness that another person is present. Advise the patient you will be asking him/her to make a simple response. Then request the patient to try to make the same response with brief priming before second, third and subsequent trials. Check with nursing staff on eye opening ability and arousability. Each side up to three repetitions if needed. Consult with nursing staff on arousability; do not judge solely on performance during testing. If patient is sleeping, repeat the assessment later.

SCORING

Level	Range (D)	Level of Awareness/Responsivity
0:	0.00–0.89:	*No coma*: consistently and readily responsive to at least 3 sensory stimulation tests (items 1–10) plus consistent responsitivity to simple commands.
1:	0.90–2.00:	*Near coma*: consistently responsive to stimulation presented to two sensory modalities and/or inconsistently or partially responsive to simple commands.
2:	2.01–2.89:	*Moderate coma*: inconsistently responsive to stimulation presented to two or three sensory modalities but not responsive to simple commands. May vocalise (in absence of tracheostomy) with moans, groans and grunts but no recognisable words.
3:	2.90–3.49:	*Marked coma*: inconsistently responsive to stimulation presented to one sensory modality and not responsive to simple commands.
4:	3.50–4.00:	*Extreme coma*: no responsivity to any sensory stimulation.

TRAINING NOTE TO NEW RATERS

While one person does the test, two, three or more observers rate each item *independently* (without discussion). Afterwards discuss ratings. If rating is changed, leave initial rating but place changed rating in parenthesis next to it. Repeat this process on 5–10 patients or until raters train themselves to place patients at least in the same category range. Thereafter single ratings can be used but, for purposes of reliabilitiy, a minimum of two independent ratings per patient is encouraged. Ratings should be done at about the same time each day if possible. Under "Comments" record special information that may have had an extraordinary effect on the ratings on a give day such as: Patient was severely ill with pneumonia; patient was vomiting; patient had known increase in intracranial pressure (viz. hydrocephalus); patient fell out of bed; etc.

NEUROPSYCHOLOGICAL REHABILITATION
2005, 15 (3/4), 454–460

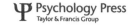

The JFK Coma Recovery Scale—Revised

Kathleen Kalmar and Joseph T. Giacino

*JFK Johnson Rehabilitation Institute, and New Jersey Neuroscience Institute,
JFK Medical Center, Edison, NJ, USA*

The JFK Coma Recovery Scale (CRS) was developed to help characterise and
monitor patients functioning at Rancho Levels I–IV and has been used widely
in both clinical and research settings within the US and Europe. The CRS was
recently revised to address a number of concerns emanating from our own clinical experience with the scale, feedback from users and researchers as well
as the results of Rasch analyses. Additionally, the CRS did not include all of
the behavioural criteria necessary to diagnose the minimally conscious state
(MCS), thereby limiting diagnostic utility. The revised JFK Coma Recovery
Scale (CRS-R) includes addition of new items, merging of items found to be
statistically similar, deletion or modification of items showing poor fit with
the scale's underlying construct, renaming of items, more stringent scoring criteria, and quantification of elicited behaviours to improve accuracy of rating.
Psychometric properties of the CRS-R appear to meet standards for measurement and evaluation tools for use in clinical and research settings, and diagnostic application suggests that the scale is capable of discriminating patients in the
minimally conscious state from those in the vegetative state.

INTRODUCTION

Specialised assessment instruments designed for use in patients with disorders of consciousness were first introduced in rehabilitation settings in
the early 1990s (Ansell & Kennan, 1989; Giacino, Kezmarsky, DeLuca, &

Correspondence should be addressed to: Kathleen Kalmar, Ph.D., JFK Johnson Rehabilitation
Institute at JFK Medical Center, Brain Trauma Unit/3 ER/Neuropsychology, 65 James Street,
Edison, NJ 08818, USA. Tel: 732-321-7762, Fax: 732-321-7921. Email: kkalmar@solarishs.org

Individuals interested in obtaining a copy of the JFK CRS-R and administration and scoring
procedures are referred to the authors.

http://www.tandf.co.uk/journals/pp/09602011.html   DOI:10.1080/09602010443000425

Cicerone, 1991; Gill-Thwaites, 1997; Horn, Watson, Wilson, & McLellan, 1992; Rader, Alston, & Ellis, 1989; Rappaport, Dougherty, & Kelting, 1992). The primary indications for use of such instruments in this patient population include diagnostic assessment, outcome prediction, projection of disposition needs, interdisciplinary treatment planning and monitoring treatment effectiveness. The JFK Coma Recovery Scale (CRS) (Giacino et al., 1991) was developed to more fully characterise and monitor patients functioning at Level I (Generalised Response) to Level IV (Confused–Agitated Response) on the Rancho Los Amigos Levels of Cognitive Functioning Scale (Hagen, Malkmus, & Durham, 1972). The original version of the CRS was comprised of six subscales addressing auditory, visual, motor, oromotor, communication, and arousal processes with the individual subscale items ordered in a hierarchical manner. The lowest item on each subscale represented reflexive activity while the highest items represented cognitively-mediated behaviours. Administration was conducted in a standardised manner and scoring was based on the presence or absence of specific elicited behavioural responses within the neurobehavioural domains identified above.

The CRS has been used widely in both clinical and research settings within the US and Europe, and its appropriateness for use in patients with disorders of consciousness has been demonstrated in a number of studies (Giacino et al., 1991; Giacino & Croll, 1991; Giacino & Kalmar, 1994, 1997; Kalmar & Giacino, 1995, 1998; Thompson, Sherer, Nick, Yablon, Hoge, Gaines, et al. (1999). The validity of the CRS as an assessment tool for detecting change in neurobehavioural responsiveness was demonstrated in an early paper by Giacino et al. (1991). That same year, Giacino and Croll (1991) found a predictive relationship between time to recovery of specific neurological signs and functional outcome based on improved Disability Rating Scale (DRS) scores in individuals with severe traumatic brain injury (TBI). Using regression analyses, these authors found that scores on the CRS motor subscale at one month post-injury were most predictive of DRS outcome at one year; motor and communication subscale scores were most predictive of 12-month outcome at three months and auditory subscale scores were most predictive at six months. In general, changes in CRS auditory, motor and communication subscale scores from months 1–3 post-injury were predictive of functional outcome at one year while CRS changes from 3–6 months were not. Using weighted CRS scores, Giacino and Kalmar (1994) explored the influence of injury aetiology (TBI and non-TBI) on rate and extent of recovery across the first year post-injury. Level of functional disability across the first year post-injury by diagnosis (vegetative state, VS, and the minimally conscious state, MCS, as determined by the CRS) and aetiology of injury (TBI and non-TBI) was studied by Giacino and Kalmar (1997). These authors also examined the incidence of selected neurobehavioural signs in VS and MCS to determine whether there were defining differences in the clinical features characterising these conditions. The CRS was also used to monitor recovery of consciousness in 25 patients undergoing rehabilitation (Thompson et al., 1999). These authors then used time to recovery of consciousness to predict change in cognitive functioning from admission to discharge from the rehabilitation setting.

DEVELOPMENT OF THE JFK COMA RECOVERY SCALE—REVISED

The purpose of this paper is to provide a summary review of the newly revised JFK Coma Recovery Scale. Readers interested in the methodology used to investigate the psychometric properties of the CRS-R, changes to subscale items, and the diagnostic utility of the CRS-R, are referred to Giacino, Kalmar, and Whyte (2004).

The CRS was recently revised to address a number of administration and scoring concerns emanating from our own clinical experience with the scale, usefulness of some of the items, feedback from other CRS users, and studies completed by outside researchers (O'Dell, Jasin, Lyons, Stivers, & Meszaro, 1996a; O'Dell et al., 1996b). Additionally, Rasch analysis, a statistical procedure that quantifies how well a test is measuring a proposed underlying dimension (i.e., neurobehavioural responsiveness) and the degree of "fit" between task difficulty and ability level of the examinee, had been conducted. These analyses indicated that although the CRS met statistical requirements for unidimensionality of neurobehavioural function and equal interval measurement, some subscales contained misfitting items (Kalmar & Giacino, 2000). The third impetus for revision of the CRS was related to the recent development of diagnostic criteria for the MCS recommended by the Aspen Workgroup (Giacino, Ashwal, Childs, Cranford, Jennett, Katz, et al., 2002). The Aspen Workgroup proposed novel behavioural criteria for differentiating MCS from VS and to establish emergence from MCS. The original CRS did not include all of the behavioural criteria necessary to diagnose MCS which limited its diagnostic utility. In view of these concerns, modifications were made to all six subscales of the CRS, yielding the 23-item JFK Coma Recovery Scale—Revised. The CRS-R Record Form is shown in Appendix 1.

Participants in the psychometric studies were 80 severely brain injured patients receiving comprehensive acute inpatient rehabilitation. Twenty of these were studied prospectively in order to obtain data for the reliability investigation. Patients had sustained traumatic, vascular and anoxic/ischaemic brain injuries and one patient was recovering from tumour resection. The CRS-R was administered to all participants by practising clinicians with 15–20 years of experience working with patients with disorders of consciousness (KK, JG). Non-parametric statistical analyses were employed due to the ordinal nature of the scale. These included Spearman ρ correlations and Wilcoxon Sign Rank tests. Cohen's κ and Cronbach's α were also used.

Modifications to the revised scale include addition of new items, merging of items found to be statistically similar in terms of their ability to differentiate patients' neurobehavioural status, deletion of items demonstrating poor fit with the underlying construct measured by the CRS, and renaming of items to provide better face validity for the behaviours they represent. Scoring criteria are more stringent and occurrences of elicited behaviours are quantified to improve accuracy of ratings. Additionally, items known to represent behaviours indicative of MCS or emergence from MCS are denoted on the response profile to facilitate accurate diagnosis once the examination has been completed and scored.

Analyses of the psychometric integrity of the CRS-R show the new scale to be a reliable and valid measure of neurobehavioural responsiveness (Giacino et al., 2004). Inter-rater and test–retest reliability for the CRS-R total score were high indicating that the scale yields reproducible findings across examiners and stability in patient performance over a brief assessment period. Analysis of internal consistency indicated that the CRS-R represents a homogeneous measure of neurobehavioural function. High concurrent validity was demonstrated between the CRS-R and the CRS total scores and between the CRS-R and the DRS (Rappaport et al., 1982) total scores. Due to the uneven data spread among items within each subscale, it was not possible to assess the reliability of the six CRS-R subscales. For this reason, individual subscale scores should be used cautiously until additional data become available. Table 1 shows the psychometric properties of the CRS-R.

A high incidence of misdiagnosis among individuals with disorders of consciousness has been reported in several studies (Tresch et al., 1991; Childs,

TABLE 1
Psychometric properties of the CRS-R

Sample Norms ($n = 80$)		
Mean	12.31	
Standard deviation	4.50	
Range	1–23	
Validity ($n = 80$)		
DRS	$r_s = -.90$	$p = .00001$
CRS	$r_s = .97$	$p = .00001$
Reliability ($n = 20$)		
Inter-rater	$r_s = .84$	$p = .001$
Test–retest	$r_s = .94$	$p = .001$
Internal consistency	Cronbach's $\alpha = .83$	
Measures of dispersion ($n = 80$)		
Skewness/SE skewness	0.41 (n.s.)	
Kurtosis/SE kurtosis	-1.34 (n.s.)	

Mercer, & Childs, 1993; Andrews, Murphy, Munday, & Littlewood, 1996). The most commonly reported error is a false positive diagnosis of VS in patients who are actually in MCS. Analyses have shown that diagnostic agreement between raters, and for the same rater over time, is high indicating that examiners can distinguish VS, MCS and emergence from MCS using the CRS-R (Giacino et al., 2004). Although diagnostic agreement between the CRS-R and DRS (Rappaport et al., 1982) has been shown to be high (87%), the CRS-R appears to be more sensitive to detecting MCS. A study of 80 patients by Giacino and associates (2004) identified 10 cases in which the CRS-R profile indicated a diagnosis of MCS while the DRS findings were indicative of VS. These preliminary data suggest that the CRS-R may improve the accuracy of differential diagnosis among this population of patients.

CONCLUSIONS

The CRS-R appears to meet the Measurement Standards for Interdisciplinary Medical Rehabilitation as set forth by the American Congress of Rehabilitation Medicine (Johnson, Keith, & Hinderer, 1992). The scale can be administered reliably by trained examiners and produces reasonably stable scores over repeated assessments. Validity analyses support use of the scale as an index of neurobehavioural function, although individual subscale scores should be used cautiously until additional data become available. Diagnostic application of the CRS-R suggests that the scale is capable of discriminating patients in MCS from those in VS; however, this will need to be confirmed by future empirical studies. Additional reliability studies with multiple rater pairs and a larger subject pool are being explored, and we are currently collecting data for Rasch analysis of the revised scale. It should be stressed that although assessment instruments such as the CRS-R used to evaluate patients with disorders of consciousness need to possess adequate psychometric characteristics and standardised administration procedures in order to prevent misdiagnosis, no diagnosis should be made on the basis of one assessment or the impressions of one examiner. Diagnostic accuracy is generally facilitated by incorporating input from other treating professionals familiar with the patient.

REFERENCES

Andrews, K., Murphy, L., Munday, R., & Littlewood, C. (1996). Misdiagnosis of the vegetative state: Retrospective study in a rehabilitation unit. *British Medical Journal, 313*, 13–16.
Ansell, B. J., & Kennan, J. E. (1989). The Western Neuro Sensory Stimulation Profile: A tool for assessing slow-to-recover head-injured patients. *Archives of Physical Medicine and Rehabilitation, 70*, 104–108.
Childs, N. L., Mercer, W. N., & Childs, H. W. (1993). Accuracy of diagnosis of persistent vegetative state. *Neurology, 43*, 1465–1467.

Giacino, J. T., Ashwal, S. A., Childs, N., Cranford, R., Jennett, B., & Katz, D. I. et al. (2002). The minimally conscious state: Definition and diagnostic criteria. *Neurology, 58,* 349–353.

Giacino, J. T., & Croll, S. (1991). Temporo-sequential neurologic markers used to predict outcome following severe traumatic brain injury (abstract). *Archives of Physical Medicine and Rehabilitation, 72,* 798.

Giacino, J. T., & Kalmar, K. (1994). Predicting outcome after brain injury with the JFK Coma Recovery Scale (abstract). *Archives of Physical Medicine and Rehabilitation, 75,* 723–724.

Giacino, J. T., & Kalmar, K. (1997). The vegetative and minimally conscious states: A comparison of clinical features and functional outcome. *Journal of Head Trauma Rehabilitation, 12,* 36–51.

Giacino, J. T., Kalmar, K., & Whyte, J. (2004). The JFK Coma Recovery Scale—Revised: Measurement characteristics and diagnostic utility. *Archives of Physical Medicine and Rehabilitation, 85*(12), 2020–2029.

Giacino, J. T., Kezmarsky, M. A., DeLuca, J., & Cicerone, K. D. (1991). Monitoring rate of recovery to predict outcome in minimally responsive patients. *Archives of Physical Medicine and Rehabilitation, 72,* 897–901.

Gill-Thwaites, H. (1997). The Sensory Modality Assessment Rehabilitation Technique—A tool for assessment and treatment of patients with severe brain injury in a vegetative state. *Brain Injury, 10,* 723–724.

Hagen, C., Malkmus, D., & Durham, P. (1972). *Levels of cognitive function.* Downey, CA: Rancho Los Amigo Hospital, unpublished measure.

Horn, S., Watson, M., Wilson, B. A., & McLellan, D. L. (1992). The development of new techniques in the assessment and monitoring of recovery from severe head injury: A preliminary report and case history. *Brain Injury, 6*(4), 321–325.

Johnson, M. V., Keith, R. A., & Hinderer, S. R. (1992). Measurement standards for interdisciplinary medical rehabilitation. *Archives of Physical Medicine and Rehabilitation, 73*(Suppl), 3–23.

Kalmar, K., & Giacino, J. T. (1995). Comparison of rates of recovery and outcome in vegetative and minimally responsive patients following traumatic vs. nontraumatic brain injury [abstract]. *Archives of Physical Medical and Rehabilitation, 76,* 597.

Kalmar, K., & Giacino, J. T. (1998). Visual tracking in the vegetative state: a predictor of eventual recovery of consciousness? (abstract). *Archives of Physical Medicine and Rehabilitation, 79,* 1322.

Kalmar, K., & Giacino, J. T. (2000). The JFK Coma Recovery Scale: An ordinal or interval measure? (abstract). *Archives of Physical Medicine and Rehabilitation, 81,* 1619.

O'Dell, M. W., Jasin, P., Lyons, N., Stivers, M., & Meszaro, F. (1996a). Standardized assessment instruments for minimally-responsive, brain-injured patients. *Neuro-Rehabilitation, 6,* 45–55.

O'Dell, M. W., Jasin, P., Stivers, M., Lyons, N., Schmidt, S., & Moore, D. E. (1996b). Interrater reliability of the Coma Recovery Scale. *Journal of Head Trauma Rehabilitation, 11,* 61–66.

Rader, M. A., Alston, J. B., & Ellis, D. W. (1989). Sensory stimulation of severely brain-injured patients. *Brain Injury, 3,* 141–147.

Rappaport, M., Dougherty, A. M., & Kelting, D. L. (1992). Evaluation of coma and vegetative states. *Archives of Physical Medicine and Rehabilitation, 73,* 628–634.

Rappaport, M., Hall, K. M., Hopkins, K., Belleza, T., & Cope, D. N. (1982). Disability Rating Scale for severe head trauma: Coma to community. *Archives of Physical Medicine and Rehabilitation, 63,* 118–123.

Thompson, N., Sherer, M., Nick, T., Yablon, S., Hoye, W., Gaines, C. et al. (1999). Predicting change in functional outcome in minimally responsive patients using the Coma Recovery Scale. *Archives of Clinical Neuropsychology, 14*(8), 790–791.

Tresch, D. D., Sims, F. H., Duthie, E. H., Goldstein, M. D., & Lane, P. S. (1991). Clinical characteristics of patients in the persistent vegetative state. *Archives of Physical Medicine and Rehabilitation, 151,* 930–932.

APPENDIX 1

CRS-R Record Form

JFK COMA RECOVERY SCALE - REVISED ©2004
Record Form

Patient: Date:									
AUDITORY FUNCTION SCALE									
4 - Consistent Movement to Command *									
3 - Reproducible Movement to Command *									
2 - Localization to Sound									
1 - Auditory Startle									
0 - None									
VISUAL FUNCTION SCALE									
5 - Object Recognition *									
4 - Object Localization: Reaching *									
3 - Visual Pursuit *									
2 - Fixation *									
1 - Visual Startle									
0 - None									
MOTOR FUNCTION SCALE									
6 - Functional Object Use †									
5 - Automatic Motor Response *									
4 - Object Manipulation *									
3 - Localization to Noxious Stimulation *									
2 - Flexion Withdrawal									
1 - Abnormal Posturing									
0 - None/Flaccid									
OROMOTOR/VERBAL FUNCTION SCALE									
3 - Intelligible Verbalization *									
2 - Vocalization/Oral Movement									
1 - Oral Reflexive Movement									
0 - None									
COMMUNICATION SCALE									
2 - Functional: Accurate †									
1 - Non-Functional: Intentional *									
0 - None									
AROUSAL SCALE									
3 - Attention									
2 - Eye Opening w/o Stimulation									
1 - Eye Opening with Stimulation									
0 - Unarousable									
TOTAL SCORE									

Denotes emergence from MCS †

Denotes MCS *

NEUROPSYCHOLOGICAL REHABILITATION
2005, 15 (3/4), 461–472

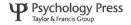

Rehabilitation practice following profound brain damage

Keith Andrews

Royal Hospital for Neuro-Rehabilitation, London, UK

The rehabilitation of the person with profound brain damage is a complex process requiring the skills of a true interdisciplinary team. The process is as much about the ability to: assess and diagnose; provide the optimal environment for recovery; prevent and treat secondary complications; support the family; and modify the environment as it is about a formal rehabilitation programme. Ideally these should be seamless but each contains many challenges, including the experience and skills of the observer, the ability to communicate with members of the family, and the ability to work within an interdisciplinary team.

INTRODUCTION

One of the problems of managing patients in vegetative or minimally conscious states has been the rarity of these conditions. This has meant that few staff see sufficient patients to gain the necessary body of experience. Rehabilitation units in the UK have been reluctant to accept patients with such profound brain damage although this is now beginning to change. For many years there was only one centre in the UK specialising in the management of people in a vegetative and minimally conscious state although, again, some units are developing a few beds specifically for this group of patients.

The potential for rehabilitation of the person in either the vegetative or minimally conscious state can seem to be an enormous task. Indeed many would argue that it is a pointless task since the person is obviously unable to contribute

Correspondence should be addressed to: Dr Keith Andrews, Director of Institute of Complex Neuro-Disability, Royal Hospital for Neuro-Rehabilitation, West Hill, Putney, London, SW15 3SW. Tel: 020 8780 4534, Fax: 020 8780 4503. Email: kandrews@rhn.org.uk

© 2005 Psychology Press Ltd
http://www.tandf.co.uk/journals/pp/09602011.html   DOI:10.1080/09602010443000326

to his or her own recovery. For this reason it is probably more appropriate to think in terms of disability management rather than rehabilitation.

This paper is not about the specific techniques of rehabilitation of the person in the vegetative state but about the concepts and principles of disability management.

There is, in fact, a considerable amount that can be achieved. It is important to recognise the objectives of the disability management programme. The first objective is to make sure that the diagnosis is correct. While this may seem to be an obvious fact there is plenty of evidence that misdiagnosis is common (Andrews, Murphy, Munday, & Littlewood, 1996; Childs, Mercer, & Childs, 1993; Tresch et al., 1991) and this is discussed elsewhere in this special issue. The second objective is to ensure an optimal level of recovery. The third objective is to ensure that once the person has reached stability that this level is maintained. Since profoundly brain damaged people can continue to show improvement over several years it is important that they are offered the opportunity to maintain whatever level of physical and mental ability they have achieved. If the levels of ability are not maintained then the disability management programme has been to some extent wasted.

ACHIEVING OPTIMAL LEVELS OF RECOVERY

In any rehabilitation programme for people with complex neurological problems there are five basic concepts to achieve the optimal level of recovery or improvement:

1. Provide the optimal environment for recovery.

2. Prevent and treat secondary complications.

3. Include in treatment physiotherapy and the other "therapies", medical, psychological and technological.

4. Support the family.

5. Modify the environment—including regulating the amount of stimulation.

These form the basis for ensuring that what potential there is for recovery is taken advantage of.

OPTIMAL ENVIRONMENT FOR RECOVERY

There is limited value in attempting rehabilitation techniques if there are factors mitigating against recovery. These can be internal to the patient or factors in the external environment.

Those internal to the patient include the general health, nutritional state, controlling infections and modifying medications.

Nutrition

A good nutritional state is essential for optimal recovery. Undernutrition results in poor healing of pressure sores, decreased resistance to infections and creates problems for carers in the physical management of the patient, such as sitting the patient out of bed, because of the risk of pressure sores.

In the early days following brain damage, especially when due to trauma, there is often a hypercatabolic state that will result in weight loss and may be difficult to make up. This can be as high as 15% of body weight per week and lack of nutritional support in the first week after brain injury increases the mortality rate (American Association of Neurological Surgeons, 2000). There is evidence (Falcao de Arruda & de Aguilar-Nascimento, 2004) that enteral feeding, especially with an enteral formula containing glutamine and probiotics, can decrease the infection rate and shorten the stay in the intensive care unit of brain injury patients. There is also evidence that starting with a good nutritional level decreases infections and other post-traumatic complications (Taylor, Fettes, Jewkes, & Nelson, 1999).

It can be very difficult to maintain a good nutritional state in someone who is unable to swallow. Nutrition in the early days following brain damage is provided by nasogastric tube in some units. However, the evidence (Akkersdijk, Roukema, & van der Werken, 1998; Annoni, Vuagnat, Frischknecht, & Uebelhart, 1998) is that percutaneous endoscopically placed gastrostomy (PEG) tube feeding has fewer complications and this is therefore now more frequently used in the early stages. PEG tube feeding has also been shown (Klodell, Carroll, Carrillo, & Spain, 2000) to be an effective and safe method of feeding patients with long-term brain damage.

One of the reasons that nutrition is still badly managed is the difficulty of weighing the patient and measuring height in a person who is deformed by contractures or spasticity—height and weight being required to assess the body mass index. Weighing requires either a weighing hoist or wheelchair weighing scales—sadly, these are rarely available in general wards.

Sphincter control

All patients with profound brain damage will be unable to control their bladder. Traditionally this has been managed by urethral catheters. The major disadvantage of this method of control is that it inevitably results in infection of the urine which, in the long term, can produce serious problems of kidney infection or encourage stones to form in the bladder or kidney. This may be due to the presence of a foreign body (the catheter) within the bladder on which bacteria can grow or it may be due to catheterisation techniques. The use of long-term antimicrobial agents in general have not been effective in preventing catheter-associated urinary tract infection in people with long-term indwelling urethral catheters and therefore, because of the complications of antibiotic therapy, should be avoided wherever possible (Trautner & Darouiche, 2004).

Urinary retention does occur in brain damage and is usually associated with diabetes mellitus or faecal impaction (Chua, Chuo, & Kong, 2003). In general it is more appropriate to use a condom-like sheath connected to a collecting bag for males. In females the use of pads to soak up the urine is considered the best compromise. These approaches seem to result in fewer long-term problems.

All patients with profound brain damage will be unable to control their bowel action. This is further complicated by the fact that immobile people (no matter how fit otherwise) tend to become constipated. In chronic immobility this can become a serious problem with loading of much of the large bowel and the risk of bowel obstruction, and it may also result in compression urinary retention.

In general both the constipation and the incontinence of faeces can be managed by giving suppositories two or three times a week. This usually results in bowel action on the day the suppository was given and continence on other days.

Bowel action is further supported by the skilled intervention of the dietician in providing a well-balanced diet containing fibre.

Prevention of infection

Maintenance of good general health is essential for optimal opportunities for recovery. There are several approaches required to prevent infections, including maintenance of good nutrition as discussed above. However, there are also other methods of preventing infections. The clinical impression is that gastrostomy tube feeding, as opposed to nasogastric feeding, has decreased the risk of chest infections. Similarly good oral hygiene, although difficult, is an essential part of preventing chest infections from inhaled bacteria.

Many patients have a clenching, or bite, reflex of the jaws when their lips or the face are touched. This constant biting, often associated with grinding of the teeth (bruxism), can wear down the surface of the teeth. Thorough brushing by carers and the use of antibacterial gels and fluoride help to prevent dental caries and gum disease. The dentist can provide special teeth guards to decrease this damage to the teeth, but they are not always effective.

Where a mouth becomes infected there is a risk of inhalation of the infected material into the lungs increasing the risk of chest infections or pneumonia.

The general maintenance of hygiene, although often seen as an unimportant basic procedure is fundamental in preventing infections. This is not only in the hygiene of the patient but also that of staff and the environment. This is seen particularly in the importance of hygiene of staff in the prevention of methicillin (or multi-) resistant staphylococcus aureus (MRSA). This is particularly relevant since most vegetative patients will have vulnerable wounds such as gastrostomy and tracheostomy sites.

It has been pointed out above that the avoidance of indwelling catheterisation of the bladder helps to decrease the risk of bladder infections which in turn may lead to kidney or blood infection.

Monitoring of drug therapy

Unfortunately many of the drugs required for brain damaged patients are to control the features of brain damage—such as epilepsy, muscle spasms, increased muscle tone or bladder function abnormalities. This means that the side effects will often also affect brain function. It, therefore, takes great skill in balancing the beneficial effect of all the drugs (separately and in combination) against the side effects and disadvantages.

Management of pre-existing conditions

Patients with brain damage are as susceptible to having had medical problems before the injury as the average man in the street. Indeed, some conditions, such as alcoholism, may be more prevalent in those who eventually have a brain injury than in the general public. Much of the medical input in the management of the brain damaged person is in controlling conditions such as diabetes mellitus, pre-existing heart or lung disease or other medical conditions. The treatment is as in the standard medical textbooks. However, if pre-existing conditions are not dealt with efficiently and with some degree of expertise then they can be a major barrier to recovery. This is particularly relevant where the profoundly brain damaged person is managed at home or in a nursing home rather than under the care of a physician.

Prevention and treatment of secondary complications

Secondary complications are those features that occur following the brain damage that are not a directly due to the brain damage or are a preventable consequence of the brain damage. Pressure sores are a good example of this; osteoporosis from disuse of limbs is another, although less preventable, condition. Contractures possibly also fall into this group although this is more debatable.

Prevention is an interdisciplinary team responsibility. Pressure sore prevention is often thought of as being a nursing staff responsibility but this is misunderstanding the cause of pressure sores. Pressure sores are rarely due to pressure—a deep sea diver has many more times the pressure on his skin that would be regarded as the cause of a pressure sore in a disabled person. The reason the diver does not develop pressure sores is because the pressure is distributed over a wide area. Pressure sores, or more appropriately decubitus ulceration, are due to distortion, stretching or abrasion of the skin exacerbated by poor nutrition and incontinence. Thus, maintaining a good nutritional state, providing supportive seating, and careful posturing and positioning of the patient by all members of the team—including families and porters—are important methods of prevention.

TREATMENT OF THE VEGETATIVE PATIENT

Having taken into account the essential prerequisites for optimal recovery there are two major functions that demand attention—the physical management of posture and positioning and the improvement in mental function. These are not separate functions but are closely intertwined. An example of this is one patient in our misdiagnosis study (Andrews et al., 1996) who was misdiagnosed for over a year, only demonstrating his awareness when he was provided with a purpose built seating system that gave support to release sufficient muscle tone for him to shrug his shoulder to indicate his awareness. The assessment of awareness is dealt with elsewhere in this special issue and therefore I will concentrate on the physical management.

Postural management

A seated posture is important for mental responses. There are two main reasons for this. The first is the arousal effect sitting or standing has on the ascending reticular formation in the brain stem. The concept of decreased activity in the ascending reticular formation has been the basis for electrical stimulation of the brain stem (Tsubokawa et al., 1990). This is a technique that has been used mainly in Japan.

The second reason is to provide optimal posturing to help release muscle spasticity, thereby giving a better chance for the patient to demonstrate any awareness. A third reason is that good postural support helps to prevent deformities and decubitus ulceration.

There are, however, problems in achieving good seating for a profoundly brain damaged person due to difficulty maintaining good posture, the risk of increasing the abnormal muscle tone patterns, and the risk of developing pressure sores if the patient is not positioned well. This takes a considerable amount of skill by several members of the team. Access to a team experienced in specialist seating of such profoundly disabled people is a major need but only a few centres around the country have developed this level of expertise.

Control of muscle tone and prevention of deformities

The degree and type of muscle tone abnormalities vary with the area(s) and site(s) of the brain damaged. Some people do not get an increase in muscle tone but most severely brain damaged people get a very marked increase in muscle tone which eventually leads to fixed deformities or contractures.

The pattern of extension or flexion abnormalities depends on the site of the lesion. The patient who has rigidity flexion of the arms, clenched fists, and extended legs (decorticate posturing) usually has damage to the corticospinal tract. The patient who has rigid extension of the arms and legs, downward pointing of the toes, and backward arching of the head (decerebrate posturing) usually has a lesion at the level of the upper brain stem or above. Decerebrate posturing has a poorer prognosis than decorticate posturing. In severe cases opisthotonos (a severe muscle spasm of the neck and back) may accompany decerebrate posture. Decerebrate posture occurs in many patterns. It can occur on one side, on both sides, or in just the arms. It may alternate with decorticate posture, or a person can have decorticate posture on one side and decerebrate posture on the other.

Several techniques can help minimise the effect of the muscle tone:

1. Avoid noxious stimulation, such as cold, heat, pain, and excess noise— all of which tend to increase the muscle tone reflexes.

2. Maintain a good supported position in bed and in a chair. This requires the skilled advice of a physiotherapist to identify the optimal position for the individual patients depending on the type of neurological damage. This also requires the provision of special seating.

3. Hydrotherapy can temporarily help control muscle tone.

The general approaches to postural management described above can help to maintain a reasonable level of positioning. However, spasticity is still difficult to control with these methods and, therefore, consideration needs to be given to other forms of treatment such as oral anti-spastic medication (such as baclofen, dantrolene sodium, clonidine or tizanidine), injection of the nerves (as with phenol, Jarrett, Nandi, & Thompson, 2002; Ward, 2003) or muscle (as with botulinum toxin), intrathecal infusion (as with baclofen) or even surgery to section nerves permanently or manage the contractures.

Oral drug therapy seems to have less effect on the spasticity of brain damage than in spinal cord injuries and therefore botulinum toxin has become one of the mainstay methods of treating severe spasticity in acquired brain damage and can be very effective (Yablon, Agana, Ivanhoe, & Boake, 1996). In some cases long-term intrathecal infusion of baclofen may be required (Becker, Alberti, & Bauer, 1997; Meythaler, Guin-Renfroe, Grabb, & Hadley, 1999) to control the spasticity and spasms. Indeed it has been suggested (Francois et al., 2001) that intrathecal baclofen be used in the early stages to decrease the autonomic effects and spasticity following brain injury.

It is impossible in a short paper to discuss all of the therapeutic skills required in the management of the vegetative patient. The work requires a considerable interdisciplinary approach. It is probably better to think in terms of functional needs rather than discipline specific functions. For instance maintaining a good nutritional state and improving swallowing requires the combined skills of the nurse (to feed the patient), dietician (to monitor the nutritional requirements), physiotherapist and occupational therapist (to provide optimal posture management), oral hygienist and dentist (to ensure effective oral management); speech and language therapist (to desensitise hyperactive oral reflexes and to assist in retraining swallowing); ENT specialist (to carry out fibro-optic investigations of swallowing), physician (to monitor and manage the medical conditions producing catabolic states and nutritional demands) and even the biomedical engineer (to provide a well-designed postural support system—for both in bed and sitting).

Similarly, postural and positional control as well as spasticity management is not something left to the nurses while waiting for therapy. It is a 24-hour management requirement by all people working with the patient, including porters and family, if only to know what actions or activities to avoid that are likely to make the spasticity worse.

The management of the mental state again requires an interdisciplinary approach. A variety of clinicians may take the lead in assessment of the mental state depending on the skills available in the various units. In our unit it has been the occupational therapists, but in other units it may well be a clinical psychologist, speech and language therapist or nurse. Irrespective of who takes the lead, all members of the team have responsibilities in ensuring optimal opportunities for demonstrating awareness if it is present. This implies recording any observations they make that will contribute to the total picture of responses throughout the 24-hour period. It also implies ensuring that the factors that inhibit responses are avoided. This includes excessive stimulation, poor positioning, and over-sedation and ensuring appropriate rest periods between treatment sessions.

There are five basic factors that influence the responses: the physical ability to respond (discussed under postural management); the desire or willingness to respond (some patients respond better to one person than another); the ability of clinicians to observe accurately; adequate time available for observation/assessment (it is time consuming if the assessment is to be carried out properly); and access to reliable assessment tools (these are discussed elsewhere in this special issue).

There are also some basic principles of assessment and treatment sessions that need to be adhered to. These include carrying out the session after a rest period (rushing in an assessment period between the nursing procedure and a physiotherapy session is unlikely to provide optimal outcome); identifying windows of opportunity (the patient rarely produces the best responses conveniently for the booked session); and keeping the sessions short, repeated and over a period of time.

FAMILY SUPPORT

The vegetative state has a devastating effect on family life. Each member of the family experiences several feelings, the degree of which varies depending on the person's isolation, abandonment, fear about the future, guilt and, most of all, incompetence in front of the complexity of the problems they may face (Mondain, 1991). Families often oscillate between acceptance and denial, with clinical presentations of sadness, exhaustion, weariness, denial, flight, excessive protection, aggressiveness, and anger.

Tasseau and his colleagues (1992) at the Centre Medical De L'Argentiere, Aveize in France has taken a lead in working with families. They have developed a programme of working with families to provide three levels of support: helping the family throughout the observation process; providing the family with a socio-administrative support; and providing the family with psychological support.

The family has the knowledge of the patient prior to the brain damage and although the majority of patients will need to be cared for long-term in a residential setting, it is the family who remains the main advocate on behalf of the patient. Equally, family members develop their own expertise, based on experience, in the management of the specific patient.

The needs of patients and their families are complex but the main areas of need are as follows.

Information

Information is by far the most important requirement listed by families. They want to know what has happened, why it has happened, what is going to happen and can anything more be done by anyone else—anywhere. Because of the rarity of the disorder and the general lack of experience it can be difficult to answer many of these questions.

Counselling

Emotional support and counselling are important because of the impact profound brain damage has on the family. Social workers, along with clinical psychologists, are able to assess for, and in some cases provide, counselling services; or provide the link into the appropriate service to help the individual patient and family.

Financial issues

Many families run into financial difficulties when they have lost a wage earner or have additional expense involved in caring for or visiting the patient. Social workers can advise families about access to benefits and grants and guide them through Court of Protection and compensation matters.

Social workers can also support by advising on access to other resources and agencies with regard to housing and travel.

Social support and continuing care

Deciding on a long-term placement which meets the needs of both the patient and the family is a difficult task both emotionally and practically. Social workers bring to families knowledge of resources and options of health and social service requirements. They can also provide the skilled support necessary to guide patients and families through the major transitions from acute care through rehabilitation into long-term care.

Ongoing and long-term emotional, practical and social support is also available from social service departments. Voluntary agencies, such as Headway, provide long-term support in local and national groups in the form of literature, advice and conferences.

One of the major needs is that of involvement. Some clinical teams are very good at working with the family but it is well recognised that many families are difficult to work with. The psychological reactions described above often make them challenging to staff who then become defensive and take avoidance action. This simply increases the family view that staff are not interested, thus exacerbating the breakdown in relationships.

CONTROLLED ENVIRONMENT

One of the more difficult concepts of care is the provision of the optimal environment for recovery. There is a natural inclination to want to "stimulate" the person to recovery—thus the constant playing of favourite music and wanting to keep the patient awake and active. Sleep is one of nature's ways of aiding recovery of tissues. Wood (1991) has argued for providing a controlled environment of sensory *regulation* to avoid sensory overload of severely damaged brain patients. Since it is likely that these patients have problems with selective attention, sensory input should be simple and interspersed with periods of rest. It is, therefore, logical to assess for cognitive responses after a period of rest rather than after a period of activity, such as being washed and dressed or after a period of physiotherapy. This requires staff and family to understand the importance of avoiding overstimulation prior to the assessment. It also has implications for the control of the ward environment. It is relatively easy in a unit dedicated to profoundly brain injured people to structure the time when there is general activity on the ward, including the playing of radios or TVs. It is much more difficult to regulate stimulation in a busy general environment.

CONCLUSION

In conclusion, profound brain damage requires considerable resources, skills and experience to manage well. It is not the domain of any single discipline but requires the skills of a well-integrated interdisciplinary team. It also requires the support and involvement of the family who will have the long-term responsibility after the formal rehabilitation programme is ended.

REFERENCES

Akkersdijk, W. L., Roukema, J. A., & van der Werken, C. (1998). Percutaneous endoscopic gastrostomy for patients with severe cerebral injury. *Injury*, *29*(1),11–4.

American Association of Neurological Surgeons (2000). The joint section on neurotrauma and critical care: Nutrition. *Journal of Neurotrauma*, *17*(6–7), 539–547.

Andrews, K., Murphy, L., Munday, R., & Littlewood, C. (1996). Misdiagnosis of the vegetative state: Retrospective study in a rehabilitation unit. *British Medical Journal*, *313*, 13–6.

Annoni, J. M., Vuagnat, H., Frischknecht, R., & Uebelhart, D. (1998). Percutaneous endoscopic gastrostomy in neurological rehabilitation: A report of six cases. *Disability and Rehabilitation*, *20*(8), 308–314.

Becker, R., Alberti, O., & Bauer, B. L. (1997). Continuous intrathecal baclofen infusion in severe spasticity after traumatic or hypoxic brain injury, *Journal of Neurology*, *244*(3), 160–166.

Chua, K., Chuo, A., & Kong, K. H. (2003). Urinary incontinence after traumatic brain injury: Incidence, outcomes and correlates. *Brain Injury*, *17*(6), 469–478.

Childs, N. L., Mercer, W. N., & Childs, H. W. (1993). Accuracy of diagnosis of persistent vegetative state. *Neurology*, *43*, 1465–1467.

Falcao de Arruda, I. S., & de Aguilar-Nascimento, J. E. (2004). Benefits of early enteral nutrition with glutamine and probiotics in brain injury patients *Clinical Science*, *106*(3), 287–292.

Francois, B., Vacher, P., Roustan, J., Salle, J. Y., Vidal, J., Moreau, J. J., & Vignon, P. (2001). Intrathecal baclofen after traumatic brain injury: Early treatment using a new technique to prevent spasticity. *Journal of Trauma-Injury Infection and Critical Care*, *50*(1), 158–161.

Jarrett, L., Nandi, P., & Thompson, A. J. (2002). Managing severe lower limb spasticity in multiple sclerosis: Does intrathecal phenol have a role? *Journal of Neurology, Neurosurgery and Psychiatry*, *73*(6), 705–709.

Klodell, C. T., Carroll, M., Carrillo, E. H., & Spain, D. A. (2000). Routine intragastric feeding following traumatic brain injury is safe and well tolerated. *American Journal of Surgery*, *179*(3), 168–171.

Meythaler, J. M., Guin-Renfroe, S., Grabb, P., & Hadley, M. N. (1999). Long-term continuously infused intrathecal baclofen for spastic-dystonic hypertonia in traumatic brain injury: 1-year experience. *Archives of Physical Medicine and Rehabilitation, 80*(1), 13–19.

Mondain, M. J. (1991). Le traumatisé crânien et sa famille (la famille traumatisée). Problèms en médecine de rééducation. *Traumatisme crânien grave et médecine de rééducation* (pp. 319–323). Paris: Masson Ed.

Tasseau, F., Berard, E., Sermet, G., Le Blay, G., & Reggad, Z. (1992). Les enjeux du diagnostic d'état végétatif chronique pour le clinicien. Problèmes en médecine de rééducation. *Traumatisme crânien et médecine de rééducation* (pp. 55–59). Paris: Masson Ed.

Taylor, S. J., Fettes, S. B., Jewkes, C., & Nelson, R. J. (1999). Prospective, randomized, controlled trial to determine the effect of early enhanced enteral nutrition on clinical outcome in mechanically ventilated patients suffering head injury. *Critical Care Medicine, 27*(11), 2525–2531.

Trautner, B. W., & Darouiche, R. O. (2004). Catheter-associated infections: Pathogenesis affects prevention. *Archives of Internal Medicine, 164*(8), 842–850.

Tresch, D. D., Farrol, H. S., Duthie, E. H., Goldstein, M. D., & Lane, P. S. (1991). Clinical characteristics of patients in the persistent vegetative state. *Archives of Internal Medicine, 151,* 930–932.

Tsubokawa, T., Yamamoto, T., Katayama, Y., Hirayama, T., Maejima, S., & Moriya, T. (1990). Deep-brain stimulation in a persistent vegetative state: Follow-up results and criteria for selection of candidates. *Brain Injury, 4*(4), 315–327.

Ward, A. B. (2003). Long-term modification of spasticity. *Journal of Rehabilitation Medicine, 41* (Suppl), 60–65.

Wood, R. L. (1991). Critical analysis of the concept of sensory stimulation for patients in the vegetative state. *Brain Injury, 5,* 401–409.

Yablon, S. A., Agana, B. T., Ivanhoe, C. B., & Boake, C. (1996). Botulinum toxin in severe upper extremity spasticity among patients with traumatic brain injury: An open-labelled trial. *Neurology, 47*(4), 939–944.

NEUROPSYCHOLOGICAL REHABILITATION
2005, 15 (3/4), 473–479

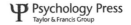

Rehabilitation outcome evaluation after very severe brain injury

Marlene Reimer and Carole-Lynne LeNavenec

Faculty of Nursing, University of Calgary, Calgary, Alberta, Canada

Few centres provide long-term therapy for survivors of very severe brain injury who continue in a minimally responsive state. We report on two outcome evaluation projects in association with one such centre in western Canada. In one project a functional scale to detect subtle changes after long-term therapy with the most severely compromised clients (Rancho levels II and III) is being tested. In the other project outcome indicators of change in quality of life after initiation of community-based rehabilitation have been generated by collecting over 400 critical incidents reported by family members, volunteers, staff and a few higher functioning clients. Our intention in this report is to highlight what can be done in terms of rehabilitation and outcome evaluation with clients who seem to be persisting in vegetative or minimally responsive states.

Correspondence should be addressed to: Marlene Reimer, Faculty of Nursing, University of Calgary, Calgary, Alberta, Canada T2N 1N4. Tel: 1 403 220-5839, Fax: 1 403 284-4803. Email: mareimer@ucalgary.ca

Neither of the research projects described in this paper would have been possible without the support of the Association for the Rehabilitation of the Brain Injured (ARBI) in Calgary, Alberta, Canada. In particular we want to acknowledge the work of Judy Stawnychko as Executive Director and the lead therapists, Mary Anne Ostapovitch, Program Director and Physical Therapist, Brenda Lee-Kemp, Physical Therapist, Sari Martin, Physical Therapist, Sharon Renton, Occupational Therapist, Arlene Lazoruk, Speech and Language Pathologist, Chamine Meghji, Speech and Language Pathologist and Ana Gollega, Occupational Therapist.

We gratefully acknowledge funding from Alberta Community Development and the University of Calgary Faculty of Nursing Research Endowment Fund. Our appreciation also goes to Patrizia Tolle from the University of Bremen, Germany who added conceptual insight in the data analysis of the second project during her study term with us.

http://www.tandf.co.uk/journals/pp/09602011.html   DOI:10.1080/09602010443000362

Few centres provide long-term, therapist supervised rehabilitation for adult survivors of very severe brain injury who continue in a state of minimal response to the environment. One such centre is the Association for the Rehabilitation of the Brain Injured (ARBI) in western Canada. In this article we briefly describe that programme and then discuss two research projects to evaluate community-based rehabilitation outcomes with this severely compromised population.

COMMUNITY-BASED REHABILITATION AT ARBI

This vision for something more, after standard publicly and insurance funded rehabilitation has been exhausted, started with the mother of a brain injured son and her friend. The son that she was told would probably remain in a vegetative state for the rest of his life now lives in his own home with minimal supervision, walks without assistance, writes legibly, speaks intelligibly, and works full-time. Most readers will be able to recount similar recovery stories. What is different about this one is that the two women went on to establish a non-profit organisation that now employs a staff of 30 that includes administrative support, therapists, support workers, and programme leaders, and engages between 60–70 volunteers weekly who contribute in excess of 10,660 hours per year working directly with clients. Most of the 21 clients in the on-site programme are brought in from their place of residence by handi-bus five half-days a week, 11½ months of the year. Another 33 clients in the outreach programme are seen in their own place of residence regularly but less frequently. All of these clients range from Level II to Level V on the Rancho Scale (Malkmus, Booth, & Kodimer, 1980). Their average length of enrolment in the on-site programme is four years.

Much of the success of this programme has been based on the recruitment and training of dedicated volunteers, most of whom provide three hours or more a week of one-on-one therapy with a particular client. Each client has an individualised programme established and monitored by the therapy team.

OUTCOME EVALUATION

Like any programme, outcome evaluation is important. Unlike most programmes, measures of functional change and quality of life with sufficient responsiveness for this severely compromised population are essentially unavailable. The existence of the programme with its concentration of clients who would otherwise be considered ineligible for further therapy, and therapists experienced in working with them, has provided a unique opportunity for research.

DEVELOPMENT OF A SEVERE BRAIN INJURY RECOVERY SCALE

Approximately half of ARBI's clients are sufficiently functional and responsive to their environment for yearly progress to be measured using existing functional measures such as the JFK Coma Recovery Scale (Giacino & Kalmar, 1997; Giacino, Kezmarsky, DeLuca, & Cicerone, 1991), Western Neuro Sensory Stimulation Profile (Ansell & Keenan, 1989), and the Chedoke-McMaster Stroke Assessment (Gowland et al., 1993). However, the other half are so severely compromised and making such slow, incremental progress that no set of existing measures have been located that are sufficiently sensitive. A team of physiotherapists and occupational and speech language therapists plus the first author, a nurse scientist, are developing and testing a composite of sub-scales to address this need.

The target population is adults who have experienced severe brain injury secondary to trauma, anoxia or cerebral vascular accident, who are clients of ARBI's community-based programme, and who currently function at Level II or III on the Rancho Scale. Responses at these levels range from inconsistent and non-purposeful reaction to stimuli, as evidenced by physiological changes or gross body movements, to vague purposeful responses such as turning the head to sound or occasionally responding to a simple command.

Using modified measurement development methods (Guyatt, Bombardier, & Tugwell, 1986), the team reviewed the literature and analysed measures currently in use. MEDLINE was searched from 1966 to the present using key words such as brain injury and recovery of function. The therapists already use an extensive battery of measures for which psychometric properties and utility were examined. Information was also sought out on additional approaches. One such approach is the Sensory Modality Assessment Rehabilitation Technique (SMART; Gill-Thwaites, 1997: http://www.rhn.org.uk) which appears to be designed for assessment of clients at a similar level. However, it is required that SMART assessors complete an intensive week of training and completion of an assessment portfolio. Such rigorous training is commendable but not feasible at this time for agencies such as ARBI that have a very limited budget. Thus it was determined that there was a need to proceed with development of a new and potentially complementary measure.

The next step was inductive. Working in pairs, drawing on their extensive professional background, the therapists addressed the question, "What change in one of these clients makes me excited?" The descriptions of those changes were then categorised into items and subscales. In spite of the exhaustive literature review there was often little evidence other than clinical experience for the expected sequence of return of responses to certain stimuli (e.g., olfactory). The variability in sequelae of the initial focal or generalised brain insult, associated trauma or deficits affecting other parts of the body, and secondary effects such as spasticity and contractures required creativity in wording and procedures to allow for individual differences.

The items and subscales so compiled were presented for discussion in regular team meetings, revised for clarity and consistency of wording and scoring, and then sent out for review by clinical experts. From early in the development process small components were pre-tested with clients. At the time of writing this comprehensive measure consists of three major subscales, each of which can be used independently or as part of the overall measure. The subscales include responses to environment (e.g., visual, olfactory), motor responses (e.g., head control, trunk control), and communication and swallowing (e.g., yes/no, vocalisation, comprehension). Components of each subscale are further subdivided into items that can be scored on a 7-point scale. A score of 1 means no response on all scales. As an example of the fine gradation for each, the first four levels for visual response are 1 = no response, 2 = blinks to light or threat; 3 = fixes gaze < 2 seconds; 4 = fixes gaze > 2 seconds. As a second example vocalisation behaviours can range from 1 = none, individual does not produce any voice/sound by mouth, not even to pain; to 7 = vocalises consistently, vocalisations begin to resemble speech sounds (vowels and consonants), are produced spontaneously (e.g., 1–5 instances over 20 minutes) or in response to commands or questions. Items are still being tested and refined but these examples suffice to show just how compromised the target population is, considering that it may take a whole year of volunteer therapy for a client to move up one or two levels. However, clinicians who have worked with this population will also recognise that progress such as being able to maintain head control with support and gaze for >2 seconds then enables more active engagement in therapy and improved quality of life for both the client and families.

Once each subscale has been through pre-testing, with further refinements as necessary, the complete measure will be piloted with approximately 40 clients. At that time initial evidence for construct validity, based on expected correlations with similar scales, test–retest and inter-rater reliability will be assessed. Our purpose has been served if this severe brain injury recovery scale allows for quantifying progress to families, health care professionals, funders and donors.

INDICATORS OF CHANGES IN QUALITY OF LIFE

The purpose of the second project has been to elicit indicators of changes in quality of life. It is commonly assumed that survivors of very severe brain injury have very little quality of life. This assumption arises from conceptual and practical sources. Conceptually, quality of life is often defined as requiring awareness of self (Kuhse & Singer, 1989; Zhan, 1992). Practically, quality of life evaluation in this population is usually based on functional abilities such as self-care and return to work, and proxy estimations by family members or health care providers.

In the project reported here, we set out to explore the quality of life of severely brain injured individuals. We used the critical incident method to elicit observed behaviours and the meanings attributed to them, rather than merely asking for proxy opinion on current quality of life (Flanagan, 1954; 1982). This approach was taken, based on an alternative conceputualisation in which quality of life is defined as the overall state of well-being; physical, psychological and social functioning; and satisfaction with important dimensions of life that cognitively impaired individuals experience, regardless of baseline (Reimer, 1997; 2001; Renwick & Brown, 1996). For this study baseline was taken as the client's status on admission to the community-based rehabilitation programme, rather than life prior to brain injury.

Using semistructured interviews with 12 clients who were able to comprehend and verbalise in short sentences, 24 family members, 18 volunteers, and 6 therapists (each interviewed about four different clients), over 400 incidents were recorded and transcribed. Using Flanagan's guidelines (1954) which call for a description of a particular incident observed by the person reporting and a judgement by that person as to what was significant about the incident, each participant was asked to describe two positive and two negative incidents which indicated changes in quality of life for a specific client since admission to ARBI. Each interview ended with a request for an incident that indicated, "What makes life good right now?", or (if the response was "nothing"), "What would have to happen to make life good right now?" For example, one mother described how her daughter can now sit propped up in a wheelchair. When asked why she saw that as important her reply was, "Now she can look people in the eye, she can make better eye contact." A higher functioning client described an incident about being able to transfer. What was important to his quality of life was that now "nobody is watching while I take a shower".

Content analysis has revealed six major themes from which emerge indicators of quality of life: behaviour, cognition, communication, emotion/ mood, physical function and capacities, and socio-environmental supports and resources (LeNavenec & Reimer, 2002). For minimally responsive clients, changes in behaviour such as decreased agitation were seen by family members, volunteers, and staff as improvements. Evidence of enhanced awareness such as visual tracking and the ability to anticipate going outside were seen as affording greater connection with people and satisfaction with self. Changes in non-verbal communication included eye contact and smiling. For example, connecting to the point of being able to smile in response to appropriate stimuli was the culmination of eight months of daily therapy for one client. Other indicators under communication included learning to use a communication device and becoming able to indicate approval and disapproval. Achieving head control and reduced spasticity were indicators under physical functioning in that these achievements were seen as important in enhancing visual stimulation. For many clients, receiving one-on-one attention was an important indicator under the social theme. Some of these clients had been receiving little more than custodial care or had come from environments prior to the brain injury in which they had seldom experienced such consistent love and care.

SUMMARY

By describing this work in progress our intention has been to highlight what can be done in terms of intervention and outcome evaluation with adults who appear to be continuing in a vegetative or minimally conscious state. The significance of these studies is two-fold. First, they have yielded methods for detecting subtle changes in function and quality of life in minimally responsive adults. Second, by demonstrating that such changes can be detected, they have provided evidence that rehabilitation efforts with this population, even long after the initial insult, can make a difference. The broader significance of this report comes in demonstrating the feasibility and effectiveness of a community-based rehabilitation programme, largely delivered by volunteers under therapist supervision, in bringing about small but significant improvements in function and quality of life.

REFERENCES

Ansell, B. J., & Keenan, J. E. (1989). The Western Neuro Sensory Stimulation Profile: A tool for assessing slow-to-recover head-injured patients. *Archives of Physical Medicine and Rehabilitation, 70*, 104–108.

Flanagan, J. C. (1954). The critical incident technique. *Psychological Bulletin, 15*, 327–358.

Flanagan, J. C. (1982). Measurement of quality of life: Current state of the art. *Archives of Physical Medicine and Rehabilitation, 81*, 56–59.

Giacino, J. T., & Kalmar, K. (1997). The vegetative and minimally conscious states: A comparison of clinical features and functional outcome. *Journal of Head Trauma Rehabilitation, 12*(4), 36–51.

Giacino, J. T., Kezmarsky, M. A., DeLuca, J., & Cicerone, K. D. (1991). Monitoring rate of recovery to predict outcome in minimally responsive patients. *Archives of Physical Medicine and Rehabilitation, 72*(11), 897–901.

Gill-Thwaites, H. (1997). The sensory modality assessment rehabilitation technique: A tool for assessment and treatment of patients with severe brain injury in a vegetative state. *Brain Injury, 11*(10), 724–734.

Gowland, C., Stratford, P., Ward, M., Moreland, J., Torresin, W., Van Hullenaar, S., Sanford, J., Barreca, S., Vanspall, B., & Plews, N. (1993). Measuring physical impairment and disability with the Chedoke-McMaster Stroke Assessment. *Stroke, 24*(1), 58–63.

Guyatt, G. H., Bombardier, C., & Tugwell, P. X. (1986). Measuring disease-specific quality of life in clinical trials. *Canadian Medical Association Journal, 134*, 889–895.

Kuhse, H., & Singer, P. (1989). The quality/quality-of-life distinction and its moral importance for nurses. *International Journal of Nursing Studies, 26*(3), 203–212.

LeNavenec, C. L., & Reimer, M. A. (2002). *Outcome indicators of quality of life changes for people with traumatic brain injury in a community rehabilitation program.* Unpublished data.

Malkmus, D., Booth, B. J., & Kodimer, C. (1980). *Rehabilitation of the head injured adult: Comprehensive cognitive management.* Downey CA: Professional Staff Association, Rancho Los Amigos Medical Center.

Reimer, M. A. (1997). *Measurement of quality of life in adult onset cognitive impairment.* Unpublished doctoral dissertation, University of Calgary, Calgary AB, Canada.

Reimer, M. A. (2001). On being human: Alterations in the sense of being. In C. Stewart-Amidei & J. A. Kunkel (Eds.), *AANN's Neuroscience Nursing: Human responses to neurologic dysfunction* (2nd ed., pp. 771–784). Philadelphia: W. B. Saunders.

Renwick, R., & Brown, I. (1996). The Centre for Health Promotion's conceptual approach to quality of life: Being, belonging, and becoming. In R. Renwick, I. Brown & M. Nagler (Eds.), *Quality of life in health promotion and rehabilitation* (pp. 75–86). Thousand Oaks, CA: Sage Publications.

Zhan, L. (1992). Quality of life: Conceptual and measurement issues. *Journal of Advanced Nursing, 17*, 795–800.

NEUROPSYCHOLOGICAL REHABILITATION
2005, 15 (3/4), 480–493

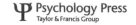

Rehabilitation interventions for vegetative and minimally conscious patients

Louise Elliott and Louise Walker

Addenbrooke's NHS Trust, Cambridge, UK

Brain injury rehabilitation is a complex and challenging task for all members of the multidisciplinary team. Medical advances have allowed more severely impaired patients to survive and consequently the number of patients in the vegetative and minimally conscious states have proportionately increased. Thus, the need for evidence-based practice and further research demonstrating the effects of specific rehabilitation interventions is required. This article reviews the current research and consensus on rehabilitation for patients in the vegetative and minimally conscious states.

INTRODUCTION

The majority of brain injuries are caused by road traffic accidents, sporting injuries or assaults and result in patients demonstrating a multitude of physical, cognitive, social, behavioural, and emotional problems (Duff, 2001; Royal College of Physicians, 2003b). Progress in intensive care medical treatment has resulted in many patients, who would previously have died, surviving severe brain injury (Jennett, 1993; Noda, Maeda, & Yoshino, 2004). This has resulted in a proportional rise in the number of such patients left severely disabled in a vegetative or minimally conscious state (Royal College of Physicians, 2003b). Patients in the vegetative state show no signs of awareness but display sleep-wake cycles and eye opening (Jennett, 2002; Jennett & Plum, 1972). Those patients that demonstrate some evidence of awareness, despite profound cognitive and physical

Correspondence should be sent to Louise Elliott, Cambridge Coma Study Group, Box 124, Addenbrooke's Hospital, Cambridge, CB2 2QQ, UK. Tel: 01223 586650. Email: louiseelliott30@ hotmail.com

© 2005 Psychology Press Ltd
http://www.tandf.co.uk/journals/pp/09602011.html   DOI:10.1080/09602010443000506

impairments, are described as being in the minimally conscious state (Giacino et al., 2002).

It has frequently been questioned whether brain injury rehabilitation is effective or whether it constitutes well-intentioned hand-holding while natural recovery takes place (Cope, 1995). Certainly, the scientific evidence demonstrating the value of rehabilitation interventions is predominantly restricted to stroke patients (Johansson, 2000; Watson, 2001). The limited evidence for vegetative and minimally conscious patients is frequently poorly described or defined (Giacino, 2001). Yet advances in neurophysio-logical research over the past 20 years has lead to dramatic changes in the understanding of the neural control of movement (Bethune, 1994). Many studies have demonstrated chemical and anatomical plasticity in the cerebral cortex and the potential ability of the brain to compensate for lesions (Bach-Y-Rita, 2003; Johansson, 2000). This work reinforces the importance of reha-bilitation for all neurologically impaired patients to assist with facilitating beneficial plastic changes within the brain (Bach-Y-Rita, 2003; Johansson, 2000; Pomeroy & Tallis, 2002; Slade, Camberlain, & Tennant, 2002; Tolfts & Stiller, 1997).

Accurately diagnosing patients as either vegetative or minimally conscious is a difficult task (Shiel et al., 2004). It is however essential that the correct diagnosis is given as this may affect the patient's long-term rehabilitation placement and his or her need for on-going treatment. Improvement from the initial stage of coma may be gradual and unless accurate assessment takes place, small gains may go unnoticed. When patients are slow to recover, professionals may be misled into believing that no recovery is occur-ring, even though slow but subtle progress is continuing over weeks or months (Shiel et al., 2000).

Even the most experienced therapist appreciates the complexity of treating brain injured patients due to the lack of a stereotypical clinical picture and the devastating consequences for the individual involved and his or her family and friends (Carr & Shepherd, 1998; Pickett-Hauber & Testant-Dufour, 2000; Slade et al., 2002). This article reviews some of the evidence and advice regarding rehabilitation interventions for vegetative and minimally conscious brain injured patients.

NEUROLOGICAL REHABILITATION

Many believe if there is no potential for recovery then there is no logical reason why rehabilitation should take place (Andrews, 1993). However many studies have shown that patients in the vegetative state can demonstrate varying degrees of recovery several years post-injury (Berrol, 1986; De Young & Grass, 1987; Levin, Saydjarin, & Eisenberg, 1991; Wales & Bernhardt,

2000; Watson, 2001). Tuel et al. (1992) found one third of a group of 49 brain injured patients considered dependent on admission to a rehabilitation unit (Bartel score below 60) achieved independence by discharge (Bartel score above 60). However, those who had a very low level of arousal benefited least. The role of rehabilitation for this patient group should however not only focus on improving function and communication, where possible, but also in maintaining existing ability and preventing deterioration (Andrews, 1993).

Unfortunately, direct evidence for the effectiveness of rehabilitation versus no treatment is only available from the 1960s, due to current ethical restrictions. Rusk et al. (1966, 1969) cited in Cope (1995) followed up 25 brain injured patients, who were not deemed appropriate for extensive rehabilitation, 5–15 years post-injury. They discovered five had died but of the 18 still alive there were hundreds of incidents of infections and respiratory complications. Contractures were evident in all patients even those initially without contractures.

EARLY VERSUS LATE INTERVENTION

Intensive care units should be deemed as early rehabilitation units (Gelling, 2004; Hough, 2001). Rehabilitation in this environment is aimed at improving patients motor and functional recovery while preventing or treating complications (Cope & Hall, 1982; Mazaux, De-S-Ze, Joseph, & Barat, 2001). Early rehabilitation has been associated with better outcomes in severely brain injured patients (Mackay, Bernstein, & Chapman, 1992; Oh & Seo, 2003). Patients in the vegetative and minimally conscious state are frequently denied early rehabilitation. This is either because of a belief that patients have to reach a specific level of responsiveness to benefit or because demand exceeds the beds available and patients therefore have to wait for a place on a specialist rehabilitation unit (Shiel et al., 2001).

Cope and Hall (1982) reported an analysis of 34 brain injured patients based upon prospectively gathered data, showing that brain injured patients, equally matched on severity of injury, co-morbidity and demographic measures, but varying on whether or not they had been referred "early" (before 35 days) or "late" (after 35 days) to a rehabilitation programme. They demonstrated that brain injured patients referred "early" had a greater than 50% reduction in total hospital treatment. However, caution is suggested when interpreting this since the "late" group had more medical problems and bilateral brain damage and were not matched for Glasgow Coma Scale Score or post-traumatic amnesia. Morgan, Chapman, and Tokarski (1988) also analysed the outcomes of 82 brain injured patients treated in the acute setting with either early rehabilitation (before seven days post-injury), against those whose rehabilitation began after seven days. The patients given early rehabilitation were reported to have significantly shortened length of hospital stay and better functional outcomes.

Mackay et al. (1992) compared matched groups of severely head-injured patients who did or did not receive formal rehabilitation during their acute care. They demonstrated substantial benefits for those patients who had received formal rehabilitation during this period, with coma length and length of stay for the rehabilitated group being approximately one-third of the length of the non-rehabilitated patients. Additionally, in the rehabilitated group, 94% were discharged home compared to only 57% of the control group. However, assessors were not blinded to the intervention, which may have resulted in the possibility of researcher bias.

These studies demonstrate the need for early rehabilitation in brain injured patients. Although not specifically based on those in the vegetative and minimally conscious state they highlight the importance of early intervention.

INTENSITY OF REHABILITATION

Intensive specialist rehabilitation programmes have been shown to be effective for the patient and cost-efficient in the long term (Shiel et al., 2001; Slade et al., 2002; Zhu, Poon, Chan, & Chan, 2001). Rehabilitation units within Europe frequently provide increased levels of rehabilitation rarely obtainable within the current National Health Service (Grieve et al., 2001). This may explain why UK rehabilitation units typically have longer periods of stay when compared to Europe, although this requires further investigation (Wolfe, Tilling, Beech, & Rudd, 1999).

A number of studies have all demonstrated the efficacy of intensive therapy on patient outcomes (Hakim & Bakheit, 1998; Kwakkel et al., 1997; Shiel et al., 2001). Shiel et al. (2001) investigated the effect of increased intensity of rehabilitation on 56 patients with moderate and severe brain injuries in a two-centre prospective, controlled study with random allocation to groups. The results supported the anecdotal view that increased intervention facilitates a more rapid improvement and has the potential to lower the incidence of early behavioural disorders and physical deformities, such as contractures. This reduces the need for later rehabilitation and community teams to spend time on correcting avoidable deficits acquired in hospital. Indeed, Slade et al. (2002) conducted a randomised controlled trial that illustrated a significant reduction in length of stay when multidisciplinary therapy was increased by 67%. From these studies it is clear to see that improved intensity of rehabilitation may be beneficial in brain injured patients, although the benefit in vegetative and minimally conscious patients requires further investigation.

PHYSIOTHERAPY APPROACHES TO REHABILITATION

There is no universally accepted treatment regime for brain injured patients (Bethune, 1994). Most physiotherapists working with neurologically impaired patients would claim to be working within the influence of a named approach, such as Bobath, Movement Science (Motor relearning) or Johnstone (Partridge & Werdt, 1995). Yet scientific evidence demonstrating the value of specific rehabilitation interventions is limited and comparisons between different methods in current use have so far failed to show that one is superior to another (Johansson, 2000). Training, experience and personal belief appear to play as much of an important role in the selection of movement therapies as the literature on current motor control theories (Lettinga, Reynders, & Mulder, 2002). Ultimately it appears, regardless of the strategy employed, the more intensive the therapy the better the outcome (Slade et al., 2002; Taub & Uswatte, 2003).

Sensory stimulation

The human brain grows and adapts through utilisation and is exquisitely responsive to external stimulation and nourishment (Bach-Y-Rita, 2003; United States Department of Health and Human Services, 1998). Evidence from studies has illustrated that sensory deprivation leads to physical deterioration of the brain in animals and humans (Bragin, Vinogradova, & Stafekhina, 1992; Grossman & Hagel, 1996). Many brain injured patients with sensorimotor impairments therefore have associated motor-related disabilities (Dobkin, 2003). Consequently, one of the many interventions currently employed with severely brain injured patients is sensory stimulation (Ansell & Keenan, 1989).

Sensory stimulation is implemented to increase the level of arousal and awareness through stimulating the reticular activating system (Candeo, Grix, & Nicoletti, 2002; Tolle & Reimer, 2003). It aims to facilitate environmental inputs through all five sensory pathways at a frequency, duration and intensity far above those in the usual hospital setting (Le Winn & Dimancescu, 1978; Davis, 1991; Doman, Wilkinson, Dimancescu, & Pelligra, 1993; Lombardi et al., 2004).

Wood (1991) and Wood et al. (1992) however believe that patients exposed to an undifferentiated bombardment of sensory information lose the ability to process information due to habituation and that the type of white matter damage to most patients will inflict information processing limitations in response to stimuli. Doman et al. (1993) demonstrated miraculous results on 200 brain injured patients with a Glasgow Coma Scale Score of less than six for up to one week following injury. They showed that 91% of patients emerged from a coma through multi-sensory stimulation as compared to none of the control group, consisting of only 33 patients. However, 56% of these remained severely impaired. Furthermore, Oh and Seo (2003) also demonstrated significant alterations in conscious levels after two weeks of sensory stimulation, composed of auditory, visual, olfactory, gustatory, tactile and physical stimulation twice a day, five days a week for four weeks. However, these results were based on only seven subjects within three months of injury where spontaneous recovery may occur.

Research has yet to clearly demonstrate the efficacy of sensory stimulation and it remains a controversial modality (Barreca et al., 2003). A Cochrane systematic review in 2004 indicated that there is still no reliable evidence to support or rule out, the effectiveness of multisensory programmes for patients in coma or vegetative state (Lombardi et al., 2004).

Facilitating postural changes

Little consensus exists concerning procedures that can be undertaken to improve arousal (Mazaux et al., 2001). However, it is known that a patient's physical position can affect his or her responsiveness (Royal College of Physicians, 2003a). There is emerging observational evidence to suggest that facilitating positional changes, by standing brain injured patients on a tilt table, may àlso positively affect arousal and awareness (Ada, Canning, & Paratz, 1990; Richardson, 1991; Weber, 1984). A study by Elliott et al. (in press) has indicated that while standing upright, patients who were vegetative or minimally conscious showed significant improvement in arousal and/or awareness, as assessed using the Wessex Head Injury Matrix. This work suggested such interventions could have a significant impact on diagnosis, rehabilitation and outcome in vegetative and minimally conscious patients.

The importance of positional changes for these types of patients has also been shown to prevent hypovolaemia, alter resting muscle length, load vertebrae, redistribute skin pressure, benefit the respiratory system and assist in improving alertness and orientation (Hough, 2001; Morgan, Cullen, Stokes, & Swan, 2003; Wenger, 1982). Standing has been shown specifically to increase ankle range of movement and reduce lower limb spasticity in neurologically impaired patients (Bohannon, 1993; Bohannon & Larkin, 1985). It also assists in reducing osteoporosis (Cybulski & Jaegar, 1986) and improves circulation (Bromley, 1985) and renal function (Duffus & Wood, 1983). Although these studies are not specifically related to brain injured patients they do illustrate the physical benefits of standing patients who are unable to achieve this position themselves.

Prevention and management of joint contractures

The development of joint contractures is a common secondary problem in the severely brain injured adult (Lehmkuhl et al., 1990; Yarkony & Sahgal,

1987). Such secondary musculoskeletal changes, as a direct sequelae to relative immobilisation imposed by neurological impairment, are associated with poor functional outcome (Ada & Canning, 1990; Herbert, 1988; Shumway-Cook & Wollacott, 2001). Therefore, it is critical that these complications are particularly addressed with vegetative and minimally conscious patients. The effects on muscle held in the shortened position are well documented, with a loss of sacromeres, a reduction in protein synthesis, an increase in protein breakdown, proliferation of collagen, and loss of extensibility in periarticular connective tissues (Ada & Canning, 1990; Bruton, 2002; Gossman, Sahrmann, & Rose, 1982; Herbert, 1988). Such adaptive changes to muscle held in a shortened position are more marked and take place more quickly than in their lengthened state (Ada & Canning, 1990).

Yarkony and Sahgal (1987), in a study of 75 brain injured adults admitted for in-patient rehabilitation, found a staggering 84% of patients presented with a contracture, which amplified proportionately with an increased duration of coma. Reasoning for such a high incidence in this population has been predominantly attributed to spasticity induced posturing (Booth, Doyle, & Montgomery, 1983; Singer, Singer, & Allison, 2001). However, this may also be due to injuries such as fractures or dislocations (Lehmkuhl et al., 1990), or heterotrophic ossification (Whyte & Glenn, 1986) and soft tissue shortening as a direct result of immobility and sustained posturing (Singer et al., 2001). The most common sites for development of contractures in the brain injured adult are hips, elbows, ankles, and shoulders (Yarkony & Sahgal, 1987). Equino-varus ankle contractures have been described to be the most common deformity associated with hypertonicity as they occur in both decorticate and decerebrate posturing (Booth et al., 1983; Conine, Sullivan, Mackie, & Goodman, 1990).

Physiotherapy plays a key role in the prevention and correction of contractures in these patients through a variety of techniques including manual stretching, positioning, weight-bearing activities, such as the tilt table, and splinting (Richardson, 2002; Singer et al., 2001). Pope (1992) made recommendations for the use of regular positional changes to help prevent contracture. For example, the use of the prone position in order to counteract the flexed posture adapted while sitting and in bed. Richardson (1991), in a single case study, looked at the effect of the tilt table to passively stretch tendo-achilles in a head injured patient and illustrated an improved foot position in the intervention period, thus facilitating further rehabilitation. It was concluded that the tilt table was an effective method for improving joint position in the neurological patient. Pope (1992) also suggested the use of the tilt-table in counteracting the flexed posture described earlier.

Manual stretching and passive movement of joints in order to maintain range of movement is a common method of contracture prevention (Lehmkuhl et al., 1990). However, there remains debate about how long a muscle needs to be stretched to prevent soft tissue shortening. Tardieu, Lespargot, Tabary, and Bret (1988) studied 10 children, all of whom had cerebral palsy, and found no evidence of progressive contractures in the soleus muscle when it was stretched for at least six hours a day. To date however, there is no research in the adult acquired brain injured population on how long muscles need to be passively stretched for, to avoid muscle shortening and this requires further investigation.

The increase in muscle length observed following stretching applied to shortened muscles does appear to be a transient occurrence and is gradually lost (Herbert, 1988). The use of splinting and in particular serial casting, is documented to be effective in the management of soft tissue contractures resulting from spasticity as the stretch is applied for a significantly longer period of time (Booth et al., 1983; Mortenson & Eng, 2003). Serial casting is a technique where a series of splints are made to progressively and continuously stretch and regain range at a joint. Each cast is worn 24 hours a day and removed after a number of days, when a new cast is made. Evidence for the use of splinting is particularly documented in the management of equinovarus ankle contractures. Booth et al. (1983) reviewed charts of 201 patients and discovered 42 were found to have had serial casting as part of their management, and in 40 of these patients an increase in range of movement had been documented. Moseley (1997) also looked at the effect of casting and stretching on passive ankle dorsiflexion in nine adults who had sustained traumatic head injuries using a cross-over design study. The results showed an increase in passive dorsiflexion in the experimental group compared to the control. In this study, as with others, the severity of brain injury is not clearly documented, with subjects ranging from being "unconscious" to standing with assistance. Singer, Jegasothy, Singer, and Allison, (2003) splinted 16 brain injured patients with equinovarus deformities and also demonstrated increased range of movement with associated improvements in function. However, some of the patients' functional abilities were not consistent with those seen in vegetative or minimally conscious patients. To date there is no paper solely looking at the effects of splinting in vegetative and minimally conscious patients.

Contracture management should be started in the acute stages following injury regardless of predicted outcome or proposed level of function (Booth et al., 1983). The need for liaison with the multidisciplinary and medical teams is imperative, especially in the acute intensive care environment (Booth et al., 1983). For patients who go on to make a good recovery, contractures can delay functional tasks such as standing, transferring or even walking (Ada & Canning, 1990). Contractures in the long-term dependent patient can hinder effective seating and hygiene needs, give rise to discomfort, and make nursing care more difficult (Edwards, 2002). However, in a study by Pohl, Mehrholz, and Ruckriem (2003) investigating serial casting in 68 patients with severe cerebral spasticity they demonstrated no difference in improvements in range of movements between those patients splinted within 90 days of injury or those splinted after 90 days. They also illustrated no difference in those who had lower levels of consciousness (GCS below or above 12). However, this was a retrospective study, not randomised and they fail to state if patients actually gained improvement in range of movement.

It is important that physiotherapy does not work in isolation for the management of spasticity in these patients. Patients need to be on suitable doses of antispasmodics, while the use of botulinum toxin in focal hypertonicity is becoming ever more widely used in facilitating physiotherapy techniques (Sheean, 1998). Guidelines for splinting of the neurologically impaired patient have been produced by the Association of Chartered Physiotherapists with an Interest in Neurology (ACPIN, 1998).

CONCLUSION

As emergency medicine and hospital care continue to make strides to save victims of trauma, therapists need to continue to meet the challenges of the traumatic brain injury population to ensure quality of life (Mackay et al., 1992; Watson, 2001). This involves ensuring intensive rehabilitation is started as soon as possible after the initial insult, and ensuring sufficient therapists are available to facilitate therapeutic handling. The Royal College of Physicians (2003b) suggests that staffing provision in terms of numbers, experience and qualification in the management of brain injury should be appropriate to the needs of the case-load. Family and friends also play an important role in assisting with rehabilitation and in motivating the patient where possible (Gleckman & Brill, 1995).

Although research evidence to support existing clinical practice is sparse, lack of evidence of effect is not evidence of lack of effect. Withholding rehabilitation from patients before research has clarified whether all or only some of its components improve outcomes for patients might be depriving them of beneficial treatment (Edwards, 2002; Watson, 2001). Funding for research needs to be increased to ensure well-defined and controlled studies into the effectiveness of rehabilitation interventions for brain-injured patients can occur (United States Department of Health and Human Services, 1998).

REFERENCES

ACPIN (Association of Chartered Physiotherapists with a Special Interest in Neurology) (1998). *Clinical practice guidelines on splinting adults with neurological dysfunction.* London: Chartered Society of Physiotherapists.

Ada, L., & Canning, C. (1990). Anticipating and avoiding muscle shortening. In L. Ada & C. Canning (Eds.), *Key issues in neurological physiotherapy* (pp. 219–236). Oxford: Heinemann Medical.

Ada, L., Canning, C., & Paratz, J. (1990). Care of the unconscious head-injured patient. In L. Ada & C. Canning (Eds.), *Key issues in neurological physiotherapy* (pp. 249–289). Oxford: Heinemann Medical.

Adams, J. H., Graham, D. I., & Jennett, B. (2000). The neuropathology of the vegetative state after an acute brain insult. *Brain, 123*, 1327–1338.

Andrews, K. (1993). Should PVS patients be treated? *Neuropsychological Rehabilitation, 3*(2) 109–119.

Ansell, B., & Keenan, J. (1989). The Western Neuro Sensory Stimulation Profile: A tool for assessing slow-to-recover head-injured patients. *Archives of Physical Medicine and Rehabilitation, 70*, 104–108.

Bach-Y-Rita, P. (2003). Theoretical basis for brain plasticity after a TBI. *Brain Injury, 17*(8), 643–651.

Barreca, S., Velikonja, D., Brown, L., Williams, L., Davis, L., & Sigouin, C. S. (2003). Evaluation of the effectiveness of two clinical training procedures to elicit yes/no responses from patients with severe acquired brain injury: A randomized single-subject design. *Brain Injury, 17*(12), 1065–1075.

Berrol, S. (1986). Evolution and the persistent vegetative state. *Head Trauma Rehabilitation, 1*, 7–13.

Bethune, D. (1994). Another look at neurological rehabilitation. *Australian Journal of Physiotherapy, 40*, 255–261.

Bohannon, R. (1993). Tilt table standing for reducing spasticity after spinal cord injury. *Archives of Physical Medicine and Rehabilitation, 74*, 1121–1122.

Bohannon, R. W., & Larkin, P. A. (1985). Passive ankle dorsiflexion increases in patients after a regime of tilt table wedge board standing: A clinical report. *Physical Therapy, 65*, 1676–1678.

Booth, B. J., Doyle, M., & Montgomery, J. (1983). Serial casting for the management of spasticity in the head-injured adult. *Physical Therapy, 63*(12), 1960–1966.

Bragin, A. G., Vinogradova, O. S., & Stafekhina, V. S. (1992). Sensory deprivation prevents integration of neocortical grafts with the host brain. *Restorative Neurology and Neuroscience, 4*, 279–283.

Bromley, I. (1985). *Tetraplegia and paraplegia*. London: Churchill Livingstone.

Brucia, J., & Rudy, E. (1996). The effect of suction catheter insertion and tracheal stimulation in adults with severe brain injury. *Heart and Lung, 25*(4), 295–303.

Bruton, A. (2002). Muscle plasticity: Response to training and detraining. *Physiotherapy, 88*, 398–408.

Candeo, A., Grix, M. C., & Nicoletti, J. (2002). An analysis of assessment instruments for the minimally responsive patient (MRP): Clinical observations. *Brain Injury, 16*(5), 453–461.

Carr, J. H., & Shepherd, R. (1998). *Neurological rehabilitation: Optimizing motor performance*. London: Heinemann Medical.

Conine, T. A., Sullivan, T., Mackie, T., & Goodman, M. (1990). Effect of serial casting for the prevention of equinus in patients with acute head injury. *Archives of Physical Medical Rehabilitation, 71*, 310–312.

Cope, D. (1995). The effectiveness of traumatic brain injury rehabilitation: A review. *Brain Injury, 9*(7), 649–670.

Cope, N. D., & Hall, K. (1982). Head injury rehabilitation: Benefits of early intervention. *Archives of Physical Medicine and Rehabilitation, 63*, 433–437.

Cope, D. (1995). The effectiveness of traumatic brain injury rehabilitation: A review. *Brain Injury, 9*(7), 649–670.

Cybulski, G. R., & Jaegar, R. J. (1986). Standing performance of persons with paraplegia. *Archives of Physical Medicine and Rehabilitation, 67,* 103–108.

Davis, A. (1991). The Visual Response Evaluation: A pilot study of an evaluation tool for assessing visual responses in low-level brain injured patients. *Brain Injury, 5*(3), 315–320.

De Young, S., & Grass, R. B. (1987). Coma recovery program. *Rehabilitation Nursing, 12,* 121–124.

Dobkin, B. (2003). Do electrically stimulated sensory inpits and movements lead to long-term plasticity and rehabilitation gains? *Current Opinion in Neurology, 16,* 685–691.

Doman, G., Wilkinson, R., Dimancescu, M. D., & Pelligra, R. (1993). The effects of intense multi-sensory stimulation on coma arousal and recovery. *Neuropsychological Rehabilitation, 3*(2), 203–212.

Duff, D. (2001). Review article: Altered states of consciousness, theories of recovery and assessment following a severe traumatic brain injury. *AXON, 23*(1), 18–23.

Duffus, A., & Wood, J. (1983). Standing and walking for the T6 paraplegic. *Physiotherapy, 69,* 45–46.

Edwards, S. (2002). *Neurological physiotherapy.* London: Churchill Livingston.

Elliott, L., Shiel, A., Coleman, M., Wilson, B., Badwan, D., Menon, D., & Pickard, J. (in press). The effect of posture on levels of arousal and awareness in vegetative and minimally conscious state patients: A preliminary investigation. *Journal of Neurology, Neurosurgery and Psychiatry.*

Gelling, L. (2004). Researching patients in the vegetative state: Difficulties of studying this patient group. *Nursing Times Research, 9,* 7–17.

Giacino, J. (2001). Revisiting the vegetative state: Major developments over the last decade. *Physical Medicine and Rehabilitation State of the Art Reviews, 15*(2), 399–415.

Giacino, J. T., Ashwal, S., Childs, N., Cranford, R., Jennett, B., Katz, D. I., et al. (2002). The minimally conscious state. Definition and diagnostic criteria. *American Academy of Neurology, 58,* 349–353.

Gleckman, A., & Brill, S. (1995). The impact of brain injury on family functioning: Implications for subacute rehabilitation programmes. *Brain Injury, 9*(4), 385–393.

Gossman, M. R., Sahrmann, S. A., & Rose, S. J. (1982). Review of length associated changes in muscle. *Physical Therapy, 62,* 1799–1807.

Grieve, R., Hutton, J., Bhalla, A., Rastenyte, D., Ryglewicz, D., Sarti, C., et al. (2001). A comparison of the costs and survival of hospital-admitted stroke patients across Europe. *Stroke, 32*(7), 1684–1691.

Grossman, P., & Hagel, K. (1996). Post-traumatic appallic syndrome following head injury. Part 2: Treatment. *Disability and Rehabilitation, 18*(2), 57–68.

Hakim, E. A., & Bakheit, A. M. (1998). A study of the factors which influence the length of hospital stay of stroke patients. *Clinical Rehabilitation, 12,* 151–156.

Herbert, R. (1988). The passive mechanical properties of muscle and their adaptations to altered patterns of use. *The Australian Journal of Physiotherapy, 34,* 141–149.

Hough, A. (2001). *Physiotherapy in respiratory care.* London: Chapman & Hall.

Jennett, B. (1993). Vegetative survival: The medical facts and ethical dilemmas. *Neuropsychological Rehabilitation, 3*(2), 99–108.

Jennett, B. (2002). *The vegetative state* (1st ed.). Cambridge: Cambridge University Press.

Jennett, B., & Plum, F. (1972). Persistent vegetative state after brain damage. *The Lancet, 1,* 734–737.

Johansson, B. B. (2000). Brain plasticity and stoke rehabilitation. The Willis lecture. *Stroke, 31,* 223–230.

Kwakkel, G., Wagenaar, R. C., Koelman, T. W., Lankhorst, G. L., & Koetsier, J. C. (1997). Effects of intensity of rehabilitation after stroke: A research synthesis. *Stroke, 28,* 1552–1556.

Lehmkuhl, D. L., Thoi, L. L., Baize, C., Kelley, C. J., Krawczyk, L., & Bontke, C. F. (1990). Multimodality treatment of joint contractures in patients with severe brain injury: Cost, effectiveness, and integration of therapies in the application of serial/inhibitive casts. *Journal of Head Trauma Rehabilitation, 5*(4), 23–42.

Lettinga, A. T., Reynders, K., & Mulder, T. H. (2002). Pitfalls in effectiveness research: A comparative analysis of treatment goals and outcome measures in stroke rehabilitation. *Clinical Rehabilitation, 16*, 174–181.

Levin, H.S., Saydjarin, C., & Eisenberg, H. M. (1991). Vegetative state after closed head injury. A traumatic coma data bank report. *Archives of Neurology, 48*(6), 580–585.

Le Winn, E. B., & Dimancescu, M. D. (1978). Environmental deprivation and enrichment in coma. *Lancet, 2*, 156–157.

Lombardi, F., Taricco, M., De Tanti, A., Telaro, E., & Liberati, A. (2004). Sensory stimulation for brain injured individuals in coma or vegetative state. *The Cochrane Library (Oxford)* no. 2. ISSN: 1464–780X.

Mackay, L. B., Bernstein, P., & Chapman, E. (1992). Early intervention in severe head injury: Long-term benefits of a formalized program. *Archives of Physical Medicine and Rehabilitation, 73*, 635–641.

Mazaux, J., De-S-Ze, M., Joseph, P. A., & Barat, M. (2001). Early rehabilitation after severe brain injury: A French perspective. *Journal of Rehabilitation Medicine, 33*(3), 99–109.

Morgan, A. S., Chapman, P., & Tokarski, L. (1988). Improved care of the traumatically brain injured. *Eastern Association for Surgery for Trauma—First Annual Conference.* Longboat Key, Florida, USA.

Morgan, C. L., Cullen, G. P., Stokes, M., & Swan, A. V. (2003). Effects of knee joint angle and tilt table incline on force distribution at the feet and supporting straps. *Clinical Rehabilitation, 17*, 871–878.

Mortenson, P. A., & Eng, J. (2003). The use of casts in the management of joint mobility and hypertonia following brain injury in adults: A systematic review. *Physical Therapy, 83*(7), 648–658.

Moseley, A. M. (1997). The effect of casting combined with stretching on passive ankle dorsiflexion in adults with traumatic head injuries. *Physical Therapy, 77*(3), 240–247.

Noda, R., Maeda, Y., & Yoshino, A. (2004). Therapeutic time window for musicokinetic therapy in a persistent vegetative state after severe brain injury. *Brain Injury, 18*(5), 509–515.

Oh, H., & Seo, W. (2003). Sensory stimulation programme to imrpove recovery in comatose patients. *Journal of Clinical Nursing, 12*, 394–404.

Partridge, C. J., & Weerdt, W. (1995). Different approaches to physiotherapy in stroke. *Reviews in Clinical Gerontology, 5*, 199–209.

Pickett Hauber, R., & Testani-Dufour, L. (2000). Living in limbo: The low-level brain injured patient and the patient's family. *Journal of Neuroscience Nursing, 32*, 22–26.

Pohl, M., Mehrholz, J., & Ruckriem, S. (2003). The influence of illness duration and level of consciousness on the treatment effect and complication rate of serial casting in patients with severe spasticity. *Clinical Rehabilitation, 17*, 373–379.

Pomeroy, V. M., & Tallis, R. C. (2002). Restoring movement and functional ability after stroke. *Physiotherapy, 88*(1), 3–17.

Pope, P. (1992). Management of the physical condition in patients with chronic and severe neurological pathologies. *Physiotherapy, 78*(12), 896–902.

Richardson, D. (1991). The use of tilt table to effect passive tendo-achilles stretch in a patient with head injury. *Physiotherapy Theory and Practice, 7*, 45–50.

Richardson, D. (2002). Physical therapy in spasticity. The modern management of adult spasticity: An evidence-based approach. *European Journal of Neurology, 9*(Suppl.1) 17–22.

Royal College of Physicians (2003a). The vegetative state: Guidance on diagnosis and management. *Clinical Medicine, 3*, 249–254.

Royal College of Physicians (2003b). *Rehabilitation following acquired brain injury—National clinical guidelines.* Sudbury, UK: Lavenham Press.

Sheean, G. L. (1998). The treatment of spasticity with botulinum toxin. In G. L. Sheean (Ed.), *Spasticity rehabilitation.* Edinburgh, UK: Churchill Communication Europe Ltd.

Shiel, A., Burn, J. P. S., Henry, D., Clark, J., Wilson, B. A., Burnett, M. E., & McLellan, D. L. (2001). The effects of increased rehabilitation therapy after brain injury: Results of a prospective controlled trial. *Clinical Rehabilitation, 15,* 501–514.

Shiel, A., Gelling, L., Wilson, B. A., Coleman, M., & Pickard, J. D. (2004). Difficulties in diagnosing the vegetative state. *British Journal of Neurosurgery, 18*(1), 5–7.

Shiel, A., Horn, S., Wilson, B. A., Watson, M., Campbell, M. J., & McLellan, D. L. (2000). The Wessex Head Injury Matric (WHIM) main scale: A preliminary report on a scale to assess and monitor patient recovery after severe head injury. *Clinical Rehabilitation, 14,* 408–416.

Shumway-Cook, A., Anson, D., & Haller, S. (1988). Postural sway biofeedback: Its effect on re-establishing stance stability in hemiplegic patients. *Archives of Physical Medicine and Rehabilitation, 69,* 395–400.

Shumway-Cook, A., & Woollacott, M. H. (2001). *Motor control theory and practical application* (2nd ed.). USA: Lippincott Williams & Wilkins.

Singer, B., Singer, K. P., & Allison, G. (2001). Serial plaster casting to correct equino-varus deformity of the ankle following acquired brain injury in adults. *Disability and Rehabilitation, 23*(18), 829–836.

Singer, B. J., Jegasothy, G. M., Singer, K. P., & Allison, G. T. (2003). Evaluation of serial casting to correct eqinovarus deformity of the ankle after acquired brain injury in adults. *Archives of Physical Medical Rehabilitation, 84,* 483–491.

Slade, A., Camberlain, M. A., & Tennant, A. (2002). A randomised controlled trial to determine the effect of intensity of therapy on length of stay in a neurological rehabilitation setting. *Journal of Rehabilitation Medicine, 34*(6), 260–266.

Tardieu, C., Lespargot, A., Tabary, C., & Bret, M. D. (1988). For how long must the soleus muscle be stretched each day to prevent contracture? *Developmental Medicine and Child Neurology, 30,* 3–10.

Taub, E., & Uswatte, G. (2003). Constraint-induced movement therapy: Bridging from the primate laboratory to the stroke rehabiltation laboratory. *Journal of Rehabilitation Medicine, 41,* 34–40.

Tolfts, A., & Stiller, K. (1997). Do patients with traumatic brain injury benefit from physiotherapy? A review of the evidence. *Physiotherapy Theory and Practice, 13,* 197–206.

Tolle, P., & Reimer, M. (2003). Do we need stimulation programs as a part of nursing care for patients in "persistent vegetative state?" A conceptual analysis. *AXON, 25*(2), 20–26.

Tuel, S. M., Presty, S. K., Meythaler, J. M., Heinemann, A. W., & Katz, R. T. (1992). Functional improvement in severe head injury after readmission for rehabilitation. *Brain Injury, 6,* 363–372.

United States Department of Health and Human Services (1998). Rehabilitation of persons with traumatic brain injury. NIH consensus statement. *Department of Health, 8*(4).

Wales, L. R., & Bernhardt, J. A. (2000). A case for slow to recover rehabilitation services following severe acquired brain injury. *Australian Journal of Physiotherapy, 46,* 143–146.

Watson, M. J. (2001). Do patients with severe traumatic brain injury benefit from physiotherapy? A review of the evidence. *Physical Therapy Reviews, 6,* 233–249.

Weber, P. (1984). Sensorimotor therapy: Its effect on electroencephalograms of acute comatose patients. *Archives of Physical Medicine and Rehabilitation, 65,* 457–462.

Wenger, N. K. (1982). Early ambulation. *Advances in Cardiology, 31,* 138–141.

Whyte, J., & Glenn, M. B. (1986). The care and rehabilitation of the patient in a persistent vegetative state. *Journal of Head Trauma Rehabilitation, 1,* 39.

Wolfe, C. D. A., Tilling, K., Beech, R., & Rudd, A. G. (1999). Variation in case fatality and dependency from stroke in Western and Central Europe. *Stroke, 30*, 350–356.

Wood, R. (1991). Critical analysis of the concept of sensory stimulation for patients in vegetative states. *Brain Injury, 4*, 401–410.

Wood, R. L., Winkowski, T. B., Miller, J. L., Tierney, L., & Goldman, L. (1992). Evaluating sensory regulation as a method to improve awareness in patients with altered states of consciousness: A pilot study. *Brain Injury, 6*, 411–418.

Yarkony, G., & Sahgal, V. (1987). Contractures: A major complication of craniocerebral trauma. *Clinical Orthopaedics, 93*, 216–219.

Zhu, X. L., Poon, W. S., Chan, C. H., & Chan, S. H. (2001). Does intensive rehabilitation improve the functional outcome of patients with traumatic brain injury? Interim result of a randomised controlled trial. *British Journal of Neurosurgery, 15*(6), 464–473.

NEUROPSYCHOLOGICAL REHABILITATION
2005, 15 (3/4), 494–502

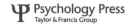

Can behaviours observed in the early stages of recovery after traumatic brain injury predict poor outcome?

Agnes Shiel[1] and Barbara A. Wilson[2]

[1]*Faculty of Medicine and Health Sciences, National University of Ireland, Galway, Ireland*
[2]*MRC Cognition and Brain Sciences Unit, Cambridge, UK*

Diagnosis of the vegetative state (VS) or minimally conscious state (MCS) is dependent on the presence or absence of behavioural variables. Diagnosis of the VS in the case of those who have had a severe head injury does not occur for several months after injury. If such outcomes could be predicted it would facilitate appropriate and timely referrals to specialist rehabilitation units. This paper describes a follow up study of patients observed prospectively after severe head injury and followed up four years later. Thirty patients had made a moderate or good recovery and eight met criteria for MCS. Analysis of early observations together with outcome data suggest that the duration of time taken to achieve some early behaviours may be predictive of poorer outcome.

INTRODUCTION

Outcome is defined as "a visible result" by the *Oxford English Dictionary* and, in the context of brain injury, has been extensively reviewed and researched. Zasler (1996) identifies four phases which he recommends should form the basis of any study of prediction: Definition of the outcome event and the time after injury when it should be assessed; identification of possible predictive factors; collection of prospective data; and statistical

---

Correspondence should be sent to A. Shiel, Faculty of Medicine and Health Sciences, NUI, Galway, Ireland. Email: agnes.shiel@nuigalway.ie

---

http://www.tandf.co.uk/journals/pp/09602011.html   DOI:10.1080/09602010443000551

analysis to evaluate the predictive power of the factors both individually and in combination. Zasler comments further that prediction of unequivocal outcome, for example death, is more accurate than prediction of "intermediate" outcomes, for example, moderate and severe disability. There are few studies of prediction, which examine both the early recovery process and later outcome in detail. It is far more common for extensive early data to be related to a single outcome measure such as the Glasgow Outcome Scale, (Jennett, Snoek, Bond, & Brooks, 1981) or for a comprehensive outcome assessment to be related to sparse acute data.

Severity of injury as measured by initial Glasgow Coma Scale (GCS; Teasdale & Jennett, 1974) and duration of coma and duration of post-traumatic amnesia (PTA), (Bishara, Partridge, Godfrey, & Knight, 1992) have been shown to be related to outcome in numerous studies. GCS scores have been used as predictors in various ways. While the majority of studies use initial summed GCS (Cowen et al., 1995; Polin et al., 1995; Quigley et al., 1997; Reeder, Rosenthal, Lichtenberg, & Wood, 1996; Salcman, Schepp, & Ducker, 1981; Sazbon, Fuchs, & Costeff, 1991; Stambrook et al., 1993), other researchers have used motor GCS (Combes et al., 1996; Spettell et al., 1991), or GCS score taken 6 hours or 24 hours after admission (Phuenpathom, Choomuang, & Ratanalert, 1993; Waxman, Sundine, & Young, 1991). Other factors which have been shown to relate to poor outcome, include abnormal pupillary responses (Teasdale, Murray, Parker, & Jennett, 1979), presence of haematoma (Waxman et al., 1991) age (Waxman et al., 1991), brainstem reflexes (Bishara et al., 1992), hypoxia (Kohi, Mendelow, Teasdale, & Allardice, 1984), hypotension (Kohi et al., 1984), raised intracranial pressure (Alberico et al., 1987) and cerebral perfusion pressure (Changaris et al., 1987).

Less attention has been given to identification or testing of possible predictors during the post-acute or rehabilitation phases. Yet, in many cases, this is when status stabilises enough to achieve reliable assessment and when decisions are made where accurate prediction could be most valuable, for example, which type of rehabilitation unit is most appropriate. There are very limited resources for rehabilitation for people in VS or MCS and if referral is too early, patients may be referred inappropriately. Alternatively, if referral is too late, secondary complications may develop affecting both accuracy of assessment and effectiveness of rehabilitation.

In a previous study, the Wessex Head Injury Matrix (WHIM; Shiel, Horn, Wilson, Watson, Campbell, & McLellan, 2000a, 2000b) was developed. The scale was developed by observing recovery after brain injury in 88 patients and dividing this into small steps or behaviours. In all, there are 62 behaviours or steps on the scale relating to social behaviour, cognition, attention, and communication. The scale is administered by observation and by presenting patients with meaningful stimuli, e.g., photographs and relevant questions (identified by the patients' families) and by observing and recording their responses to these. Clinical recovery is divided into small steps. All items require ability to make some kind of response and items are fine grained enough to show small increments.

The aim of this paper is to evaluate whether the behaviours observed in a cohort of patients during the post-acute stages of recovery from head injury contribute to prediction of cognitive outcome three to four years after head injury with specific reference to poorer outcome. Of particular interest is whether any of the early signs or behaviours are suggestive of poorer outcome, i.e., whether the duration taken to achieve a behaviour or its presence or absence can contribute to prediction of VS or MCS.

METHOD

In a previous study prospective observations of behaviour were made on a cohort of patients recovering from severe head injury (Shiel et al., 2000a). The characteristics of the cohort have been described in detail elsewhere (Shiel et al., 2000a, 2000b). Four years later, patients who participated in this first study, who could be traced, were contacted and invited to participate in the follow up study. Of those not contacted, 6 were untraceable, 2 had died, and initial data on the remaining 14 were restricted to age and GCS score only.

From the original sample of 88, 66 patients were contacted. Fourteen refused to participate and 11 failed to reply. Forty one agreed to participate or agreement to participate was obtained from next of kin. The group was retrospectively divided into those who met the criteria for the minimally conscious state (MCS) and those who did not.

Eight of the sample were very severely impaired and met the criteria for the MCS as described by Giacino et al., (2002). All were resident in nursing homes and four had been diagnosed as being in a vegetative state at least three years previously and had not been re-assessed. This group were reassessed using the Wessex Head Injury Matrix.

The other 30 patients had all had severe brain injury. Although the levels of recovery varied, all were capable of carrying out at least some of the cognitive tests. Data from these were examined to evaluate the relationships between early behaviours and outcome. The tests used are described in Table 1.

The prospective data used were the number of days taken from insult to achieving each behaviour. The behaviours identified as having potential predictive value were evaluated to ascertain whether there were any differences between the MCS group and the other group.

RESULTS

The patients in the prospective study (Shiel et al., 2000a) ranged in age from 14 to 67 years with a mean age of 30.3 years. Coma duration and duration of

TABLE 1
List of functions tested and outcome measures used in the study

Function	Test
General cognitive function	Wechsler Intelligence Test—Revised (WAIS-R)
Premorbid intelligence	National Adult Reading Test (NART)
Memory	Wechsler Memory Test—Revised (WMS-R)
	Rivermead Behavioural Memory Test (RBMT)
Executive functions	Behavioural Assessment of Dysexecutive Function (BADS)
	Modified Card Sorting Test (MCST)
Visual perception	Visual Object and Space Perception Battery (VOSP)
Language	Token test—Revised
	Graded naming test (GNT)
Attention	Speed of information processing
Motor	Rivermead Mobility Index (RMI)
	Grooved pegboard

post-traumatic amnesia were measured prospectively. Mean coma duration was 14.67 days and mean duration of PTA was 56.94 days.

In the follow up sample ($n = 41$), age range was 17–71 years with a mean age of 34.6 years. There was no significant difference between the group who were followed up ($n = 41$) and the group who declined ($n = 14$) or the group who could not be traced ($n = 6$) with regard to severity of injury as measured by coma duration ($w = 1075, p = .36$). The group who met the criteria for the MCS ($n = 8$) had a median age of 25 years and median coma duration of 56 days. They did not differ significantly from the less severely impaired group ($n = 30$) in terms of age but had a significantly longer duration of coma ($w = 118.5, p = .01$).

Relationship between outcome measures and early behaviours

The two datasets—early and outcome data—were analysed to evaluate whether any behaviours predictive of better or poorer outcome could be identified.

Four of the cognitive tests correlated significantly at the 1% level with early behavioural data. These were the WAIS-R Full-Scale IQ, Verbal IQ and Performance IQ and the Rivermead Behavioural Memory Test (RBMT). In each case, the dependent variable was the outcome measure identified as significant in the initial analysis and the independent variables were those early behaviours of which were significantly associated with it.

The WAIS-R Full-Scale IQ score was significantly associated with eye pointing. Time taken to achieve this explained 38% of the variance in IQ score. Verbal IQ was associated with a combination of four behaviours (alerting, removing cloth from face, eye pointing and volitional vocalisation) and this combination gave an r^2 of .36.

Performance IQ was associated with a combination of seven items of early behaviour (expletive utterance, eye contact, focusing on person giving attention, initiating conversation, looking at person giving attention, eye pointing, watching person giving attention) explaining 66% of the variance. The RBMT was associated with five items of early behaviour (age at injury, coma duration, eye pointing, turning head to look at someone talking, watching someone giving attention), which, together, explained 71% of the variance.

Differences between the group tested and the MCS group

The time taken to achieve the behaviours identified above was examined to evaluate whether there were differences between the two groups during the early stage of recovery using Mann–Whitney U tests. The results are summarised in Table 2. Items where the difference in time was significantly different between the groups are highlighted in bold.

It was not possible to evaluate the significance of several other behaviours as either none or very few of the severely injured group had been observed to achieve these. Thus behaviours which were not included in the regression analysis were also tested but only two significant findings were identified— "eyes open" ($U = 150, p = .01$) and "attention held by a dominant stimulus" ($U = 94.5, p = .008$). In the case of some, there were too few data to carry out the analysis and in all cases, this was because the severe group had never been observed to carry out the behaviours.

DISCUSSION

The results suggest that recovery of certain behaviours observed in the early stage may be predictive of better outcome after severe traumatic brain injury. Better outcome was related to early return of attention, particularly visual attention. Surprisingly, neither age nor coma duration was related to any of the cognitive outcomes nor was duration of PTA associated with cognitive outcome. It is difficult to explain these findings but the duration of coma in both groups (which was measured using Glasgow Coma Scale scores) indicated that both groups had had very severe head injuries. Therefore, these results may relate to recovery rather than severity of injury. Furthermore, it may indicate that those patients who show signs of early recovery of attention and cognition have greater spontaneous recovery, or alternatively, it may be that those patients whose attentional and cognitive skills recover quickly are better able to benefit from rehabilitation, thereby having a better outcome.

TABLE 2

Differences in time taken (days) to achieve predictor variables between patients able to carry out cognitive tests and the severely injured group unable to carry out cognitive tests

Variable	Mean		Median		Minimum		Maximum		U	p
	Group 1	Group 2	Group 1	Group 2	Group 1	Group 2	Group 1	Group 2		
Age	30	32	25	28	14	17	56	67	ns	ns
Coma	56	14	54	7	32	1	84	97	118.5	**.005**
Removes cloth from face (2)		24		9	27	4	91	103	n/a	n/a
Obey command to verbal request	55	18	54	10	31	1	83	106	107	**.01**
Watches someone move in line of vision	71	21	73	14	26	3	112	88	73	**.009**
Looks at person giving attention	80	19	92	11	27	3	112	88	94	**.004**
Alerts to familiar voice (2)		37		38	34	6	112	63	n/a	n/a
Turns head to look at person talking	67	16	66	11	27	4	112	75	70.5	**.007**
Focus on person talking	49	20	31	14	27	4	91	67	57.0	**.03**
Make eye contact (2)		30		19	27		91	151	n/a	n/a
Eye pointing (1)		29		24		7		105	n/a	n/a
Frown to express displeasure	72	20	72	10	13	5	133	75	ns	ns
Expletive utterance (0)		22		17		4		49	n/a	n/a
Speech fluent (0)		23		27		7		38	n/a	n/a
Remembers something earlier in the day (1)		40		24		8		109	n/a	n/a
Initiates conversation (0)		35		29		8		105	n/a	n/a

Group 1: Minimally Conscious state at follow up, Group 2: Able to participate in cognitive testing at follow up.

Some of the behaviours significantly associated with better outcome showed significant differences between the MCS group and the other group. The majority of these behaviours were early attentional behaviours. These results are open to a number of interpretations. Perhaps the significant differences between the groups on the time taken to achieve the behaviours, which were associated with outcome, confirmed their importance as predictors. Alternatively, it may be argued that many of these were the early behaviours, which the majority of patients achieved. The severely injured patients did not achieve many of the later behaviours making comparisons of these impossible. Therefore, the possible significance of failure to achieve behaviours must not be overlooked either. It may be that in the case of the early behaviours, time to achievement is significant whereas whether the behaviour is achieved at all is more significant for the later behaviours.

Although these results may indicate that early recovery of attentional behaviours may be an important predictor of better outcome, this cannot be considered conclusive at present. There are several reasons for this. First, there were only eight patients in the severely impaired group. Neither all of these nor all of the 30 in the main study group were observed to carry out all behaviours. The reason why this was so may have been different in that the severely injured group may have been unable to or have not recovered the behaviour whereas the missing data in the main patient group may be explained because some patients recovered rapidly, "skipping" over some of the behaviours. A second reason to exercise caution is that the time taken to achieve the behaviours may merely reflect severity of injury, which can be gauged by GCS score and duration of coma. It is unlikely that this is the case however as, first, GCS score on admission did not predict either outcome, and, second, duration of coma was significantly associated with only the RBMT score but did not differentiate between groups. Thus neither GCS score nor coma duration would have predicted whether these patients would have made a good or moderate recovery or remained in MCS.

These findings also raise important questions regarding accurate assessment of patients diagnosed as being in VS or MCS. The Royal College of Physicians have issued guidelines for withdrawal of artificial nutrition and hydration. In terms of predicting outcome the behaviours, where significant differences between the groups were observed, none fully meet the criteria for diagnosis of VS. This could be taken to suggest that none of these patients were in VS at the time of initial assessment. Yet, four had been diagnosed as being in VS by the time the follow up study took place. This may be explained by the fact that the patients in the prospective study were seen daily, sometimes for several hours, by the research team. This meant that patients were observed both in responsive and unresponsive states and more accurate assessment of optimum function was obtained. It may be that the later diagnosis of vegetative state was made on the basis of a short or one off assessment when the patient was unresponsive.

The results suggest that the time taken to achieve five behaviours—obeying commands, watching someone moving in the line of vision, looking at a person giving attention, turning head to look at a person talking, and focusing on a person talking may be predictive of overall outcome. These behaviours—with the exception of obeying a command—may be perceived as falling into a "grey" area in terms of whether patients displaying such behaviours may be defined as being in VS or MCS. For example, brief eye tracking and fixation are consistent with a diagnosis of VS. Further evaluation of this needs to be carried out, particularly in relation to a more robust definition of terms such as "brief". In the Wessex Head Injury Matrix all such terms are defined.

In conclusion, it should be noted that these results are speculative at present. The sample sizes are small and there is a possibility of both Type 1 and Type 2 errors. Therefore, it is strongly recommended that a further prospective study to test this hypothesis is undertaken.

REFERENCES

Alberico, A. M., Ward, J. D., Choi, S. C., Marmarou, A., & Young, H. F. (1987). Outcome after severe head injury. Relationship to mass lesions, diffuse injury, and ICP course in pediatric and adult patients. *Journal of Neurosurgery, 67*, 648–656.

Bishara, S. N., Partridge, F. M., Godfrey, M. P. D., & Knight, R. G. (1992). Post-traumatic amnesia and Glasgow Coma Scale related to outcome in survivors in a consecutive series of patients with severe closed head injury. *Brain Injury, 6*, 373–380.

Changaris, D. G., Mcgraw, C. P., Richardson, J. D., Garretson, H. D., Arpin, E. J., & Shields, C. B. (1987). Correlation of cerebral perfusion pressure and glasgow coma scale to outcome. *Journal of Trauma, 27*, 1007–1013.

Combes, P., Fauvage, B., Colonna, M., Passagia, J. G., Chirossel, J. P., & Jacquot, C. (1996). Severe head injuries: An outcome prediction and survival analysis. *Intensive Care Medicine, 22*, 1391–1395.

Cowen, T. D., Maythaler, J. M., Deviro, M. J., Ivie, C. S., Lebow, J., & Novack, T. A. (1995). Influence of early variables in traumatic brain injury on functional independence measures scores and rehabilitation length of stay and charges. *Archives of Physical Medicine and Rehabilitation, 76*, 797–803.

Giacino, J. T., Ashwal, S, Childs, N., Cranford, R., Jennett, B., Katz, D. I., et al. (2002). The minimally conscious state: Definition and diagnostic criteria. *Neurology, 58(3)*: 349–353.

Jennett, B., Snoek, J., Bond, M. R., & Brooks, N. (1981). Disability after severe head injury: Observations on the use of the Glasgow Outcome Scale. *Journal of Neurology, Neurosurgery and Psychiatry, 44*, 285–293.

Kohi, Y. M., Mendelow, A. D., Teasdale, G. M., & Allardice, G. M. (1984). Extracranial insults and outcome in patients with acute head injury—relationship to the Glasgow Coma Scale. *Injury, 16*, 25–29.

Phuenpathom, N., Choomuang, M., & Ratanalert, S. (1993). Outcome and outcome prediction in acute subdural hematoma. *Surgical Neurology, 40*, 22–25.

Polin, R. S., Shaffrey, M. E., Phillips, C. D., Germanson, T., & Jane, J. A. (1995). Multivariate analysis and prediction of outcome following penetrating head injury. *Neurosurgery Clinics of North America, 6*, 689–699.

Quigley, M. R., Vidovich, M. D., Cantella, R. N., Wilberger, J. E., Maroon, J. C., & Diamond, D. (1997). Defining the limits of survivorship after very severe head injury. *Journal of Trauma: Injury, Infection and Critical Care, 42*, 7–10.

Reeder, K. P., Rosenthal, M., Lichtenberg, P., & Wood, D. (1996). Impact of age on functional outcome following traumatic brain injury. *Journal of Head Trauma Rehabilitation, 11*, 22–31.

Royal College of Physicians (1996). The Permanent Vegetative State: Review of a Working Party. Convened by the Royal College of Physicians and endorsed by the conference of Medical Royal Colleges and their faculties of the United Kingdom. *Journal of the Royal College Physicians London, 30*, 119–121.

Salcman, M., Schepp, R. S., & Ducker, T. B. (1981). Calculated recovery rates in severe head trauma. *Neurosurgery, 8*, 301–308.

Sazbon, L., Fuchs, C., & Costeff, H. (1991). Prognosis for recovery from prolonged post-traumatic unawareness: Logistic analysis. *Journal of Neurology, Neurosurgery and Psychiatry, 54*, 149–152.

Shiel, A., Horn, S. A., Wilson, B. A., Watson, M. J., Campbell, M., & McLellan, D. L. (2000a). The Wessex Head Injury Matrix (WHIM) main scale: A preliminary report on a scale to assess and monitor patient recovery after severe head injury. *Clinical Rehabilitation, 14*(4): 408–416.

Shiel, A., Horn, S. A., Wilson, B. A., Watson, M. J., Campbell, M., & McLellan, D. L. (2000b). *The Wessex Head Injury Matrix (WHIM)*. Thames Valley Test Company.

Spettell, C. M., Ellis, D. W., Ross, S. E., Sandel, E., O'Malley, K. F., Stein, S. C., et al. (1991). Time of rehabilitation admission and severity of trauma: Effect on brain injury outcome. *Archives of Physical Medicine and Rehabilitation, 72*, 320–325.

Stambrook, M., Moore, A. D., Lubusko, A. A., Peters, L. C., & Blumenschein, S. (1993). Alternatives to the Glasgow Coma Scale as a quality of life predictor following traumatic brain injury. *Archives of Clinical Neuropsychology, 8*, 95–103.

Teasdale, G., & Jennett, B. (1974). Assessment of coma and impaired consciousness: A practical scale. *Lancet i*, 81–84.

Teasdale, G., Murray, G., Parker, L., & Jennett, B. (1979). Adding up the Glasgow Coma Score. *Acta Neurochiruga Supplement Wien, 28*, 13–16.

Waxman, K., Sundine, M. J., & Young, R. F. (1991). Is early prediction of outcome in severe head injury possible? *Archives of Surgery, 126*, 1237–1243.

Zasler, N. (1996). Nomenclature: Evolving trends. *Neurorehabilitation, 6*, 3–8.

NEUROPSYCHOLOGICAL REHABILITATION
2005, 15 (3/4), 503–513

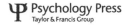
Psychology Press
Taylor & Francis Group

Vegetative and minimally conscious states: How can occupational therapists help?

Ros Munday

Royal Hospital for Neuro-disability, London, UK

There is little documentation about the role of occupational therapy specifically for the vegetative and minimally conscious patient. This paper sets out to clarify the role using one model of occupational therapy, namely that of Reed and Sanderson (1992), and proposes occupational therapy assessment and treatment for this patient group. It explores how patients are affected in the performance components of motor, sensory, cognitive, intrapersonal, and interpersonal skills, which are explored through assessment. The paper then explains how these skills impact upon occupational performance (functional ability) and suggests methods occupational therapists will use in treatment planning. Throughout the manuscript, a person-centred approach, which is vital to occupational therapy, is demonstrated.

INTRODUCTION

The term vegetative state (VS) was initially introduced by Jennett and Plum in 1972 to describe patients who demonstrate a sleep-wake cycle but do not demonstrate behaviour indicating awareness of self or their environment. Patients whose behaviours demonstrate an inconsistent awareness are diagnosed in a minimally conscious state (MCS). The behaviours indicating awareness include: following simple instructions; yes/no responses, although these do not need to be accurate; appropriate emotional responses to the situation/environment; and eye tracking (Giacino et al., 2002).

Correspondence should be sent to Ros Munday, Occupational Therapy Department, Royal Hospital for Neuro-disability, West Hill, Putney, London SW15 3SW, UK. Tel: 020 8780-4500 extension 5108, Fax: 020 8780-4501. Email: rmunday@rhn.org.uk

© 2005 Psychology Press Ltd
http://www.tandf.co.uk/journals/pp/09602011.html   DOI:10.1080/09602010443000533

This paper uses the authors' clinical experience as an occupational therapist to explore the role of occupational therapy (OT) with this complex patient group using the Reed and Sanderson model of OT (Reed & Sanderson. 1992). This model was initially selected by the Royal Hospital for Neuro-disability OT department due to the diverse and differing clinical needs of the patient population and the requirement for an adaptable model of practice. The flexibility of the model has since been corroborated by Chapparo and Ranks (1997). Another well-know, model was considered (the model of human occupation developed by Kielhofner, 1985). However, this is reliant on volition and was not felt to be appropriate for the patient group. This paper will address the areas of OT assessment and OT intervention rationale for treatment. In addition it will link patients' abilities and/or deficits to occupation by suggesting intervention and will propose a hierarchical model of OT intervention with severe brain injury.

OT PRACTICE MODEL

With the severity of impairment, those in a VS or MCS present a challenge to all clinical staff, including OTs. However, there is little written about the role of OT with this patient group. This paper is based on 14 years personal experience working in the UK with patients in VS/MCS. In the author's experience, OTs in acute district hospitals concentrate at a biomechanical level, i.e., splinting to prevent development of contractures, and wheelchair seating when there is an active duty of care. However, on many occasions patients have been admitted to a rehabilitation unit without OT intervention due to patients in VS/MCS not being classified as high priority. Griffin (2002) identified improving self-care independence, preventing contractures, and discharge planning as the core interventions for acute neurology OTs.

Central to OT is the belief that engagement in an occupation (which differs according to individuals' roles, interests and the importance they place upon these) is essential for human beings. For an OT, an occupation encompasses all purposeful activity engaged in a lifetime. This can be divided into three areas: self-maintenance, e.g., skills necessary for personal care; productivity, e.g., work, job roles; and leisure. Environmental and sociocultural issues are considered within these three occupational areas. OTs will use meaningful activities to assess how motor, sensory, cognitive, intrapersonal and interpersonal skills (performance components) impact upon ability within occupational areas (Reed & Sanderson, 1992). OTs either adapt the environment, provide equipment and teach patients to use the adaptations to carry out activities (compensation technique), or use activities and tasks to address impaired abilities impacting upon performance (remediation technique). With either technique, assessment of the abilities required for an activity is analysed by breaking it down into the component steps and skills required (activity and task analysis). Intervention can then be devised to further develop patients" abilities. Both compensation and remediation approaches are implemented with individuals who have sustained severe brain injury.

The VS and MCS patient is affected in all performance components. As with all clinicians, it is essential that OTs are able to distinguish between reflexive and meaningful responses. By linking motor, sensory and cognitive skills, OTs make an invaluable contribution to the assessment process, which establishes the impact of deficits in any component and the resulting effect on functional ability. As VS and MCS patients cannot contribute to goal planning, the OT will need to obtain information regarding the patient's pre-injury interests, roles, and cultural and social background to ensure a person-centred approach to assessment and treatment. Where the patient is disassociated from family and friends, the OT must make a judgement about the patient's perceived pre-injury occupational lifestyle.

THE AIMS OF OT

As previously highlighted, OT assessment will normally focus on the abilities required to participate in functional activities relevant to a patient's pre-injury role and interests. However, with patients in VS/MCS, OTs will initially focus on assessment at an impairment level, due to the high degree of disability experienced in all performance components. Broad aims of intervention are suggested in Table 1. Following assessment, treatment and further

TABLE 1
Initial occupational therapy aims of intervention

Domain	Aim
Overall aim	To establish the patients rehabilitation potential
Motor	To establish physical management programme
	To prevent development of secondary complications, e.g., contractures, skin breakdown
Sensory	To establish level of sensory responses
Cognition	To establish meaningfulness of behavioural responses
	To establish the level of function through assessment of awareness levels
	To develop purposeful behaviours which can be used functionally
Interpersonal/intrapersonal	To establish contingency of behavioural/emotional responses
	To establish patient's ability to communicate
Self-maintenance/leisure	Enhancing abilities and improving function
	To develop purposeful behaviours which can be used functionally
	To establish disability management programmes
Environmental	To educate families/carers

assessment will be carried out at an activity and ability level of occupation, to further explore behaviours demonstrated in assessment sessions. Therefore, the OT systematic process of information gathering, assessment, analysis of assessment planning, goal setting, treatment planning and re-evaluation applies with patients in VS/MCS.

Many of the aims listed in Table 1 will be carried out jointly with other multidisciplinary team (MDT) members, with the OTs contributing their unique perspective of integrating physical, psychosocial and mental processes.

OT INTERVENTION

Performance components are the building blocks (skills) required in the development/execution of any activity. Therefore careful evaluation of performance components is required to establish the impairments and abilities impacting on activity engagement. In order to devise treatment blocks, areas of ability are analysed in terms of self-maintenance, e.g., to develop a consistent yes/no response, switch access to computer/environmental controls, grooming and feeding tasks, and leisure.

Apart from the areas mentioned above there are two areas important at any stage of OT intervention: communication with family, friends or carers and risk assessment. Family/friends and carer liaison will be mentioned in more detail later in this paper. In the UK, the advent of clinical governance (NHS Executive, 1999) has identified that risk assessment (and identifying methods to reduce risk), is an integral part of clinical practice. For an OT, risk assessment includes relatives' use of the wheelchair, the patient going outdoors, travelling in a vehicle, and seating and bed-positioning guidelines to minimise any risk identified. Although patients should be medically stable before sensory and cognitive responsiveness is established, intervention may be required earlier to ensure secondary complications are prevented. These interventions will focus on motor/physical management, i.e., guidelines for positioning in bed, and splinting regimes should be created to prevent development of contractures and pressure areas.

PERFORMANCE COMPONENTS

The assessment and intervention in the five performance component areas are discussed in more detail.

Motor skills

Patients with profound brain injury can present with primitive reflexes and altered muscle tone and strength, which impact on a patient's ability to participate in a functional task. Giacino et al. (1997) suggested that the minimum intervention required with severe brain injury is range of movement exercises, positioning, and management of altered tone. Able-bodied people automatically change their postural control when voluntary movement is carried out to enable performance of functional tasks. However, with neurological impairment this ability is lost, with muscles being recruited to maintain posture, and therefore not available for use in function. To reduce gravity effects, poor postural control and abnormal tone it is essential that equipment providing postural support is used. Positioning in a wheelchair is claimed to increase arousal levels by stimulating the vestibular systems. Supportive wheelchair positioning can also inhibit abnormal muscle tone and reduce the risk of developing secondary complications (pressure sores, contractures, abnormal tone) (Radomski, 2002), while allowing the patient to interact and gain a more normal view of the environment.

Joint OT and physiotherapy assessment is conducted to establish range of movement, postural control and muscle tone. This allows development of bed and wheelchair positioning guidelines to ensure that alignment is maintained on a 24 hour basis; that the effects of gravity on body segments are reduced; that postural support is provided to ensure less effort is required to maintain balance; and that risk of secondary complications is minimised. Such postural management reduces the possibility of limited functional ability due to motor impairment (Pope, 2002). The Royal College of Physicians (2003) acknowledged the effect positioning might have on an individual's responses, suggesting in the recent guidelines that assessments be carried out in different positions.

When joints are held in a shortened position this can lead to adaptive shortening, poor skin hygiene and development of spasticity. OTs use regular passive range of movement alongside splinting and casting to maintain passive range of movement, reduce risk of secondary complications, maintain skin hygiene, decrease risk of abnormal muscle tone, and increase or maintain a patient's functional movement. However, research evidence is not clear on the efficacy of this treatment approach (Lannin, 2003). OTs can advise the MDT on the patient's functional movement and the impact of any tone treatment on functional ability.

Sensory/cognition skills

Through the use of standardised objective measures it is possible to establish the behavioural repertoire demonstrated by a patient to sensory stimuli. A number of assessments have been developed for this purpose including the Western Neuro-Sensory Stimulation Profile (Ansell & Keenan, 1989), the Disability Rating Scale (Rappaport et al., 1982), the Wessex Head Injury Matrix (Shiel et al., 2000), and the Sensory Modality Assessment and

Rehabilitation Technique (SMART; Gill-Thwaites & Munday, 1999). It is beyond the remit of this paper to address all the assessments available, instead it will concentrate on SMART, which was developed by OTs to provide an assessment sensitive enough to detect small behavioural responses and changes in patients' responses.

SMART is a 10 session assessment process consisting of observing the patient's behaviour for 10 minutes in a non-stimulating environment. This is immediately followed by an assessment of behavioural responses (sensory and cognitive) to different stimuli in the five senses and also motor function, communication, and level of wakefulness. A five-point hierarchical scoring system categorises responses from no response, to those indicating a non-meaningful response through to cognitively mediated responses (Gill-Thwaites & Munday, 1999). For example, a patient may respond in a reflexive manner in the visual modality with pupils constricting to light and repetitive blinking to threat. Or they may demonstrate the cognitive ability to visually discriminate between two words and follow written one-step instructions. This detailed multi-observational assessment enables evaluation to be based on the quality and quantity of patient responses in each of the modalities, thus assisting in the differential diagnosis of VS and MCS. Relatives' observations of responses are also incorporated into the process, as patients may respond differently to family and MDT members. Information from the therapist assessments and family observations allows for a broad picture to be built of the patient's responses (Gill-Thwaites & Munday, 1999).

Intrapersonal/interpersonal

Patients in VS and MCS may present with emotional responses, such as crying or laughter. While a patient in VS may demonstrate laughter and crying for no apparent reason, a patient in MCS will only laugh or cry dependent upon the situation, e.g., when a certain relative visits. Following administration of an assessment, such as SMART, the OTs will have developed an understanding of the patient's behavioural repertoire. Through joint sessions with the family and behaviours observed when the family is not present, the OT will be able to provide valuable information for the MDT to assist in identifying the cause of the behaviour. For example, in one case members of the MDT reported that whenever the family visited and said the patient's name the patient would laugh. This response could indicate the patient was aware. However, on assessment with SMART, the OT noticed that, with a repeated loud sound, the patient consistently demonstrated a startle response and laughed. On further assessment, the MDT discovered the family would shout the patient's name, resulting in a startle and laughter response. This response was therefore felt to be part of the patient's reflexive response repertoire.

OCCUPATIONAL AREAS

Following assessment of the performance components, the OT will link abilities and limitations observed into the treatment of occupational areas. Self-maintenance and leisure are described below. Due to the nature of the productivity occupational area (i.e., domestic skills, child care, work) this area is not appropriate with VS/MCS patients and will not be covered.

Self-maintenance

One role of OTs is to carry out a sensory programme for patients responding at a reflexive/sub-cortical level. This programme will not be based at an impairment level (as with the assessment) but will use responses observed during the assessment with the aim of increasing the consistency and complexity of the tasks/responses. For example, a treatment programme using an errorless learning approach may be developed for a patient who inconsistently follows one-step motor instructions during assessment, with the aim to achieve a consistent response. This response is then linked to a method for yes and no, which is upgraded to answering biographical yes/no questions. The sensory programme may consist of continuing to explore all senses (multimodal) or may focus on one sense that demonstrates a higher level of response (uni-modal). The OT will use information gained from relatives and friends about the patient's pre-injury interests and incorporate familiar stimuli into treatment sessions. For example, if a patient demonstrates inconsistent visual tracking of an unfamiliar picture in the assessment, the treatment session can compare responses to unfamiliar and familiar pictures, establishing whether the patient shows increased awareness of familiar stimuli. Other areas the OT may wish to incorporate in the treatment sessions include providing cues (visual, tactile, auditory), using approaches of errorless learning, and chaining. However, with tactile cues the OT needs to be aware of the possibility that responses are due to the physical contact and not the initial stimulus.

Alternatively, for patients who have very limited movements, the OT may choose to explore the use of assistive technology. This can range from exploring the most appropriate method of using a switch, and type of switch, based on information gained on the patient's movement patterns in assessment, e.g., head, foot, and thumb. Once the response is considered consistent, sessions can be upgraded to using the switch with radios or computers to assess cause and effect, and subsequently linked to environmental controls or method of communication.

Following assessment, the OT will have identified any potential abilities that can be used or explored further. Patients who have active movement, and without severely limited range of movement in upper limbs, can be assessed with pre-learnt functional tasks such as face-washing, hair-combing, bed-rolling (dependent upon cultural beliefs and past lifestyle). Using guided movement or verbal or visual prompts it is possible to use a task analysis approach to establish preservation of skills over a series of sessions. These sessions will also establish learning ability within a session and carryover between sessions of pre-learnt skills. Use of physical facilitation movement techniques will allow the therapist to inhibit tone increase and enable the patient to select movements to enable participation in functional activities. However, while facilitating, the therapist must minimise the assistance provided and encourage the patient's active participation.

A number of nursing homes in the UK utilise a multi-sensory room with this patient group. The OT can assess and advise on those stimuli that provide maximum benefit to the patients, risk assess the activity and provide guidelines.

Leisure

Using information pertaining to a patient's pre-injury interests it is possible to devise a daily leisure programme incorporating rest periods. Knowledge gained in the assessment and sensory treatment session provides valuable information about the patient's activity and stimulation tolerance. Wood, Winkowski, and Miller (1993) suggested a sensory regulation approach where the environment is controlled to prevent over-stimulation and enable selective attention. The patient's daily programme should provide a balance of activity with rest, preventing over-stimulation and allowing for all patients, the possibility of making sense of their environment while incorporating leisure interests.

Many patients who have sustained profound brain injury will not have left a hospital/institution environment since the time of onset. Assessing behavioural responses to trips in the ambulance, behaviour in different environments (parks, shopping centres, pubs, sporting events) allows development of guidelines for families and future placements to enable pre-injury leisure interests to be pursued.

ENVIRONMENT

Some families wish for patients to return home for day visits or to be discharged home. In these cases it is essential links are made with community services, and assessment made to ensure that the property is suitable for wheelchair accessibility. OTs will also recommend equipment required within the home environment. Training the family in areas of care required and in use of equipment is essential. If feasible, a trial period of the family caring for the patient in a flat within the hospital grounds provides invaluable information about further training required and assists families in realistic assessment of the patient's potential.

FAMILY

To enable development of assessment and treatment that is meaningful to the patient, information from relatives and friends is essential regarding pre-injury interests, roles and culture and the patient's social background.

VS and MCS are difficult concepts for relatives, and families often do not understand altered consciousness (Springer, Farmer, & Bouman, 1997). Although OTs do not work as counsellors they can support the families by answering any questions objectively and realistically and not becoming emotional if family anger is directed towards them. We need to accept that families are under stress and grieving. Information needs to repeated when required and individuals' methods of coping must be respected.

Relatives are often the patient's best advocates; they know what was important to the patient pre-injury. Hauber, Testani-Dufour, and Coleman (2002) reported that families have a need to share the information and knowledge they have with the treating teams. To assist their understanding of the OT perspective joint sessions should be carried out and feedback from relatives used to assist development of treatment plans. Clinical experience shows that some families and friends may interpret a patient's lack of response as laziness, being bored in sessions, or a dislike of the therapist. Although relatives may interpret behaviour they observe optimistically as meaningful, it must be recognised patients may respond differently to family members.

Joint sessions allow exploration of the interaction between patient and family members. Using the concept of activity analysis and sensory regulation (Wood et al., 1993) OTs can assist families in appropriate interaction styles, thereby allowing patients the best chance to respond if able, and make sense of their environment. This can be introduced and explored in detail with families where the patient has not demonstrated awareness in order to redirect attention from the patient's responses, or lack of them, and towards quality time for the family. For example, with a family that assists in grooming the patient, the OT can assist in structuring these tasks. Using task analysis it is possible to break the activity into the component parts exploring the senses being stimulated. Subsequently, tasks can be structured to ensure only one sense is stimulated at a time and the environment is conducive to the task.

Watanabe et al. (2001) reported families requested training and this is particularly important for those who are considering caring for their relative, even for day leave at home. OTs can introduce a graded programme of addressing what knowledge and skills are required in areas of care such as moving and handling, positioning guidelines, use of equipment provided, and splint application. As part of the process for day trips or discharge home, a home visit is required to establish suitability of the environment, equipment required (including bath, hoists, and vehicles) and access to the property.

SUMMARY

This paper has highlighted the wide-ranging skills that OT brings to the assessment and treatment of patients in VS and MCS. As stated, this article is based on the author's clinical experience. The lack of published research demonstrates the need for research into the role of OT with this patient group.

The combination of skills and knowledge OTs possess in motor, sensory, cognitive, interpersonal and intrapersonal skills within functional tasks makes OTs invaluable team members in the assessment and treatment of this rare patient group. Using a person-centred approach, OTs will involve family and friends closely in the process.

REFERENCES

Ansell, B. J., & Keenan, J. E. (1989). The Western Neuro Sensory Stimulation Profile: A tool for assessing slow to recover head injured patients. *Archives of Physical Medicine and Rehabilitation, 70*, 104–108.

Chapparo, C., & Ranks, J. (1997). *Towards a model of occupational performance: Model development.* Retrieved 4 December 2004 from http://www.occupationalperformance.com/origin00.html.

Giacino, J. T., Ashwal, S., Childs, N., Cranford, R., Jennett, B., Katz, D. I., et al. (2002). The minimally conscious state. Definition and diagnostic criteria. *Neurology, 58*, 349–353.

Giacino, J. T., Zasler, N., Katz, D., Kelly, J., Rosenberg, J., & Filley, C. (1997). Development of practice guidelines for assessment and management of the vegetative and minimally conscious states. *Journal of Head Trauma Rehabilitation, 12*(4), 79–89.

Gill-Thwaites, H., & Munday, R. (1999). The Sensory Modality Assessment and Rehabilitation Technique (SMART): A comprehensive and integrated assessment and treatment protocol for the vegetative state and minimally responsive patient. *Neuropsychological Rehabilitation, 9*(3/4), 305–320.

Griffin, S. (2002). Occupational therapy in acute care neurology and orthopaedics. *Journal of Allied Health, 31*(1), 35–42.

Hauber, R. P., Testani-Dufour, L., & Coleman, K. (2002). Better care for low-level brain injured patients and their families. *Journal of Neuroscience Nursing, 34*(1), 20–24.

Jennet, B., & Plum, F. (1972). Persistent vegetative state after brain damage. A syndrome in search of a name. *Lancet, 1*, 734–737.

Kielhofner, G. (1985). *A model of human occupation theory and application.* Baltimore: Williams and Wilkins.

Lannin, N. A. (2003). Is hand splinting effective for adults following stroke? A systematic review and methodological critique for published research. *Clinical Rehabitiation, 17*, 807–816.

NHS Executive (1999). *Clinical governance: Quality in the new NHS,* Leeds, UK: NHSE.

Pope, P. (2002). Posture management and special seating. In S. Edwards (ed.), *Neurological physiotherapy. A problem-solving approach.* (pp. 189–217) (2nd ed.). Edinburgh, UK: Churchill Livingstone.

Radomski, M. V. (2002). Traumatic brain injury. In C. A. Trombly & M. V. Radomski (Eds.) *Occupational therapy for physical dysfunction* (5th ed.). Philadelphia: Lippincott, Williams & Wilkins.

Rappaport, M., Hall, K. M., Hopkins, K., Belleza, T., & Cope, D. N. (1982). Disability rating scale for severe brain trauma: Coma to community. *Archives of Physical Medicine and Rehabilitation, 63*, 118–123.

Reed, K., & Sanderson, S. (1992). *Concepts of occupational therapy*, (3rd ed.). Baltimore: Williams & Wilkins.

Royal College of Physicians (2003). *The vegetative state: Guidance on diagnosis and management.* London: Royal College of Physicians.

Shiel, A., Horn, S. A., Wilson, B. A., Watson, M. J., Campbell, M. J., & McLellan, D. L. (2000). The Wessex Head Injury Matrix (WHIM) main scale: A preliminary report on a scale to assess and monitor patient recovery after severe head injury. *Clinical Rehabilitation, 14*, 408–416.

Springer, J. A., Farmer, J. E., & Bouman, D. E. (1997). Common misconceptions about traumatic brain injury among family members of rehabilitation patients. *Journal of Head Trauma, 12*(3), 41–50.

Watanabe, Y., Shiel, A., McLellan, L. D., Kurihara, M., & Hayashi, K. (2001). The impact of traumatic brain injury on family members living with patient: A preliminary study in Japan and the UK. *Disability and Rehabilitation, 23*(9): 390–378.

Wood, R. L., Winkowski, T. B., & Miller, J. L. (1993). Sensory regulation as a method to promote recovery in patients with altered states of consciousness. *Neuropsychological Rehabilitation, 3*(2): 177–190.

NEUROPSYCHOLOGICAL REHABILITATION
2005, 15 (3/4), 514–521

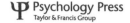

Considerations for the use of assistive technology in patients with impaired states of consciousness

Karen Naudé and Matthew Hughes

Royal Hospital for Neuro-disability, London, UK

While there is limited literature addressing the application of assistive technology in patients in persistent vegetative state (PVS) and minimally conscious state (MCS), it is believed that it can assist with the assessment, diagnosis and treatment as well as management of these patients. The use of technology to assist in PVS and MCS is mostly limited to the application of simple binary switch devices to determine whether a motor response is consistent or otherwise. However, the application of such technology is often undermined due to a lack of established protocols for use by the multidisciplinary team (MDT), as well as a lack of available technical resources. Therefore the ongoing development of assessment instruments as well as effective outcome measures used by an MDT is imperative. This article aims to discuss some key aspects to consider in the use of assistive technology when assessing and treating people in impaired conscious states. Possible considerations and suggestions will be discussed through this paper and a case study will be used to demonstrate some of these interventions.

It has been argued that advancing medical technologies and associated means of sustaining life have led to a greater proportion of brain-injured people surviving and hence requiring long-term intervention despite significant disability (Piguet, King, & Harrison, 1999). Some of these patients present as minimally conscious, which is a relatively new diagnostic classification in the spectrum of consciousness disorders following the Multi-Society Task Force on PVS (Giacino & Kalmar, 1997). This classification is

---

Correspondence should be sent to Karen Naudé, Department of Occupational Therapy, Royal Hospital for Neuro-disability, West Hill, Putney, London SW15 3SW, UK. Tel: 020 8946 1472. Email: karennaude@hotmail.com

---

© 2005 Psychology Press Ltd
http://www.tandf.co.uk/journals/pp/09602011.html   DOI:10.1080/09602010443000470

proving especially beneficial in the diagnosis and management of patients, in particular by distinguishing between PVS and MCS. This is a condition of severely altered consciousness in which the person demonstrates minimal but definite evidence of self or environmental awareness. Historically it has been speculated that such patients may have some internal awareness but no ability to demonstrate it as such. However, despite the development of a diagnostic classification there are difficulties with its successful application, primarily due to the very nature of the clinical features, namely the inconsistent response style of these patients and often severe motor and sensory impairments, making assessment somewhat complex.

Despite the complexity of these patients, several standardised assessment measures (O'Dell, Jasin, Lyons, Stivers, & Meszaros, 1996) have been developed to assess the potential transition between states of consciousness. These include the Western Neuro Sensory Stimulation Profile (Ansell & Keenan, 1989), the Coma Near Coma Scale (Rappaport, Doughtery, & Kelting, 1992), and the Sensory Stimulation Assessment Measure (Rader & Ellis, 1994). Additional measures such as the Sensory Modality Assessment and Rehabilitation Technique (SMART; Gill-Thwaites & Munday, 1999), and the Wessex Head Injury Matrix (Shiel et al., 2000) highlight the importance of collaborative work within the MDT, in order to record any behavioural changes that may influence the "level" of the intervention (Canedo, Grix, & Nicoletti, 2002). Some of these instruments go on to suggest treatment interventions, which are based on sensory stimulation, although this is not conclusively supported in the literature. The SMART, however, suggests the use of a buzzer to determine a person's ability to respond to auditory stimuli and follow verbal commands by eliciting a purposeful movement. This is possibly one of the only examples of the use of assistive technology to help with assessment and treatment intervention.

Assistive technology encompasses any device used to demonstrate, increase, maintain, or improve interaction and functional capabilities of individuals with disabilities. Assistive technology solutions improve an individual's ability to learn, compete, work, interact with family and friends, achieve greater independence, and enjoy a better quality of life. Therefore, areas to consider for the use of assistive technology, such as simple binary switches, include assessment and diagnosis, family involvement, communication and application.

ASSESSMENT AND DIAGNOSIS

Switch use has been successfully applied in the identification of misdiagnosis due to visual deficits (Andrews, Murphy, Munday, & Littlewood, 1996), neuropsychological assessment of a potential "euthanasia" case (McMillan,

1996; McMillan & Herbert, 2000), and a lack of potential for further recovery (Watson, Horn, & Wilson, 1999). Switch use is also suggested in assessment and treatment protocols such as the SMART (Gill-Thwaites, 1997). Successful use may lead to functional implications for the individual, such as the possibility of controlling the environment or facilitating basic communication.

FAMILY

Family involvement and adjustment to change has been sighted as an integral part of treating a patient with a severe head injury (Kreutzer, Kolakowsky-Hayner, Demn, & Mead, 2002). One way in which families interact with patients demonstrating inconsistent responses in MCS is through the use of low level technological interventions, such as a plate switch connected to a latched timer to operate an electronic device. In exceptional circumstances more advanced, and often custom made switches, including blink and muscle activated switches, are considered for patients with very limited motor ability. These switches can additionally be used to access further integrated systems such as those used to facilitate both communication and mobility needs concurrently.

COMMUNICATION

The use of assistive technology has greater potential application in those patients who progress beyond the MCS. A single switch or buzzer can be used to express an established yes/no response, develop a simple communication system to express basic needs, or even assist in determining mental capacity. This may be done either through the use of a scanning device or by activating switches directly. The provision of technology at this stage can consequently facilitate the use of environmental controls, powered mobility, and complex communication devices known as augmentative alternative communication (AAC). Currently, the use of these communication aids to assist with memory impairment in complex disability remains an explorative topic for further research.

FURTHER CONSIDERATIONS AND APPLICATION

Although establishing a person's ability to elicit a motor movement is essential, it is also important to be aware of the factors affecting the use of a single switch. Angelo (2000), completed a study in which she identified 11 considerations that therapists regarded as important for switch access.

Some of these include the reliability of motor movement, endurance and ability to perform timed response, hence, highlighting the complex nature of such interventions.

Environmental adaptations are also important to compensate for patients' limited and restricted movement due to their impairment in neuromotor systems (Gentile, 1998). Therefore, appropriate posture and seating and accurate mounting of devices are required to ensure matches between the environment and motor ability of the patient (Gentile, 1998).

Much work has been done by Cook and Hussey (2002) regarding the interdisciplinary approach and the effectiveness of the use of technology with patients with severe disability. They adapted the model used by Bailey (1989) to define the application of assistive technology. The Human Activity Assistive Technology (HAAT) model focuses on the interaction of the human/technology interface, the activity output, and the environmental interface when determining the appropriate use of assistive technology. This, however, has not necessarily been generalised to the population of MCS and PVS patients.

Some specialist neurorehabilitation units have technology clinics where a variety of the approaches described above are used. Where appropriate, these models need to be considered to develop an effective assistive technology service. One such example is the technology clinic at the Royal Hospital for Neuro-disability, London, UK.

In this clinic a systematic approach is followed to establish the potential for the use of assistive technology, which includes a variety of assessment criteria such as sensory abilities, posture, and seating and motor function. These clinics are ideally run by an interdisciplinary team to ensure a patient's problems are holistically identified and their needs analysed to guarantee a cohesive multi-sensory and collaborative approach to therapeutic intervention.

The following case of Mr M is used to demonstrate the successful application of some of the above considerations.

CASE STUDY

Mr M is in his 20s and sustained a severe closed head injury as a result of a high speed single vehicle collision. His initial Glasgow Coma Scale (GCS) score was 3/15. A cerebral computed tomography scan was reported to reveal diffuse cerebral damage; a subarachnoid haemorrhage, blood in his right ventricle, diffuse cerebral oedema, multiple haemorrhages, and contusions, specifically in the frontal and parietal regions. His right pupil remained dilated and non-reactive, he spent three weeks in ITU and his GCS score remained 3/15 although more spontaneous eye opening was noted at approximately 25 days.

He was subsequently admitted to the Royal Hospital for Neuro-disability 70 days post-injury. On admission it was evident that he had severe physical management issues that needed to be addressed. In particular he presented with severe increased tone throughout, flexed neck and no active movement in his limbs. Physical management included upper and lower limb serial casting, medication for tone management, and complex postural assessment including bed and wheelchair positioning. He remained nil by mouth, was Percutaneous Endoscopic Gastrostomy (PEG) fed and decannulation commenced 120 days post-injury.

Mr M was assessed over four weeks, between days 80–115, using the SMART. The assessment was complicated by complex physical management issues and pyrexia. The overall impression from the SMART indicated that Mr M was functioning on a

- *Reflex level* (level 2) for visual, motor and tactile stimuli.

- *Withdrawal level* (level 3) for auditory stimuli.

- *Optimal arousal level* (level 5) for wakefulness, which suggested that he could have some underlying awareness but expression of this was limited by his physical problems.

A multi-modal SMART sensory treatment programme was (Gill-Thwaites & Munday, 1999) commenced on day 120 and focused on visual and auditory modalities based on the assessment results and behavioural observations. The overall aim was to provide modulated sensory stimulation in a structured way, in order to improve eye and head control, as well as consistency and reliability of localising to stimuli. Localisation to stimuli was measured as either eye gaze or head movement towards stimuli.

The visual modality consisted of use of familiar visual stimuli (photos of rally cars, family and girlfriend, and mechanical tools) and unfamiliar stimuli (colour cards) with the objective of establishing a consistent localising and tracking response (SMART level 4) in all visual fields.

The auditory modality incorporated familiar auditory stimuli (favourite music, voice of therapist, voice of family members) to achieve consistent localising to the left and right, observing gaze or head movement (SMART level 4).

Treatment sessions continued from day 120 to day 150. He continued to experience severe increased tone; however, purposeful movement and his level of awareness remained questionable. His eye movements to visual and auditory stimuli were uncontrolled and inconsistent and his arousal levels fluctuated and were often low. At this time the team considered the benefits of increasing his tone medication and the associated effect this would have on his level of arousal versus the benefits of improved physical management. His legs underwent serial casting and despite using removable elbow casts he was losing range at his wrists, which became more flexed.

He started showing improved responses around day 160. He turned his head in response to auditory and visual stimuli in all visual fields, and demonstrated improved head control, lifting it to command on several occasions. His eye movement was more sustained and controlled and arousal levels were often optimal during sessions. Due to improved responses, differentiating exercises were introduced into the sensory programme. The aim was to assess the potential to use eye gaze responses to express a choice or preference. Pictures, colour cards and yes/no words were used and visual gaze following a verbal command was observed. Verbal commands were introduced to improve consistency of simple motor responses, e.g., "raise your eyebrows", "move your finger", etc. Facilitated movement of his head, left index finger and thumb was used to assess his ability to carry over motor control in order to press a switch to command. Feedback from the MDT and Mr M's mother regarding his behaviour was very important at this stage, in particular as consistency of purposeful responses could determine he had progressed from MCS and had the potential to interact more purposefully with his environment.

Switch work progressed and at day 210 goals changed to establish Mr M's ability to follow motor commands using a switch and to move his left index finger and thumb, as well as his head. Several different switches were trialed including a Toby Churchill switch, a small plate switch and a micro-lite switch from Toby Churchill Ltd, 20 Panton St, Cambridge CB2 1HP.

Consequently, a single switch was positioned in his left hand, between his left index finger and the dorsal aspect of his thumb, and connected to a radio and a latched timer. Mr M was instructed to press the switch to make his music play. Should he do this, it would only play for 20 seconds and then he had to press the switch again for the music to continue. The aim of this intervention was to establish his understanding of cause and effect relationships. This is the stage where assistive technology would be appropriate for patients in low awareness states. Should the use of low technology aids such as those described above be successful, it would indicate that the individual is no longer in a low awareness state, and may have the potential to access more complex assistive technology such as environmental controls. It is important to note that the technology is not used in isolation to diagnose such patients but to assist them to access their residual function after a severe injury.

In the case of Mr M, the auditory and visual treatment interventions were successful and by day 240 following correct hand positioning he was able to activate a radio using a single switch. Treatment progressed to sessions in the specialised computer therapy room, which focused on his ability to further conceptualise cause and effect using a microlite switch to participate in target shooting games on the computer and looking at familiar photos on a power point presentation. Mr M was subsequently referred to the hospital-based technology clinic for further assessment and integration of assistive devices and he continues to progress in his interaction with the environment and use of assistive technology.

CONCLUSION

To date there have been limited studies reporting the use of assistive technology in patients in low awareness states. However, there is scope for the use of binary switches to assist with the assessment and management of patients in low awareness states. The literature offers valuable insights highlighting the factors affecting the use of a single switch (Angelo, 2000), models that look at movement classification namely the skills acquisition model (Gentile, 1997) and models that describe how assistive technology impacts the end-user such as that of HAAT (Cook & Hussey, 2002), all of which are important to consider when using assistive technology.

While recommendations for the management of patients in PVS and MCS have been developed (Royal College of Physicians, 2003), there are currently no standards of care to guide the selection of rehabilitation assessments and treatment procedures for patients with disorders of consciousness (Giacino & Trott, 2004), let alone the development of protocols for the use of assistive technology with PVS or MCS patients. However, the case study presented demonstrates the use of assistive technology and in particular how the application of switches assisted in the identification of consistent levels of responses and hence the emergence from MCS.

REFERENCES

Andrews, K., Murphy, L., Munday, R., & Littlewood, C. (1996). Misdiagnosis of the vegetative state: Retrospective study in a rehabilitation unit. *British Medical Journal, 313,* 13–16.

Angelo, J. (2000). Factors affecting the use of a single switch with assistive technology devices. *Journal of Rehabilitation Research and Development, 37,* 591–598.

Ansell, B. J., & Keenan, J. E. (1989). The Western Neuro Sensory Stimulation Profile: Tool for assessing slow-to-recover head injured patients. *Archives of Physical Medicine and Rehabilitation, 70,* 104–108.

Bailey, W. R. (1989). *Human performance engineering: Using human factors/ergonomics to achieve computer system usability* (2nd ed.). Englewood Cliffs, NJ: Prentice Hall.

Canedo, A., Grix, M. C., & Nicoletti, J. (2002). An analysis of assessment instruments for the minimally responsive patient (MRP): Clinical observations. *Brain Injury, 16,* 453–461.

Cook, A. M., & Hussey, S. M. (2002). *Assistive technologies, principles and practice* (2nd ed.). St. Louis, MO: Mosby Inc.

Gentile, A. M. (1997). Skills acquisition: Action, movement and neuromotor processes. In J. Carr & R. Shepherd (Ed.), *Movement science: Foundations for physical therapy in rehabilitation*. Rockville, MD: Aspen.

Gentile, A. M. (1998). Implicit and explicit processes during acquisition of functional skills. *Scandinavian Journal of Occupational Therapy, 5*, 7–16.

Giacino, J. T., & Kalmar, K. (1997). The vegetative and minimally conscious states: A comparison of clinical features and functional outcome. *Journal for Head Trauma Rehabilitation, 12*, 36–51.

Giacino, J. T., & Trott, C. T. (2004). Rehabilitative management of patients with disorders of consciousness. *Journal of Head Injury Trauma, 19*, 254–265.

Gill-Thwaites, H. (1997). The Sensory Modality Assessment and Rehabilitation Technique: A tool for the assessment and treatment of patients with severe brain damage in a vegetative state. *Brain Injury, 11*, 723–734.

Gill-Thwaites, H., & Munday, R. (1999). The sensory modality assessment and rehabilitation technique (SMART): A comprehensive and integrated assessment and treatment protocol for the vegetative state and minimally responsive patient. *Neuropsychological Rehabilitation, 9*, 305–320.

Kruetzer, J. S., Kolakowsky-Hayner, S. A., Demn, S. R., & Meade, M. A. (2002). A structured approach to family intervention after brain injury. *Journal of Head Trauma Rehabilitation, 17*, 349–364.

McMillan, T. M. (1996). Neuropsychological assessment after extremely severe head injury in a case of life and death. *Brain Injury, 11*, 483–490.

McMillan, T. M., & Herbert, C. M. (2000). Neuropsychological assessment of a potential "euthanasia" case: A 5 year follow up. *Brain Injury, 14*, 197–203.

O'Dell, M. W., Jasin, P., Lyons, N., Stivers, M., & Meszaros, F. (1996). Standardised assessment instruments for minimally-responsive, brain-injured patients. *NeuroRehabilitation, 6*, 45–55.

Piguet, O., King, A. C., & Harrison, D. P. (1999). Assessment of minimally responsive patients: Clinical difficulties of single-case design. *Brain Injury, 13*, 829–837.

Rader, M. A., & Ellis, D. E. (1994). The sensory stimulation assessment measure (SSAM): A tool for elderly evaluation of severely brain-injured patients. *Brain Injury, 8*, 309–321.

Rappaport, M., Doughtery, A. M., & Kelting, D. L. (1992). Evaluation of coma and vegetative state. *Archives of Physical Medicine and Rehabilitation, 72*, 628–634.

Royal College of Physicians (2003). The vegetative state: Guidance on diagnosis and management. London: Royal College of Physicians.

Shiel, A., Horn, S. A., Wilson, B. A., Watson, M. J., Campbell, M. J., & McLellan, D. L. (2000). The Wessex Head Injury Matrix (WHIM) main scale: A preliminary report on a scale to assess and monitor patient recovery after severe head injury. *Clinical Rehabilitation, 14*, 408–416.

Watson, M., Horn, S., & Wilson, B. (1999). Assessing a minimally responsive brain injuries person. *British Journal of Therapy and Rehabilitation, 6*, 436–441.

NEUROPSYCHOLOGICAL REHABILITATION
2005, 15 (3/4), 522–536

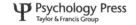

Music therapy with patients in low awareness states: Approaches to assessment and treatment in multidisciplinary care

Wendy L. Magee

Institute of Complex Neuro-disability, Royal Hospital for Neuro-disability and University of Sheffield

This paper outlines the rationale for and role of music therapy as a clinical intervention and diagnostic tool in multidisciplinary (MDT) rehabilitation programmes for patients in low awareness states. A review of the literature indicates that music is a useful clinical tool in stimulating a range of behavioural, physiological and expressive responses in patients in low awareness states. Referral criteria for music therapy with this patient group are provided, along with suggested methods for collaborative multidisciplinary work. A case vignette is presented of a client whose diagnosis of vegetative state (VS) was contradicted by her purposeful responses within music therapy assessment, contributing towards a changed diagnosis to minimally conscious state (MCS). The case illustrates the particular role of music therapy in assisting with diagnosis in complex cases. Music therapy provides a clinical forum in which recovery of function can be assessed in an informal way, using a medium which does not rely on language, is non-evasive and elicits emotional responses.

Correspondence should be sent to Dr. Wendy Magee, International Fellow in Music Therapy, Institute of Complex Neuro-disability, Royal Hospital for Neuro-disability, West Hill, London SW15 3SW. Tel: 020 8780 4500 ext 5146, Fax: 020 8780 4569.
Email: drwmagee@rhn.org.uk

The author would like to thank the patient and family whose case vignette has been included in this paper, and Barb Daveson, Head of Music Therapy at the Royal Hospital for Neuro-disability for her helpful comments on this paper.

The Royal Hospital for Neuro-disability received a proportion of its funding to support this paper from the NHS Executive. The views expressed in this publication are those of the authors and not necessarily those of the NHS Executive.

---

http://www.tandf.co.uk/journals/pp/09602011.html   DOI:10.1080/09602010443000461

BACKGROUND

Music therapy is a clinical intervention that can be defined as the planned and intentional use of music to meet an individual's social, psychological, physical, and spiritual needs within an evolving therapeutic relationship (Magee, 2002). Therapeutic intervention is structured upon clinical goals which aim to improve both an understanding of the client from a holistic perspective, and address the individual's health needs (Bruscia, 1998). Using a range of clinical methods, all of the interactions within therapeutic contacts are based on the client's own musical utterances or musical preference. Therefore, the client most usually is involved in actively making music in dialogue with the therapist (Magee, 2002). Music's independence from language function means that it is a useful medium in work with individuals who are not able to communicate verbally for pathological, emotional or cultural reasons (Sergent, Zuck, Tenial, & MacDonald, 1992). Music therapy is used with populations across the age spectrum with a range of communication, psychological and medical conditions in hospital, school, community and secure settings (Fachner & Aldridge, 2004). Music therapy requires specialist training on recognised tertiary courses and, within the UK, music therapy is a state registered allied health profession with training at a post-graduate level only.

A range of empirical studies demonstrate the effectiveness of music therapy as a treatment modality in brain injury rehabilitation. In particular, it has been shown to improve expressive communication in cases of neuro-communication disorders (Baker, 2000; Cohen, 1988, 1992; Cohen & Masse, 1993; Pilon, McIntosh, & Thaut, 1998). Functional gains have been demonstrated through applying music therapy within gait retraining programmes following stroke and traumatic brain injury (TBI) (Hurt, Rice, McIntosh, & Thaut, 1998; McIntosh, Thaut, Rice, & Prassas, 1993, 1995; Prassas, Thaut, McIntosh, & Rice, 1997; Thaut & McIntosh, 1992; Thaut, Hurt, McIntosh, 1997; Thaut, McIntosh, Prassas, & Rice, 1993; Thaut, Rice, & McIntosh, 1997; Thaut, Rice, McIntosh, & Prassas, 1993; Thaut, McIntosh, & Rice, 1997; Thaut, McIntosh, Rice, & Miller, 1995). Music therapy with people with post-traumatic amnesia following TBI was found to significantly reduce agitation and enhance orientation (Baker, 2001). In neurological patients it is an effective treatment for improving self-esteem (Purdie, Hamilton, & Baldwin, 1997), mood states (Magee & Davidson, 2002), and, when included in neuro-rehabilitation programmes, has been shown to improve social interaction skills and increase patients' participation in other therapies (Nayak, Wheeler, Shiflett, & Agnostinelli, 2000).

Music therapy and other music-based methods in the treatment of low awareness states

In recent years, reviews and clinical case reports have been published of music therapy interventions with patients in either VS or MCS, often under the umbrella term of "coma" (Tamplin, 2000). The methods described in all of these publications involve only live music, reporting a range of physiological responses including changes in respiration and heart rate (Aldridge, Gustorff, & Hannich, 1990; Kennelly & Edwards, 1997; Rosenfeld & Dun, 1999; Tamplin, 2000). Behavioural changes are also reported including increased body movements, eye opening, tracking, and orienting towards the therapist and source of music (Gustorff, 2002; Jochims, 1995; Kennelly & Edwards, 1997; Rosenfeld & Dun, 1999; Tamplin, 2000). One study reports the patient regaining consciousness as a consequence of music therapy intervention (Gustorff, 2002). Gustorff sang to her patient while he was unconscious, using the rhythm of his breathing to guide her non-verbal singing. When he emerged into consciousness, he described having the sensation of being on a battlefield and wanting to die, but that "...when he heard music for the first time, he sensed there was somebody there who wanted him to live. He realised that the music was meant for him" (Gustorff, 2002, p. 372). Increased communicative responses are frequently described, including vocalisations (Kennelly & Edwards, 1997; Magee, 1999; Rosenfeld & Dun, 1999), and non-verbal interaction (Jochims, 1995; Magee, 1999).

Many of these music therapy case reports suggest that the fundamental elements of music such as pulse, tempo and rhythm effect physiological change through rhythmic entrainment of the cardiovascular and respiratory systems. Most of the literature describes both the inherent emotional and non-verbal nature of the stimulus as being the primary factors which result in dramatic behavioural responses. This is supported by the number of descriptive studies providing accounts of emotional responses to music in patients emerging from VS. While it may be debated whether people in VS or MCS have the cognitive capacity to process stimuli in an emotionally meaningful way, it is also essential to consider the evidence of self-reports from people who have emerged from these states. These indicate that fear and pain are central to the emotional experience of emerging from coma and that not being able to make oneself understood can lead to feelings of anger (Wilson, Gracey, & Bainbridge, 2001). Given this, finding a non-verbal medium which can prompt, enable and support emotional expression, including "difficult" feelings such as fear and anger, should be of priority to the MDT wishing to gain optimum engagement from the patient.

Another music-based method, entitled "musicokinetic therapy" (MKT), is reported as having some success with patients with prolonged consciousness disturbances. MKT combines live music with physical stimulation for short intensive bursts followed by extended periods of no stimulation. Reported improvements include increased arousal and responsiveness to commands (Mochizuki, Noda, & Maeda, 2002; Oyama et al., 2003; Sato et al., 2002), evidence of purposeful functional movement and communication (Sato et al., 2002; Yamamoto, Osora, Noda, & Maeda, 2003), and increased emotional expression (Mochizuki et al., 2002; Mochizuki, Nishikawa, Noda, & Maeda, 2003; Oyama et al., 2003; Sato et al., 2002; Yamamoto et al., 2003). The responsiveness noted in these reports may result from the combination of musical and intense physical stimuli used in this method. It is outside the remit of this paper to compare music-based methods which play music "to" the patient with music therapy methods which are inherently interactive in nature. However, it should be noted that across disciplines, music has been noted to elicit increased responsiveness in this patient group where this is the primary clinical goal.

There are only a few empirical studies to date that have examined the effects of music on patients in VS or MCS. These are characterised by small sample sizes ($n = 4-26$) and varying methodological approaches, including whether the music used is live or recorded. Dependent variables include arousal (Tsunakawa et al., 2000; Wilson, Cranny, & Andrews, 1992), awareness (Boyle, 1995; Noda, Maeda, & Yoshino, 2004), cardio-respiratory and neurological responses (Aldridge, 1991; Ito et al., 2000), purposeful response to verbal requests (Boyle & Greer, 1983), and purposeful learnt behaviours (Boyle, 1995).

Studies examining the effect of music have shown mixed results within and across studies. One study examined EEG traces during live music, finding desynchronisation from theta rhythm to alpha rhythm or beta rhythm suggesting arousal and perceptual activity, which faded after the music had stopped (Aldridge, 1991). Noda et al. (2004) linked optimal responses to MKT with causes of brain damage, finding that those with injury caused by trauma or subarachonoid haemorrhage were most likely to show change. More significantly, changes were found in these groups even when intervention was introduced more than 12 months post-injury. Wilson et al. (1992) provided additional observations indicating that music stimulated not only behaviours suggesting increased arousal, but also stimulated emotional responses in one of their subjects. While the available literature indicates positive effects of music with patients in low awareness states, the main methodological differences observed are in the use of live music or recorded music.

The content of this paper is based on the author's experience of working on a unit for patients in low awareness states over a period of 14 years. The following sections outline working practices which have integrated music therapy into multidisciplinary treatment programmes where its value can be optimised.

MUSIC THERAPY IN THE DIAGNOSIS AND TREATMENT OF VS AND MCS

Rationale for using music as a treatment medium in neurorehabilitation

There are four simple reasons why music can be an effective treatment medium for patients in low awareness states who may have severely compromised receptive and expressive language faculties, and who may be experiencing a range of emotional responses to their immediate and ongoing situation. First, all early communication relies on musical parameters such as pitch, dynamics, melodic contour, articulation, timing and phrasing (Papousek, 1996; Trevarthen, 1999, 2002). Long before language development, infants communicate immediate feeling states through vocalisations. Music is an innate ability in all human beings. Second, music is a powerful social medium cross-culturally and throughout the lifespan (Blacking, 1976). It motivates and provides an organisational framework through which individuals can interact and respond. Third, music elicits emotional responses and conveys feeling states (Sloboda, 1991a, 1991b). Lastly, there is growing neurological evidence that music assists with neuroplasticity, thereby enabling connections to be made between healthy and damaged centres of the brain in populations with acquired brain injury (O'Callaghan, 1999).

What does music therapy offer a MDT rehabilitation programme?

The music therapist has a unique contribution to make to MDT rehabilitation of the profoundly brain-injured patient. Although the patient is likely to be surrounded by uncontrolled sounds in the ward environment, the manipulation of acoustic parameters within a music therapy assessment can provide specific information for the team about how the patient is experiencing the acoustic environment, thereby assisting with the assessment of sensory abilities. For example, musical sound can be manipulated in terms of pitch (high or low), volume (soft or loud), attack (sudden or gradual), form (repetition, novel, or familiar material), and so on. This type of information can assist in the development of communication strategies with patients with receptive communication disorders, making suggestions for the most appropriate pitch, volume and melodic contour of voice to use. For example, patients with receptive communication disorders present a considerable challenge for staff providing personal care. Recommendations from music therapy assessment can be made about emphasising and manipulating the musical parameters of verbal communication (e.g., pitch and volume of voice; direction of spoken intonation to convey reassurance). In doing so, the communicative intent of the carer is enhanced.

Second, music therapy can assist with the rehabilitation of social functioning and the ability to develop relationships with others. Music is a social activity, and the tasks within sessions involve pragmatic communication skills such as listening, turn-taking, imitation, repetition and development of ideas, rather than passive listening. In this way, social skills can be addressed without the use of language.

The emotional nature of the medium facilitates social and emotional adjustment to the changed circumstances of the patient's condition, as demonstrated amply in the published clinical reports. Vocalisation of immediate feeling states through non-verbal, musical parameters is innate in the human condition across all cultures (Papousek, 1996; Trevarthen, 1999, 2002). A music therapist is skilled at interacting with the patient on this non-verbal level, both enabling the patient to express his or her immediate feeling states, and providing a supportive intervention for exploration of these states. The music therapy session is typically one which is not based on formal tests, but instead encourages play and creativity, enabling a range of emotional expression through musical parameters. It is often a welcome relief from other therapies where the patient may feel "tested". It provides a forum for the whole team to observe the patient responding in a more spontaneous way, offering opportunities for rehabilitation of function in a more creative environment.

Burke et al. (2000) illustrate this in a case study of a young woman emerging from a low awareness state receiving multidisciplinary rehabilitation. They state that music therapy validated emotional expression as well as addressing functional communication through singing activities, and physical goals through bilateral activities with instrument playing.

Referral criteria, treatment techniques and potential for multidisciplinary collaboration

Table 1 provides criteria which have been found useful for promoting appropriate referrals on the profound brain injury unit at the Royal Hospital in London. Broadly, these fall under the clinical areas of communication, cognition, behaviour, emotional expression, physical health, and occupation and leisure needs. This last criterion may indicate work which can be undertaken with the family to provide them with ideas for shared leisure activities. This can assist relatives in spending time with a loved one who can no longer engage actively in shared activities of a personally meaningful nature. Although musical ability is not a prerequisite, those patients who have premorbid experience as a musician should be considered a priority for music therapy assessment, as the personal meaning of this medium may increase motivation and enhance engagement in therapy. Similarly, care should be

TABLE 1

Referral criteria, treatment techniques and tasks used in assessment and/or treatment and multidisciplinary collaborators

Referal criteria	Examples of music therapy techniques and tasks used in assessment and/or treatment	Potential MDT collaborators
Communication		
Patient's responses to verbal material are unknown or inconsistent	Development of communication strategies using music-related stimuli such as familiar musical instruments or pictures of known favourite musical artists. Stimuli to be presented in concrete form (i.e., instruments) or symbolic representation (i.e., pictures) dependent on current communication strategy. Activities range from visual discrimination tasks, through to choice-making employing current communication strategies, e.g., eye pointing, use of "yes/no" gesture, matching pictures to real objects, use of communication devices, etc. Reinforcement of "choice" through live presentation of "chosen" song on "chosen" instrument.	SLT Psychology OT
Patient is aware but cannot interact verbally due to language impairment	Interactive musical tasks to assess interaction and social awareness, such as turn-taking or clinical improvisation. All tasks involve live music, with therapist using voice or instrument, and client using vocal sounds and/or musical instrument which is responsive to client's physical abilities, i.e., touch sensitive and accessible. Musical tasks assess for evidence of patient's ability to directly imitate or develop melodic or rhythmic fragments or other parameters such as tempo (speed) and dynamics (velocity) of music given by therapist and/or in interaction with therapist.	SLT OT
Patient does not have a consistent yes/no	Choice-making employing current communication strategy with known preferred and disliked music-related stimuli: Reinforcement of choice with live presentation of chosen musical stimuli.	SLT
Patient is developing voice or speech	Interactive and/or structured musical tasks using client's vocalisations. Breathing and oro-motor exercises within song activities using familiar or improvised music.	SLT
Cognition		
Patient's awareness is unknown	Behavioural observation pre, during and post-presentation of auditory and visual musical stimuli to all sides. Particular focus on breathing rates, eye opening, attempts to vocalise, tracking, localising, changes in movements and facial gestures and changes to these during musical stimuli/no stimuli. Use of familiar music of personal meaning as well as novel musical material with familiar structural forms.	OT Psychology

Behaviour Patient has agitated behaviour from environmental stimuli	Assessment of responses to auditory stimuli with manipulation of parameters such as pitch, volume, attack/accent, tempo, timbre, melodic contour, duration with behavioural observations. Compare use of live and recorded music.	OT Psychology
Emotional expression Patient is demonstrating behaviours thought to be emotionally driven	Behavioural observations (particularly of facial gesture and spontaneous behaviours) during conditions of music vs. no music; music of personal meaning vs. novel musical material. Use of clinical improvisation techniques to match emotional expression of vocalisations. Presentation of musical stimuli of differing and varied mood contents, e.g., "lively" vs. "sad". Use of face charts for patient to identify subjective mood state, reinforced through musical stimuli played by therapist to match/reflect identified subjective mood state.	Psychology
Physical Patient has active movement but the purpose of this movement is unclear	Presentation of musical instruments requiring contrasting motor patterns, e.g., guitar (downward strum with finger extension); windchimes (lateral arm movement); shaker or beater with drum (hand grasp with repeated downward movement); lightweight blowing instrument (hand grasp, hand to mouth, exhalation). Interactive musical tasks to assess musical responses, such as turn-taking or clinical improvisation, in which ability to provide controlled musical response can be "seen" and "heard".	OT PT
Patient has difficulty with initiating or organising motor/speech patterns	Musical tasks using strong rhythms to facilitate motor entrainment. Musical tasks using structures to prompt participation, e.g., use of musical lead-in (anacrusis); use of musical gaps; use of repetition. Musical tasks with strong formal elements, e.g., clear beginning and endings.	OT PT
Occupation and leisure Relatives/carers are having difficulty interacting due to the patient's awareness/communication	Development of guidelines for shared music listening leisure activities, aiming to enhance time spent with significant others.	Family Psychology OT SLT Nursing
Requirements for optimum sensory environment unknown	Assessment techniques as for cognition and behaviour (see above). Guidelines for use of music and auditory stimuli as part of overall sensory programme which can be used by family or carers.	

529

taken with patients who were previously musicians, as the use of music may enhance difficulty with adjustment to their current ability level.

Music therapy should be fully integrated into multidisciplinary working at both direct and indirect levels of care, from goal-planning through to intervention and evaluation of rehabilitation progress. Table 1 provides suggestions for MDT collaborators which may prove fruitful for all members of the team. Appropriate music therapy techniques and tasks to address multidisciplinary goal areas are also outlined.

The following case vignette illustrates music therapy's contribution to multidisciplinary assessments of patients with complex disabilities stemming from profound brain damage.

CASE VIGNETTE: "MRS P"

Mrs P was a woman in her early 50s who experienced a severe anoxic brain injury following a cardiac arrest. She was admitted with a diagnosis of VS. The aim for the MDT was to complete an assessment of her awareness, in order to confirm or contradict her diagnosis. She had no consistent active movement and presented with high tone spastic quadraplegia, muscle shortening and a posture involving left-sided rotation, left-sided flexion and extension of her neck. This prevented the team achieving a well-supported head position in midline for her, despite considerable wheelchair adaptations and specialist skills. In a well-supported position she was able to look and turn slightly towards midline. Postural management was a constant challenge in her care. She was hypersensitive to touch making all physical interventions difficult. Cognitive assessment using SMART (Gill-Thwaites, 1997) was complicated due to the difficulty of achieving optimal physical positioning, her hypersensitivity to tactile stimulation, and the frequent spasms throughout her body. Her cognitive function remained unclear for a period of time. At the time of music therapy referral within SMART she showed inconsistent localising and differentiating responses within the auditory modality but did not follow verbal commands, and showed no response within the visual modality. The available standardised test therefore was not sensitive enough to demonstrate awareness. However, there were contradictory reports from family and some members of the team concerning her responsiveness observed within informal situations. Although the team had difficulty finding active responses using formalised tests, her family reported that she responded to them and cried each time they ended visits.

Reasons for referral to music therapy

Mrs P was referred for music therapy by speech and language therapy (SLT) and occupational therapy (OT) to "assess behavioural responses to non-verbal stimuli" and to provide more information about her responses to a wider range of stimuli.

Assessment methods

Assessment examined Mrs P's responses to auditory and visual stimuli by presenting a range of musical stimuli in varying positions around her midline. All music presented was live, being played and sung by the music therapist. Musical material had been selected considering written information about Mrs P's personal lifestyle provided by her family on admission on a "lifestyle history" questionnaire. The session took place in Mrs P's bedroom, which was a quiet, private space where there were no interruptions. Mrs P was in her wheelchair, and the therapists moved around her.

Behavioural observations were conducted by the OT prior to the introduction of visual and musical stimuli. The OT then observed Mrs P's responses during musical stimuli from one side for the rest of the session. The music therapist placed the guitar within Mrs P's line of vision and moved it slowly across her midline in both directions, before beginning to play the guitar in a midline position. Single notes were played on her exhalations, gradually building to a simple chordal progression based on familiar Western harmonic style. The tempo of the music followed the rate of her exhalations closely. The therapist improvised a simple non-verbal hummed melody, which then gradually grew into a phrase of "Hello (patient's first name)" modelled on the intonation of speech, i.e., with a falling major third on "hello". This phrase was repeated four times in a typical song structure with slight developments of each phrase, and then repeated with some musical modification. Following this, a familiar song by one of Mrs P's favourite singer/songwriter's ("Lady in red" by Chris de Burgh) was played on the electric piano to her left. To finish, a simple well-known folk song ("Greensleeves") was played on the flute to her right.

Responses

Mrs P's responses to the musical stimuli were clearly observable. In immediate response to visual presentation of the guitar, Mrs P's facial gesture changed completely. Her face tightened, her eyes closed, and she looked "upset". Following this, in the initial musical activity, her head moved repeatedly in an upward direction as she attempted to raise her head to look towards the guitar. Her breathing rate was noted to increase during the initial music activity. When the song was played on the piano, it was noted that she attempted to lift her head repeatedly to look towards the piano. In discussion with Mrs P's husband after this initial session it emerged that both the guitar and the familiar song held greater personal meaning than first realised. The therapist had not known that one of the patient's children was a keen guitarist, and that "Lady in red" was a song of particular significance to the patient and her husband.

The responses in this initial session were noted again in a following session in which the SLT carried out behavioural observations. A period of treatment followed in which the music therapist used specific songs and music known to be meaningful to Mrs P. All behavioural responses were noted. In particular it was found that the music which was known to be most personally meaningful to Mrs P elicited the most notable responses, where she tried to lift her head, or showed changes in her facial gesture. Stimuli of lesser significance did not prompt such responses. A period of intervention followed, including work with her family on leisure activities using music which could potentially be shared together.

Outcomes of treatment

Mrs P's responses in music therapy demonstrated that she was able to show purposeful consistent responses to her environment. That is, she showed emotional responses to particular pieces of music and instruments within and across different sessions. Her responses in music therapy were the major contributing factor in a change of diagnosis from VS to MCS as it was the only intervention where her responses could be determined to be purposeful, that is, "including movements or affective behaviours that occur in contingent relation to relevant environmental stimuli and not . . . reflexive" (Giacino et al., 2002, p. 349).

Feedback from the referring OT identified the role of music therapy in this case, stating, "Music therapy offered qualitative analysis of [the patient's] responses which contrasted with other multidisciplinary assessments. The responses seen in music therapy contributed to her diagnosis—contradicting the diagnosis of VS". Her family also validated the contribution made by music therapy to her care, by saying, "We knew that she was in there, but music therapy was able to show that in a consistent way. Music therapy indicated that (her) cognitive function was there. More importantly, music therapy established that there were emotional responses there. It was absolutely vital that music therapy was involved. Input from music therapy was indispensable. We regard music therapy as so important for her."

CONCLUSION

The overview given by published case reports and empirical studies concerning the use of music and, more specifically, clinical music therapy with patients in low awareness states indicates that it is a viable intervention in multidisciplinary assessment and intervention with this very challenging patient group. In particular, its value is to provide the team with a non-invasive medium which promotes an informal clinical setting in which the patient's broader functions can be examined and addressed. It provides a means of enablement for very profoundly disabled patients and for expressing a range of emotional states, including unbearable feelings which may be experienced by the person who is emerging into an aware state. The self-report provided by Gustorff (2002) provides evidence for this.

Music therapy seems to engender hope for the family, the team caring for the patient, and possibly for the patient her or himself. When working with this patient group, where progress is slow and very small, and motivation difficult to maintain, hope might be the most important thing that the music therapist has to offer as part of the MDT. Malec (1996) proposes that "effectiveness should be taken to mean that the treatment will improve the quality of the patient's relationships" (Malec, 1996, p. 788). This paper puts forward the case that music therapy is a highly effective intervention in enabling the patient to relate to others within the clinical and social forums, bearing wider impact on their rehabilitation overall.

REFERENCES

Aldridge, D. (1991). Creativity and consciousness: Music therapy in intensive care. *The Arts in Psychotherapy, 18,* 359–362.

Aldridge, D., Gustorff, D., & Hannich, H.-J. (1990). Where am I? Music therapy applied to coma patients. *Journal of the Royal Society of Medicine, 83,* 345–346.

Baker, F. A. (2000). Modifying the melodic intonation therapy program for adults with severe non-fluent aphasia. *Music Therapy Perspectives, 18,* 110–114.

Baker, F. A. (2001). The effects of live, taped, and no music on people experiencing posttraumatic amnesia. *Journal of Music Therapy, 38,* 170–192.

Blacking, J. (1976). *How musical is man?* (2nd ed.). London: Faber and Faber.

Boyle, M. E. (1995). On the vegetative state: Music and coma arousal interventions. In C. Lee (Ed.), *Lonely waters: Proceedings of the international conference music therapy in palliative care* (pp. 163–172). Oxford: Sobell Publications.

Boyle, M. E., & Greer, R. D. (1983). Operant procedures and the comatose patient. *Journal of Allied Behaviour Analyses, 16,* 3–12.

Bruscia, K. (1998). *Defining Music Therapy* (2nd ed.). Gilsum, NH: Barcelona Publishers.

Burke, D., Kirrily, A., Baxter, M., Baker, F., Connell, K., Diggles, S. et al. (2000). Rehabilitation of a person with severe traumatic brain injury. *Brain Injury, 14*(5), 463–471.

Cohen, N. S. (1988). The use of superimposed rhythm to decrease the rate of speech in a brain-damaged adolescent. *Journal of Music Therapy, 25*(2), 85–93.

Cohen, N. S. (1992). The effect of singing instruction on the speech production of neurologically impaired persons. *Journal of Music Therapy, 29*(2), 87–102.

Cohen, N. S., & Masse, R. (1993). The application of singing and rhythmic instruction as a therapeutic intervention for persons with neurogenic communication disorders. *Journal of Music Therapy, 30*(2), 81–99.

Fachner, J., & Aldridge, D. (2004). *Dialogue and debate: Proceedings of the 10th World Congress of Music Therapy.* Witten, Germany: MusicTherapyWorld.Net.

Giacino, J. T., Ashwal, S., Childs, N., Cranford, R., Jennet, B., Katz, D. I. et al. (2002). The minimally conscious state: Definition and diagnostic criteria. *Neurology, 58,* 349–353.

Gill-Thwaites, H. (1997). The Sensory Modality Assessment Rehabilitation Technique—A tool for assessment and treatment of patients with severe brain injury in a vegetative state. *Brain Injury, 10,* 723–734.

Gustorff, D. (2002). Beyond words: Music therapy with comatose patients and those with impaired consciousness in intensive care. In D. Aldridge & J. Fachner (eds.), *info cd rom iv, university witten herdecke: witten* (pp. 353–377). Witten: Witten University.

Hurt, C. P., Rice, R. R., McIntosh, G. C., & Thaut, M. H. (1998). Rhythmic auditory stimulation in gait training for patients with traumatic brain injury. *Journal of Music Therapy, 35,* 228–241.

Ito, S., Tsuda, Y., Kafuku, T., Suzuki, M., Obonai, T., Kanno, A. et al. (2000). Effects of music therapy in patients with prolonged consciousness disturbance—A study focusing on heart rate changes. *Proceedings of the 9th Annual Meeting of the Society for Treatment of Coma, Tokyo: Vol. 9* (pp. 25–29). Tokyo: Neuron Publishing Co. Ltd.

Jochims, S. (1995). Emotional processes of coping with disease in the early stages of acquired cerebral lesions. *The Arts in Psychotherapy, 22*(1), 21–30.

Kennelly, J., & Edwards, J. (1997). Providing music therapy to the unconscious child in the paediatric intensive care unit. *Australian Journal of Music Therapy, 8,* 18–29.

Magee, W. (1999). Music therapy within brain injury rehabilitation: To what extent is our clinical practice influenced by the search for outcomes? *Music Therapy Perspectives, 17*(1), 20–26.

Magee, W. L. (2002). Identity in clinical music therapy: Shifting self-constructs through the therapeutic process. In R. MacDonald, D. J. Hargreaves, & D. Miell (Eds.), *Musical identities* (pp. 179–197). Oxford: Oxford University Press.

Magee, W. L., & Davidson, J. W. (2002). The effect of music therapy on mood states in neurological patients—A pilot study. *Journal of Music Therapy, 39*(1), 20–29.

Malec, J. F. (1996). Ethical conflict resolution based on an ethics of relationships for brain injury rehabilitation. *Brain Injury, 10*(11), 781–795.

McIntosh, G. C., Thaut, M. H., Rice, R. R., & Prassas, S. G. (1993). Auditory rhythmic cuing in gait rehabilitation with stroke patients. *Canadian Journal of Neurological Sciences, 20,* 168.

McIntosh, G. C., Thaut, M. H., Rice, R. R., & Prassas, S. G. (1995). Rhythmic facilitation of gait kinematics in stroke patients. *Journal of Neurologic Rehabilitation, 9,* 131.

Mochizuki, E., Nishikawa, E., Noda, R., & Maeda, Y. (2003). Improvement in cognitive ability of a patient with disturbance of consciousness by playing music. *Proceedings of the 12th Annual Meeting of the Society for Treatment of Coma, Tokyo: Vol. 12* (pp. 117–120). Tokyo: Neuron Publishing Co. Ltd.

Mochizuki, E., Noda, R., & Maeda, Y. (2002). Synchronized music-kinetic therapy (SMK) as a home care rehabilitation for patient with prolonged disturbance of consciousness—A case report. *Proceedings of the 11th Annual Meeting of the Society for Treatment of Coma, Tokyo: Vol. 11* (pp. 69–71). Tokyo: Neuron Publishing Co. Ltd.

Nayak, S., Wheeler, B. L., Shiflett, S. C., & Agnostinelli, S. (2000). The effect of music therapy on mood and social interaction among individuals with acute traumatic brain injury and stroke. *Rehabilitation Psychology, 45,* 274–283.

Noda, R., Maeda, Y., & Yoshino, A. (2004). Therapeutic time window for musicokinetic therapy in a persistent vegetative state after severe brain damage. *Brain Injury, 18*(5), 509–515.

O'Callaghan, C. (1999). Recent findings about neural correlates of music pertinent to music therapy across the lifespan. *Music Therapy Perspectives, 17*(1), 32–36.

Oyama, A., Arawaka, Y., Oikawa, A., Owada, H., Oimatsu, H., Obonai, T. et al. (2003). Trial of musicokinetic therapy for traumatic patients with prolonged disturbance of consciousness: Two case reports. *Proceedings of the 12th Annual Meeting of the Society for Treatment of Coma, Tokyo: Vol. 12* (pp. 121–126). Tokyo: Neuron Publishing Co. Ltd.

Papousek, H. (1996). Musicality in infancy research: Biological and cultural origins of early musicality. In I. Deliege & J. Sloboda (Eds.), *Musical beginnings: Origins and development of musical competence* (pp. 37–55). Oxford: Oxford University Press.

Pilon, M. A., McIntosh, K. W., & Thaut, M. H. (1998). Auditory vs. visual speech timing cues as external rate control to enhance verbal intelligibility in mixed spastic-ataxic dysarthric speakers: A pilot study. *Brain Injury, 12*, 793–803.

Prassas, S., Thaut, M. H., McIntosh, G. C., & Rice, R. (1997). Effect of auditory rhythmic cueing on gait kinematic parameters of stroke patients. *Gait & Posture, 6*, 218–223.

Purdie, H., Hamilton, S., & Baldwin, S. (1997). Music therapy: Facilitating behavioural and psychological change in people with stroke—A pilot study. *International Journal of Rehabilitation Research, 20*, 325–327.

Rosenfeld, J. V., & Dun, B. (1999). Music therapy in children with severe traumatic brain injury. In R. Rebello Pratt & D. Erdonmez Grocke (Eds.), *MusicMedicine 3* (pp. 35–46). Parkville: University of Melbourne.

Sato, Y., Yoshimoto, S., Kobayashi, Y., Katoka, E., Yoshida, A., Matsuzuki, M. et al. (2002). Successful treatment by music kinetic therapy for a patient in a vegetative state: A case report. *Proceedings of the 11th Annual Meeting of the Society for Treatment of Coma, Tokyo: Vol. 11* (pp. 73–76). Tokyo: Neuron Publishing Co. Ltd.

Sergent, J., Zuck, S., Tenial, S., & MacDonald, B. (1992). Distributed neural network underlying musical sightreading and keyboard performance. *Science, 257*, 106–109.

Sloboda, J. (1991a). Music structure and emotional response: Some empirical findings. *Psychology of Music, 19*, 110–120.

Sloboda, J. (1991b). Empirical studies of emotional response to music. In M. R. Jones & S. Holleran (eds.), *Cognitive bases of musical communication* (pp. 33–46). Washington: American Psychological Association.

Tamplin, J. (2000). Improvisational music therapy approaches to coma arousal. *Australian Journal of Music Therapy, 11*, 38–51.

Thaut, M. H., Hurt, C. P., & McIntosh, G. C. (1997). Rhythmic entrainment of gait patterns in traumatic brain injury rehabilitation. *Journal of Neurologic Rehabilitation, 11*, 131.

Thaut, M. H., & McIntosh, G. C. (1992). Effect of auditory rhythm on temporal stride parameters and EMG patterns in normal and hemiparetic gait. *Neurology, 42*, 208.

Thaut, M. H., McIntosh, G. C., Prassas, S. G., & Rice, R. R. (1993). Effect of rhythmic cuing on temporal stride parameters and EMG patterns in hemiparetic gait of stroke patients. *Journal of Neurological Rehabilitation, 7*, 9–16.

Thaut, M. H., McIntosh, G. C., & Rice, R. R. (1997). Rhythmic facilitation of gait training in hemiparetic stroke rehabilitation. *Journal of Neurological Sciences, 151*, 207–212.

Thaut, M. H., McIntosh, G. C., Rice, R. R., & Miller, R. A. (1995). Rhythmic auditory-motor training in gait rehabilitation with stroke patients. *Journal of Stroke and Cerebrovascular Disease, 5*, 100–101.

Thaut, M. H., Rice, R. R., & McIntosh, G. C. (1997). Rhythmic facilitation of gait training in hemiparetic stroke rehabilitation. *Journal of Neurological Sciences, 151*, 7–12.

Thaut, M. H., Rice, R. R., McIntosh, G. C., & Prassas, S. G. (1993). The effect of auditory rhythmic cuing on stride and EMG patterns in hemiparetic gait of stroke patients. *Physical Therapy, 73*, 107.

Trevarthen, C. (1999). Musicality and the instrinsic motive pulse: Evidence from human psychobiology and infant communication in rhythms, musical narrative and origins of musical communication. *Musicae Scientiae, Special Issue (1999–2000)*, 155–215.

Trevarthen, C. (2002). Origins of musical identity: Evidence from infancy for musical social awareness. In R. MacDonald, D. J. Hargreaves, & D. Miell (Eds.), *Musical identities* (pp. 21–38). Oxford: Oxford University Press.

Tsunakawa, K., Nakamura, A., Yamaguchi, K., Tanaka, M., & Mizunari, T. (2000). An attempt to establish sleep-awaking rhythm using music therapy for patients with disturbed consciousness. *Proceedings of the 9th Annual Meeting of the Society for Treatment of Coma, Tokyo: Vol. 9* (pp. 31–35). Tokyo: Neuron Publishing Co. Ltd.

Wilson, B. A., Gracey, F., & Bainbridge, K. (2001). Cognitive recovery from 'persistent vegetative state': Psychological and personal perspectives. *Brain Injury, 15*(2), 1083–1092.

Wilson, S. L., Cranny, S. M., & Andrews, K. (1992). The efficacy of music for stimulation in prolonged coma—Four single case experiments. *Clinical Rehabilitation, 6,* 181–187.

Yamamoto, K., Osora, M., Noda, R., & Maeda, Y. (2003). The importance of effective music selection for synchronized musico-kinetic therapy in patients with disturbance of consciousness. *Proceedings of the 12th Annual Meeting of the Society for Treatment of Coma, Tokyo: Vol. 12* (pp. 109–116). Tokyo: Neuron Publishing Co. Ltd.

NEUROPSYCHOLOGICAL REHABILITATION
2005, 15 (3/4), 537–547

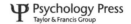

Nutrition and hydration for the vegetative state and minimally conscious state patient

Helen Finch

Royal Hospital for Neuro-disability, London, UK

This paper presents nutritional issues particular to patients in the vegetative state (VS) or minimally conscious state (MCS). It assumes that such patients would be tube fed and it examines suitable ways of assessing and monitoring their nutrition. It covers problems frequently encountered such as undernourishment, high fluid requirements, bowel management, and vomiting. It also looks at the practicalities of long-term tube feeding.

Once medical stability has been achieved, feeding these patients is almost always successful with the patient's body weight restored to being within normal limits.

INTRODUCTION

Patients who are in a vegetative state (VS) or minimally conscious state (MCS) will almost all be unable to take food and drink orally. Any oral intake is likely to be insignificant, therefore nutrition and fluid must be given through a feeding tube. Nutrition by this method is called enteral tube feeding (ETF).

This paper makes the assumption that patients with a diagnosis of VS or MCS are medically stable enough to be cared for out of an acute hospital setting (typically a nursing home) where administration of intravenous infusions is not normal practice. Therefore this method cannot be used to supplement hydration. Usual practice for ETF, as described in Bowling (2004), Thomas (2001), and Todorovic and Micklewright (1997), does

---

Correspondence should be sent to Helen Finch, Head of Dietetics, Royal Hospital for Neurodisability, West Hill, London SW15 3SW, UK. Tel: 020 8780 4500 extension 5080, Fax: 020 8780 4503. Email: hfinch@rhn.org.uk

---

© 2005 Psychology Press Ltd
http://www.tandf.co.uk/journals/pp/09602011.html   DOI:10.1080/09602010443000542

apply but there are particular nutritional problems associated with VS and MCS patients. The aim of this paper is to present the nutritional challenges particular to VS and MCS patients and how to address them. Although this is an interesting group of patients in regards to nutrition support, little evidence is published to inform clinical practice. Therefore this article is based on the author's clinical experience.

It is assumed that ETF has been started at the acute hospital and this article will discuss the nutritional care of these patients once they have passed the critical care stage.

The ethics of artificially feeding or withdrawing feeding in VS and MCS patients is not discussed here as this is a highly complex issue and a subject in itself beyond the scope of this paper. Some guidance on this issue can be found in publications by the British Medical Association Medical Ethics Committee (2001) and the General Medical Council (2002).

Good nutrition is essential for the maintenance of health. The effects of under-nutrition on immune function, wound healing, cardiac and respiratory health are thoroughly described by Stratton, Green, and Elia (2003).

NUTRITIONAL ASSESSMENT

The objective of the initial assessment is to identify if any nutritional problems are present and to form the basis of nutritional goals. In this patient population it is likely that the patient has some contractures which will confound assessment of some anthropometric measurements that might normally be used. Increased muscle tone may lead to asymmetric and misleading anthropometry. The patient will not be able to co-operate, this again may make measuring difficult, probably inaccurate, and even impossible.

The most useful measurements in this patient population are body weight and body mass index (BMI). BMI relates body weight to height; it is the weight in kilograms divided by the height in metres squared. Prolonged immobility has the effect of reducing fat free mass, which weight and BMI do not measure. However, measurement of total body weight and BMI provide an approximate estimation of nutritional status to form a reasonably firm basis for nutritional care. Body weight is useful as a baseline and if an accurate series of weights is obtained, this is useful for monitoring progress. VS and MCS patients need to be weighed either in a hoist scale or wheelchair scale as they are not able to stand or sit safely, making normal scales or sitting scales unsuitable. BMI gives an idea of how the patient's weight relates to the normal population (Garrow & Webster, 1985) but because of inevitable muscle wasting as a result of immobility, the desirable BMI range would be lower than for normal, ambulant individuals.

It is necessary to obtain the height of the patient in order to calculate the BMI. A standing height is impossible in the VS or MCS patient, however, reported height from relatives has been shown to be within 1% of actual height (Reed & Price, 1998) and, in practice, this is the most practical and usually reliable method. Measuring ulna length is possible in this patient population but is not a very accurate surrogate method of measuring height due to individual differences in ulna length and actual height (Elia, 2003). Other derivative measurements like knee height (Han & Lean, 1996) and demispan (Bassey, 1986) are almost always impossible to assess due to contractures or high muscle tone. Recumbent height can be measured in a contracted patient when side lying but this method has not been validated.

Mid upper arm circumference (MUAC) is possible to do and may be useful as a check along with weight. However, it is likely that normal values (Thomas, 2001) may not apply in many patients because of high and varying muscle tone in the upper arm. Skinfold thickness (Durnin & Wormsley, 1974) measurements require skill and training to perform accurately (Garrow, James, & Ralph, 2000) even with a co-operative subject in an optimal position, but a VS or MCS patient will not be able to help and would almost always be in bed or a very supportive seating system making measurement difficult.

Due to immobility, oedema is often present in these patients, usually in the feet and ankles, but it also can be in the hands and arms. It may be useful to make an assessment of the oedema and to monitor for any change. There are estimates for weight of peripheral oedema (Bowling, 2004; Madden & Wicks, 1994) but since these figures are only estimates, it may be better not to deduct the weight of the estimated oedema, since lower limb oedema, the more common form, is likely to remain fairly constant. However, these estimates may be useful to help interpret the patient's weight if there is any discernable change in the oedema. Changes in weight will guide nutritional care rather than absolute weights. Therefore, if the oedema is fairly consistent, it will not influence nutritional decisions.

An adapted subjective global assessment (SGA) is also essential. The full assessment described by Detsky et al. (1987) is probably not necessary but it is useful to assess subcutaneous fat and muscle wasting subjectively to help verify other measurements and build a better picture. Relatives can be a useful source of subjective information as they can give an opinion on whether the patient looks thinner or heavier than before the brain injury. A subjective assessment can be used to help confirm or question the measurements of height, weight and BMI. For example, if the patient looks overweight, and the measured weight is accurate, and the patient's BMI comes out at 20 kg/m^2, it is likely that the height measurement was incorrect.

The nutritional assessment carried out by a registered dietitian would also cover a review of the type, condition and suitability of the feeding tube for long-term use. Nasogastric tubes are not a good option for long-term feeding as they commonly become misplaced putting the patient at increased risk of aspiration, and multiple insertions are distressing for the patient, staff and relatives. In addition, they are not aesthetically pleasing for the patient or relatives. The most satisfactory and most common feeding tube used for long-term ETF is a gastrostomy tube, with percutaneous endoscopic gastrostomy (PEG) being the most common method of insertion. Medium sized diameter tubes are most suitable for VS and MCS patients. Fine bore tubes (≤ 10 French gauge) are more prone to blocking and large (>18 French gauge) were shown on an audit at the Royal Hospital for Neuro-disability (RHN) to result in more problems (hypergranulation and infection) with the gastrostomy site. Most VS and MCS patients need to be fed and hydrated for many hours throughout the day and night so a low profile/button gastrostomy tube would not be advantageous as a feeding extension tube would need to be connected most of the time making it no more discrete than a conventional gastrostomy tube. Low profile gastrostomy tubes also have the disadvantage of needing to be changed for a longer shaft length if the patient gains weight. If problems occur with feeding tubes advice can be sought from specialist nurses or from senior doctors or nursing staff in endoscopy units.

NUTRITIONAL CHALLENGES AND HOW TO OVERCOME THEM

Undernourishment

During the critically ill phase after a severe brain injury, nutritional requirements are often very high and difficult or even impossible to meet (Weeks & Elia, 1996) resulting in weight loss. This was supported by a recent audit study conducted at RHN between 2001 and 2003 on 227 patients. It was found that about 30% of patients admitted from acute hospitals to the RHN were undernourished as defined by McWirter and Pennington (1994). On admission 14% were mildly undernourished (BMI $18.1-20 \, \text{kg/m}^2$), 11% were moderately undernourished (BMI $16.1-18 \, \text{kg/m}^2$), and 5% severely undernourished (BMI $\leq 16 \, \text{kg/m}^2$). Other factors that contribute to the increased energy requirements that persist after the acute care phase are high muscle tone, frequent infections and agitation. In addition the patient is often a young male who would have inherently high requirements. All or some of these factors may contribute to the patient having become underweight.

To correct under-nourishment, it is our usual practice to continue the feeding regimen started at the acute hospital, to weigh the patient on admission and at two weekly intervals thereafter. If the patient gains weight then the regimen is continued. If the patient is not gaining weight then the amount is increased, usually in increments of about 200 to 300 kcal, until a suitable weight gain is achieved.

Overweight

Some VS/MCS patients present at the non-acute setting overweight. They may have been overweight prior to the brain injury and although some weight may have been lost, due to the reasons outlined above, they might still be overweight or their nutritional requirements have been overestimated and they have gained weight.

Weight monitoring would indicate whether reduction of intake is required. If the patient is not losing weight then a reduction of intake would be needed while ensuring intake of micronutrient and protein intakes are in accordance with dietary reference values (Department of Health, 1991).

Tissue viability

Because of immobility all VS/MCS patients are at high risk of skin break-down. If a pressure ulcer develops and has a large exudate, higher nutritional demands may be imposed on the patient. Thin patients with bony prominences are at very high risk of skin breakdown. In general these patients require a high calorie intake to enable them to gain weight and a high intake of protein, vitamins and minerals which would ensure their additional nutritional requirements would be met. However, an overweight patient may also develop pressure ulcers. To avoid further weight gain, it is necessary to provide relatively small volumes of feed which may put these patients at risk nutritionally. It is our practice in overweight patients with exudating wounds to aim at keeping their weight stable and to give at least 1 – 1.5 g of protein per kilo body weight until the skin has healed. This is in accordance with the upper safe limit set by the COMA report on dietary reference values (Department of Health, 1991). In a patient who has very low energy requirements it may be necessary to use a protein supplement; a vitamin and mineral supplement may also be considered. This would need to be soluble to enable it to be administered via the gastrostomy tube. Care should be taken to use a supplement that brings any shortfall of micronutrient up to reference nutrient intake levels as described in the dietary reference values book (Department of Health, 1991).

Vomiting

Vomiting is frequently a problem in these patients and can have serious consequences as they are at high risk of aspiration. Vomiting may be due to slow gastric emptying or could be vestibular in origin. Prokinetic and anti-emetic medications can be useful, however, some changes in the way the feed is administered can be helpful. Reducing the pump rate, especially while the patient is in bed, can help; the patient might be able to tolerate a higher rate while seated. Avoiding feeding at a time when the patient is being moved (e.g., when being showered, dressed or having physiotherapy) and reducing the number of hours for feeding by using a more energy dense feed may help.

Diarrhoea

Diarrhoea can be problematic in patients who are tube fed and frequently taking antibiotics (Bartlett, 2002). In addition these patients are at increased risk of developing *Clostridium difficile* toxin enteritis (Yassin, Young-Faddock, Zein, & Pardi, 2001). Once treated medically (i.e., with an antibiotic) it may help promote a non-pathogenic gut flora by giving the patient a fibre feed containing fructo-oligosaccharide (FOS) as a prebiotic (Garleb et al., 1996). It may also help to give a liquid probiotic; typically a fermented milk product, in an attempt to normalise the gut flora. Although this is the author's preference there is no evidence to support its use.

Constipation

Constipation can also be a problem, possibly due to lack of mobility, poor gut peristalsis, some medications, or lack of fluid or fibre. A fibre-containing feed may help along with other bowel management strategies. It is important that bowel care is approached with a co-ordinated multidisplinary strategy using fibre, fluid and medications to best effect. If available, it may be helpful to include the advice of continence specialist nurses and pharmacists as well as the ward nurses, doctors and dietitians.

Fluid requirements

In a non-acute hospital environment all fluid for the VS/MCS patient will be given through the feeding tube. In an acute hospital, fluid given by tube may have been supplemented with intravenous fluids, therefore, handover information to the non-acute facility should be scrutinised. Patients under 60 years old need at least 35 ml of fluid per kg body weight (Kleiner, 1999; Todorovic & Micklewright, 1997). Many VS and MCS patients have larger than normal fluid losses thus increased requirements. Often they have a tracheostomy, which may need frequent suctioning. Since these patients are usually unable to swallow their own saliva, fluid is lost from their mouths. Additionally excessive sweating commonly occurs probably due to autonomic disturbances as an indirect result of severe brain injury. Occasionally the sweating can be extreme and is sometimes referred to as "autonomic storming". All these losses have to be replaced consistently via the feeding tube. Blood tests for urea and electrolytes can be a useful intermittent check on hydration status but typically will not be done sufficiently frequently in the non-acute setting to be relied on. Observations by the nursing staff of quantity and appearance of urine output can provide a practical day-to-day measure of hydration status.

Urinary tract infections (UTIs) are common in this patient population, which is an additional reason for a high fluid intake. Cranberry juice may be helpful in preventing UTI (Kontiokari et al., 2001) although its effectiveness is uncertain. The dose usually given at the RHN is 300–400 ml of 25% cranberry juice drink and, since effectiveness is uncertain, it is our practice to evaluate after about three months of use. Renal calculi are often found and flushing the urinary system with plenty of fluid may help to reduce their formation (Klugman & Favus, 1995).

Diabetes

Treating VS/MCS patients with types 1 and 2 diabetes who require insulin can be particular challenging. Often VS/MCS patients with Type 1 diabetes may exhibit very erratic blood sugar levels in spite of being in a very controlled environment where food intake is very regular and insulin is given systematically. As these patients may suffer hypoglycaemia asymptomatically, blood glucose monitoring should be done at least 6 hourly. It is essential that a well-documented, practical procedure is in place to give clear direction on treating low blood glucose. Fibre-containing feed is probably preferable as it has a lower glycaemic index than standard feeds. Intake of feed and insulin need to be administered at times to co-ordinate blood glucose control so it is important that the doctor and dietitian work together to devise a regimen most likely to achieve good control. Advice may also be sought from a diabetes specialist team.

Medication

Certain medications are incompatible with enteral feeds as described by the BAPEN Working Party (2003). Dose frequency and timing of the medication in relation to feeding will prevent problems occurring. Medications commonly used in VS/MCS patients that need to be considered when planning an enteral feeding regimen are phenytoin, rifampicin to treat TB meningitis, alendronic acid, or disodium etidronate which may be used to be help treat heterotrophic ossification. The feeding regimen needs to be planned taking incompatible medications into account, e.g., stopping feeding two hours before a dose of phenytoin and recommencing two hours afterwards. If breaks are not accounted for, then the feeding regimen no longer fits in 24 hours resulting in incomplete amounts being given.

GOAL SETTING

The main nutritional goals will be to ensure the patient reaches, or remains at, a suitable body weight, and to minimise ETF-related complications. It is helpful to have an idea of the patient's premorbid weight, build and probable BMI to guide towards a suitable BMI that should form the basis of the goal weight. For example, if a young woman was very slender premorbidly, a goal weight based on a BMI of 19 to 20 kg/m^2 would probably be appropriate. Whereas for a big built man, a target BMI of 23 to 24 kg/m^2 may be suitable. Photographs taken of the patient before the brain damage can be useful as well as talking to relatives. If the patient has very involved relatives it is helpful to include them in goal weight setting. They often have useful information but also may have strong opinions on how heavy their relative should be. In artificial feeding, professionals have total control over how much the patient is fed, therefore if relatives are included in setting the goal weight, they may feel more included. Since body weight is part of an individual's identity, it is especially important to help restore this aspect of an extremely damaged patient. Taking the relatives' points of view into consideration can be of great emotional benefit.

It is important to ensure the feeding regimen is practical for the patient's individual therapy schedule and for the normal ward routine. Consideration should also be given to activities the patient's relatives may want to do.

PROGRESS AND MONITORING

The main nutritional monitoring tool is regular and frequent weighing, usually at 2–3 week intervals. The nutritional intake needs to be reviewed in the light of the patient's weight and changes made, usually in small increments of about 200–300 kcal. In a severely undernourished VS/MCS patient it may take many months for the goal weight to be achieved. Once the goal weight is achieved it is very important to continue to monitor weight because, frequently, energy requirements reduce significantly and if the patient is not weighed frequently and reductions of intake are not made accordingly, the patient's weight will quickly increase above target. This effect is usually seen once the patient becomes more medically stable with fewer infections and when many of the problems mentioned above have resolved.

In the very long-term (several years post-injury), energy requirements will continue to diminish with slow muscle wasting due to immobility. It is not unusual for a VS or MCS patient to be weight stable on an intake of just 1000 kcal/day. Unfortunately there is only one feed available in this country that meets the recommended intakes for all nutrients at 1000 kcal. A few patients need less than 1000 kcal for which there is no proprietary product, so a supplement of protein, vitamins and minerals will be necessary.

In the non-acute setting envisaged in this paper, blood tests would only be done if the patient were unwell or for some other specific purpose. Blood testing would not be as frequent as in an acute unit so cannot be relied upon to detect dehydration or overhydration. Urine output is usually the most practical way of monitoring hydration. VS/MCS patients are likely to be fed artificially for many years so it is our practice to have an annual blood test for full blood count, urea and electrolytes, liver function test, magnesium, zinc, copper, calcium, phosphate, vitamin B_{12} and red cell folate. However, in many VS patients it is extremely difficult to take blood due to contractures and poor peripheral perfusion so the full testing may not be possible. Occasional abnormalities found are low zinc and raised B_{12} and red cell folate. The low zinc may be accounted for because the blood sample was taken at the beginning of the day after the patient had ETF overnight (Baldwin, Dewit, & Elia, 2004). The raised B_{12} and folates are probably due to high intakes from the enteral feeds and since these nutrients have low toxicity (Expert Group on Vitamins and Minerals, 2003) are very unlikely to be a problem.

A speech and language therapist may assess some MCS patients as being able to take small tastes of semi-solid food orally. This is usually given in the expectation of improving the patient's quality of life. However, some would disagree that an MCS patient would be able to appreciate the food and would question if the risk is worth taking. It may be recommended as a positive interaction for the patient's relatives to give tastes of suitable foods.

CONCLUSION

ETF is a very effective way of feeding VS and MCS patients and almost always the patients reach their goal weight. Nourishment is a very emotive area; being able to nourish the VS patient to approximately their premorbid size can be a small comfort for relatives. It can be reassuring to relatives to see measurable progress of the patient's weight to the agreed goal, and for them to be included in evaluating whether the patient looks right once the goal weight is achieved can be a positive contribution. Body weight is part of a person's identity so its restoration may have emotional benefits for relatives. The physical health benefits of good nutrition have been well documented (Stratton et al., 2003). Good nutrition underpins good nursing and medical care; fortunately this is almost always achievable in the VS and MCS patient.

REFERENCES

Baldwin, C., Dewit, O., & Elia, M. (2004). Changes in circulating concentrations of vitamins and trace elements after cessation of nocturnal enteral tube feeding. *Clinical Nutrition*, *23*, 249–255.

546   FINCH

BAPEN Working Party (2003). *Drug administration via enteral feeding tubes.* Maidenhead UK: BAPEN.

Bartlett, J. G. (2002). Antibiotic-associated diarrhea. *New England Journal of Medicine, 346*(5), 334–339.

Bassey, J. E. (1986). Demi span as a measure of skeletal size. *Annals of Human Biology, 13,* 499–502.

BMA Medical Ethics Committee (2001). *Withholding and withdrawing life-prolonging medical treatment; a guidance for decision making.* London, UK: BMJ Books.

Bowling, T. (2004). *Nutritional support for adults and children.* Oxford, UK: Radcliffe Medical Press.

Department of Health (1991). *Dietary reference values for food energy and nutrients for the United Kingdom. COMA Report 41.* London: HMSO.

Detsky, A. S., McLaughlin, J. R., Baker, J. P., Johnson, N., Whittaker, S., Mendelson, R. A., & Jeejeebhoy, K. N. (1987). What is subjective global assessment of nutritional status? *Journal of Parenteral and Enteral Nutrition, 11,* 8–13.

Durnin, J. V. G. A., & Wormsley, J. (1974). Body fat assessed from body density and its estimation from skinfold thickness: Measurement on 481 men and women from 16–72 years. *British Journal of Nutrition, 32,* 77–97.

Elia, M. (2003). *The 'MUST' Report. Nutritional screening of adults: A multidisciplinary responsibility.* Maidenhead, UK: BAPEN.

Expert Group on Vitamins and Minerals (2003). *Safe upper levels for vitamins and minerals.* Food Standards Agency.

Garleb, K. A., Snook, J. T., Marcon, M. J., Wolf, B. W., & Johnson, W. A. (1996). Effect of fructossoligosaccharide containing enteral formulas on subjective tolerance factors, serum chemistry profiles and faecal bifidobacteria in healthy adult male subjects. *Microbial Ecology in Health and Disease, 9,* 279–285.

Garrow, J. S., James, W. P. T., & Ralph, A. (2000). *Human nutrition and dietetics.* London, UK: Churchill and Livingstone.

Garrow, J. S., & Webster, J. (1985). Quetelet's Index (W/H^2) as a measure of fatness. *International Journal of Obesity, 9,* 147–153.

GMC (2002). Withholding and withdrawing life-prolonging treatments: good practice in decision-making. Retrieved 12. December 2004 from: http@//www.gmc-uk.org/standards/whwd.htm

Han, T. S., & Lean, M. E. J. (1996). Lower leg length as an index of stature in adults. *Internationl Journal of Obesity, 20,* 21–27.

Kleiner, S. M. (1999). Water: An essential but overlooked nutrient. *Journal of the American Dietetic Association, 99,* 200–206.

Klugman, V., & Favus, M. J. (1995). Diagnosis and treatment of kidney stones. *Advances in Endocrinology and Metabolism, 6,* 117–142.

Kontiokari, T., Sundqvist, K., Nuutinen, M., Pokka, T., Koskela, M., & Uhari, M. (2001). Randomised trial of cranberry-lingonberry juice and Lactobacillus GG drink for the prevention of urinary tract infection in women. *British Medical Journal, 322,* 1571–1577.

Madden, A., & Wicks, C. (1994). *Liver interest group of the British Dietetic Association. A practical guide to nutrition in liver disease.* Birmingham, UK: British Dietetic Association.

McWirter, J. P., & Pennington, C. R. (1994). Incidence and recognition of malnutrition in hospital. *British Medical Journal, 308,* 945–948.

Reed, D. R., & Price, R. A. (1998). Estimates of heights and weights of family members: Accuracy of informant reports. *International Journal of Obesity and Related Disorders, 22,* 827–835.

Stratton, R. J., Green, C. J., & Elia, M. (2003). *Disease-related malnutrition: An evidence-based approach to treatment.* Oxford, UK: CABI Publishing.

Thomas, B. (2001). *Manual of dietetic practice* (3rd ed.). London, UK: Blackwell Science.

Todorovic, V. E., & Micklewright, A. (1997). *A pocket guide to clinical nutrition* (2nd ed.). Birmingham, UK: British Dietetic Association.

Weeks, E., & Elia, M. (1996). Observations on the patterns of 24 hour energy expenditure, changes in body composition and gastric emptying in head injured patients receiving nasogastric tube feeding. *Journal of Parenteral and Enteral Nutrition, 20,* 31–37.

Yassin, S. F., Young-Faddock, T. M., Zein, N. N., & Pardi, D. S. (2001). *Clostridium difficile* – associated diarrhea and colitis. *Mayo Clinic Proceedings, 76,* 725–730.

NEUROPSYCHOLOGICAL REHABILITATION
2005, 15 (3/4), 548–555

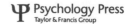

Psychological needs of patients in low awareness states, their families, and health professionals

Sarah Crawford and J. Graham Beaumont

Department of Clinical Psychology, Royal Hospital for Neurodisability, London, UK

Patients who have emerged from low awareness states may present with psychological needs that can be addressed via adapted formal clinical psychological interventions, or by behavioural techniques. Families of these patients may experience similar psychological reactions to relatives of any patients with severe brain injury, but there are also additional factors that are unique to patients in low awareness states. These sources of psychological distress for relatives are discussed. The needs of clinicians working with these clients are also discussed. It is important that services attending to the needs of clients in low awareness states also have adequate support for both relatives and clinicians.

INTRODUCTION

Improvements in medical techniques over recent decades have led to increased numbers of survivors of all types of brain injury. In addition to their medical, physical and cognitive needs, many survivors of moderate to severe brain injury also have psychological needs. Up to 50% of patients who have suffered a traumatic brain injury (TBI) will suffer subsequently from depression (Fleminger, Oliver, Williams, & Evans, 2003) and over one-third of carers of people who have suffered severe TBI experience significant symptoms of anxiety and depression (Marsh, Kersel, Havill, & Sleigh, 1998). For patients in low awareness states and their relatives and carers,

Correspondence should be sent to Dr. S. Crawford, Department of Clinical Psychology, Royal Hospital for Neurodisability, West Hill, Putney, London, SW15 3SW, UK. Tel: 020 8241 4566. Email: sazcrawford@hotmail.com

© 2005 Psychology Press Ltd
http://www.tandf.co.uk/journals/pp/09602011.html   DOI:10.1080/09602010543000082

there may be additional factors contributing to psychological distress, some of which are discussed below. Given the relatively limited published research in this area, many of the points made derive from our clinical experience in a specialist unit for the assessment, rehabilitation and disability management of patients in vegetative (VS) and minimally conscious states (MCS; the diagnostic criteria for these conditions appear elsewhere in this volume). This paper will inevitably focus more on the needs of relatives, carers and clinicians as we have very limited access to the psychological status of the patients and restricted opportunities to engage in a therapeutic process with them.

PSYCHOLOGICAL NEEDS OF PATIENTS WHO HAVE EMERGED FROM VS

It is assumed that patients in VS cannot possess the self-awareness necessary to experience psychological distress, although some studies have examined psychological functioning in patients who have emerged from VS. McMillan and Herbert (2000) described a patient who had been in VS for approximately 4–5 months. Some years after the injury, and still in MCS, she was able to communicate "yes" and "no" by means of a response button, and it was established that she experienced low mood and perceived her future as hopeless. However, despite this, she consistently expressed a desire to carry on living, and was able to participate in psychological therapy addressing her thoughts about death and dying. Another patient was in VS and then a minimally responsive state for approximately 6 months (MacNiven et al., 2003). She was subsequently able to communicate, and described the pain and distress she suffered during routine care tasks. At the time, her only means of communicating distress had been via screaming, and she expressed anger that clinicians did not routinely explain what they were doing and why. She subsequently benefited from psychological therapy including anger management and cognitive therapy techniques, which helped her to focus more optimistically on her present and future.

These studies have demonstrated that even when patients have extremely limited communicative skills it is possible to adapt psychological interventions to help improve mood and adjustment. However, few patients who emerge from VS will develop a high enough level of communicative skill for formal therapeutic techniques to be employed. Nevertheless, behavioural principles can still be applied. The appropriate behavioural techniques rely upon conditioning procedures which are designed to increase the frequency of "desirable" behaviours at the expense of other incompatible behaviours. Learning without awareness has been unequivocally established by psychologists, but the implications of this have commonly not been recognised by those working with low awareness states. For example, thorough multidisciplinary team (MDT) assessments will establish whether patients are able to make any consistent choices, e.g., using pointing to make concrete decisions such as what to wear or eat. These choices can then be reinforced by the team, enabling the patient to have some, albeit limited, control over decision-making. In more severely impaired patients, a detailed functional analysis of behaviour may be necessary in order to determine whether any "challenging behaviours" such as hitting out or screaming are serving to communicate distress, and whether aspects of the care environment can be altered in order to reduce the distress experienced by patients (we infer) and so the frequency of these behaviours. The over-riding principle must nevertheless remain that at all times patients must be treated with dignity and respect.

PSYCHOLOGICAL NEEDS OF RELATIVES/CARERS OF PEOPLE IN LOW AWARENESS STATES

Relatives of patients in low awareness states have been reported to experience a range of emotional reactions including shock, anxiety, guilt, denial, depression and hostility towards staff caring for the patient (Tzidkiahu, Sazbon, & Solzi, 1994; Jacobs, Muir, & Cline, 1986). Many factors may contribute to these reactions including loss of the person they care about, changes in roles and/or social circumstances and the complex medical and ethical decisions in which they may become involved. All these factors can in turn impact on their relationships with staff caring for the patient, although issues such as the hostility which may be expressed to staff are more appropriately regarded as firstly a problem for the relative, and not simply a problem for the staff.

Loss without death

Many patients do not emerge from VS, and recovery is rare more than 12 months after traumatic brain injury and more than 6 months after non-traumatic brain injury (Royal College of Physicians, 2003). When there is little expectation of recovery, the loss for a family of a patient with severe brain injury has been compared with bereavement since the patient is no longer the person they previously were, although the family may be unable to mourn and adjust to their loss given that the body remains alive (Lezak, 1988). In addition, the patient also receives an expensive care package provided by highly skilled staff. Thus, clinicians may indicate hope of recovery by their actions, even if not by their words.

In our clinical experience, some relatives maintain hope of a significant recovery in the absence of any evidence of improvement over long periods of time. Media portrayals may contribute to this. For example, a recent newspaper article claimed that a man had recovered from VS after a period of

18 years, accompanied by emotive reports of how his mother "refused to give up on him" and how "her faith was repaid" (The Guardian, 11 July, 2003). While a matter of great joy for the family in question, reports such as this can give the message not only that there is always hope, but also that recovery is more likely the more time and devotion family members give to the injured person. In addition, the internet is increasingly a source of information for relatives. While the internet can provide people with extremely valuable information, many relatives do not have the knowledge and experience that would enable them to judge the quality and reliability of the information they obtain. They may also understandably be biased towards any information that fosters hope, regardless of its source. By contrast, relatives who believe there is little hope of recovery may wish to visit less frequently. This can lead to feelings of guilt and blame, which are among the most common emotional reactions of relatives of people in VS (Tzidkiahu et al., 1994).

Changes in roles and social circumstances

Family members may experience unexpected role changes when someone has suffered a severe brain injury, for example, by taking on a caring role for the patient, or suddenly becoming the sole earner in the family at a time when they have also lost their main source of emotional support. This may occur in conjunction with a loss of other sources of support. Thus, in a recent study, over 70% of primary caregivers of people diagnosed as being in a persistent vegetative state reported being socially isolated and having low levels of engagement in their previous recreational activities (Chiambretto, Rossi Ferrario, & Zotti, 2001). In the longer term, some relatives may wish the patient to return home with themselves in the role of primary carer. While this may be a viable option for some, it should be balanced against the best interests of both patient and the whole family since even with a 24-hour supportive care package, the burden of care is likely to be considerable.

Psychological distress in family members can be exacerbated when relatives of the same patient experience different reactions. For example, if a patient's partner and parents had different opinions about the prognosis, the parents may perceive a reduction in visiting by the partner not only as a betrayal of the patient, but even detrimental to their chances of recovery. Such conflicts can only add to the distress experienced by all concerned.

Although these factors are possible sources of psychological distress, for some people the changes in roles may actually have a positive psychological outcome, at least in the short term; some relatives appear to draw strength from developing a caring role for the patient, and may form a new social network with relatives of other patients in a similar state.

Family involvement in withdrawal of feeding decisions

Once recovery is assessed as unlikely, it is possible that relatives may be asked to give their opinion on issues such as resuscitation status, active treatment and withdrawal of feeding. Irrespective of the extent of involvement of relatives in these decisions, such highly emotive issues can lead to psychological distress, primarily in terms of feelings of guilt and responsibility. Within our clinical experience, several relatives have expressed openly that they think it would be better for the patient to be dead than in VS. Many relatives become upset when they express these thoughts because they do not want to abandon hope of recovery, and feel guilty at such open expression.

Sources of difficulty between relatives and clinicians

Sources of difficulty or disagreement between relatives and professionals may exacerbate the distress of either. One common source of such difficulties is misunderstanding by relatives about the diagnosis of vegetative state. One study reported that 31 out of 33 relatives interviewed believed their family member was aware of at least some external stimuli (Tresch, Sims, Duthie, & Goldstein, 1991). In particular, the degree of cognitive impairment can be very hard for relatives to appreciate, especially if patients exhibit nonpurposeful movements or noises. Patients in VS can demonstrate behaviours that are associated in nonbrain injured individuals with emotional experience, such as crying, grimacing, smiling, or laughing (Royal College of Physicians, 2003). When the patient fulfils diagnostic criteria for VS, these behaviours must reflect subcortical functions and are not indicative of subjective distress. Not surprisingly, this can be difficult for relatives to understand, and many families reasonably perceive these behaviours as signs that the patient is intentionally trying to "wake up" (Jacobs et al., 1986).

In our experience, it is very common for relatives to report that the patient is making meaningful responses when these have not been observed by the professionals who have been assessing the patient. Usually, it can be shown that while the relative believes the behaviour to be purposeful or environmentally driven, objective evidence indicates it is not. However, it is possible for patients' behaviours to be genuinely different when their relatives are present. When relatives are reporting behaviours not observed by professionals, staff should consider observing the patient with the relatives and involving the relatives in some of the formal assessment sessions in order to gain a more comprehensive view of the patient's behaviour. This can also be advantageous when the relatives have overestimated the patient's level of awareness as they may come to revise their opinion.

Another source of potential tension between relatives and staff occurs when relatives request the continuation of treatment that will not benefit the patient. Requests for physical treatments such as physiotherapy or occupational therapy may reflect an underlying belief that recovery might be possible if only enough treatment is received. Relatives may believe that physiotherapy will enable the patient to walk again; a belief based on a failure to appreciate the role of the brain in planning physical activities. Others may be denying the extent of the patient's impairments and the poor prognosis; denial is commonly reported in relatives of people in VS (Tzidkiahu et al., 1994; Jacobs et al., 1986). This may be unintentionally promoted by therapists' reports of good progress. For the therapist, the goals of prevention of contractures or maintenance of range of motion are being achieved; but for the relatives, the goal of recovery is not being achieved.

It has been argued that hostility and complaints from relatives towards staff caring for the patient can be framed as emotional reactions to poor adjustment to the prognosis (Tzidkiahu et al., 1994). Relatives not uncommonly make seemingly minor complaints, for example about nursing tasks or cleaning standards on the ward. We believe that, if complaints seem unfounded, it is helpful to interpret them as a wish by relatives to do something tangible to assist. There is little they can do for the patient, so they tend to focus on the only tasks over which they can have some control, seemingly becoming fixated on such issues as whether or not the patient's water was given at exactly at the expected time, or how frequently the ward is cleaned. If professionals take this behaviour at face value, it can be a source of continual frustration at the relatives' failure to accept the explanations offered by staff.

Misunderstandings may arise from a lack of clarity by professionals when explaining the diagnosis to the relatives; in part from the uncertainty of the prognosis. There is no definitive test of whether or not a patient will emerge from VS. Current guidelines for diagnosis of persistent VS are based on the low probability of the condition improving after specified time periods, but not on a certainty that it will not. Professionals may communicate their own lack of certainty when giving the diagnosis and prognosis, leading to false hope by the relatives. Professionals would be advised to refer explicitly to the relevant statistics, so explaining the lack of certainty of outcome, and also the professional's range of opinion. It may also be useful to provide appropriate literature, which has the added advantage of de-personalising the issue.

Intervention with families

In many cases it may be appropriate for teams working with these families to encourage them to seek psychological support from external sources such as their GP or voluntary sector organisations. Interventions in the form of cognitive behaviour therapy are likely to be effective for depression, guilt and bereavement reactions, and generic counselling approaches for the wider problems of psychological adjustment. Although there is no formal evidence to support such interventions in this context, their efficacy may be inferred from applications in other clinical settings. However, it may also be appropriate to offer support within the service. It has been argued that while there is little formal scientific evidence to date supporting the efficacy of intervention with families of people with brain injury, although there is informal clinical evidence that it may be of benefit, there is stronger evidence showing the impact that brain injury has on the whole family. This can be used to plan appropriate interventions such as provision of information and education, involvement in rehabilitation and decision-making, setting up of family support groups, and individual or group family therapy (Oddy & Herbert, 2003). Any unit caring for individuals in VS or MCS needs to have good access to clinical psychology, social work and counselling services, and to ensure their local provision for relatives who may be resident at some distance from the unit.

PSYCHOLOGICAL NEEDS OF CLINICIANS WORKING WITH PEOPLE IN LOW AWARENESS STATES

Clinicians working with patients in low awareness states may encounter situations that are unique to this client group. One of the contentious issues in working with patients in VS is the possibility that withdrawal of artificial nutrition and hydration may be requested. This may have a psychological impact on the clinicians who have been caring for the patient over a considerable period of time, and there is likely to be considerable individual differences based on cultural and religious beliefs and the attitude of staff members towards death and the vegetative state. In our clinical experience, it may be particularly problematic for the most junior health care staff, who may have had the most immediate contact with the patient during the caring stage, but who may lack formal training in caring for the dying patient. Staff should be given the choice as to whether or not they will participate; some staff members may see this role as an important part of their duty towards the patient.

Another problem for staff is the source of their job satisfaction. Many of these patients will not show any signs of improvement, and most are unlikely to be able to express gratitude to staff. It is important that professionals working with these patients are able to have pride and satisfaction in providing anticipatory, maintenance and palliative care.

SUMMARY

In summary, there are several potential sources of psychological distress for patients, relatives and professionals working with this client group. Not all these factors are unique to this patient group. There are some common reactions, but there is no set and predictable pattern; every family is different and factors such as cultural and religious beliefs are likely to contribute to the type of reaction seen. It is important for health care organisations to be aware of the range of psychological reactions, and to have adequate support systems in place for their staff. Organisations should also have a structure in place for supporting relatives, whether this is via in-house professionals such as psychologists, counsellors or social workers, or by linking the relatives to other organisations, in the public or voluntary sectors.

REFERENCES

Chiambretto, P., Rossi Ferrario, S., & Zotti, A. M. (2001). Patients in a persistent vegetative state: Caregiver attitudes and reactions. *Acta Neurologica Scandinavica, 104*, 364–368.

Fleminger, S., Oliver, D. L., Williams, W. H., & Evans, J. (2003). The neuropsychiatry of depression after brain injury. *Neuropsychological Rehabilitation, 13*, 65–87.

Jacobs, H. E., Muir, C. A., & Cline, J. D. (1986). Family reactions to persistent vegetative state. *Journal of Head Trauma Rehabilitation, 1*, 55–62.

Lezak, M. D. (1988). Brain damage is a family affair. *Journal of Clinical and Experimental Neuropsychology, 10*, 111–123.

MacNiven, J. A., Poz, R., Bainbridge, K., Gracey, F., & Wilson, B. A. (2003). Emotional adjustment following cognitive recovery from 'persistent vegetative state': Psychological and personal perspectives. *Brain Injury, 17*, 525–533.

Marsh, N. V., Kersel, D. A., Havill, J. H., & Sleigh, J. W. (1998). Caregiver burden at 1 year following severe traumatic brain injury. *Brain Injury, 12*, 1045–1059.

McMillan, T. M., & Herbert, C. M. (2000). Neuropsychological assessment of a potential 'euthanasia' case: A 5 year follow up. *Brain Injury, 14*, 197–203.

Oddy, M., & Herbert, C. (2003). Intervention with families following brain injury: Evidence-based practice. *Neuropsychological Rehabilitation, 13*, 259–273.

Royal College of Physicians (2003). *The vegetative state: Guidance on diagnosis and management*. London: Royal College of Physicians.

Tresch, D. D., Sims, F. H., Duthie, E. H., & Goldstein, M. D. (1991). Patients in a persistent vegetative state: Attitudes and reactions of family members. *Journal of the American Geriatric Society, 39*, 17–21.

Tzidkiahu, T., Sazbon, L., & Solzi, P. (1994). Characteristic reactions of relatives of post-coma unawareness patients in the process of adjusting to loss. *Brain Injury, 8*, 159–165.

Subject Index